C·A·N·C·E·R THERAPY

THE INDEPENDENT CONSUMER'S GUIDE
To Non-Toxic Treatment & Prevention

Vitamins ❧ Minerals ❧ Herbs ❧ Diets ❧ Immune Boosters ❧ Less Toxic Drugs ❧ Ways to Reduce Side Effects of Chemotherapy ❧ Research from Around the World ❧ Resources to Help You Make Choices

RALPH W. MOSS, PhD

AUTHOR OF
THE CANCER INDUSTRY

What the Experts Are Saying About *Cancer Therapy*

"Combining scholarship and readability, Moss comprehensively surveys innovative cancer therapies. **This book is a must** for cancer patients and their families who want to be involved in their own treatment."
> — *Samuel S. Epstein, M.D., Professor of Occupational and Environmental Medicine, The University of Illinois at Chicago*

"This carefully researched and objective presentation respects the capacity of people to make their own judgments about cancer. The choices offered in this book permit the exercise of human rights. Its panoramic view is **a service not just to people with cancer but to science itself.**"
> — *Paul W. Scharff, M.D., Medical Director Rudolf Steiner Fellowship Foundation, Inc.*

"This book is remarkable in revealing the existence of so many high-quality peer-reviewed studies on natural and innovative approaches to cancer....*Cancer Therapy* points the way to promising directions for resolving the disease. The book is **a milestone for the enlightenment of the public** and of the scientific and medical communities..." —*Robert G. Houston, author,* Repression and Reform in the Evaluation of Alternative Cancer Therapies

"After looking at the first few pages of *Cancer Therapy: The Independent Consumer's Guide,* I found myself reading every word. This book contains very practical information for the person interested in taking positive steps to recover from, or prevent, cancer. **I intend to recommend it to every patient!**"
> — *Jack O. Taylor, M.S., D.C., Wellness Center, Inc. Arlington Heights, Illinois*

"Reading *Cancer Therapy* is like standing on a mountain top surveying the entire landscape of cancer treatment. This landmark book is **an incredible feat of research and reporting**....Here is everything you need to know about cancer fighters—from the latest discoveries to little-known healers from the past ....*Consumer's Guide* is rightly named; the Resources section, found in every chapter, brings every product, treatment and cancer center as close as your telephone....Here is no 'slash and burn' discussion of conventional medicine or breathless claims for alternative treatment; **Moss, possibly the best science writer in our midst,** lets the scientific facts speak for themselves....*Cancer Therapy* is a model of organization and research. Moss's crisp compelling style should arouse awe and envy in every journalist ....My advice to every cancer patient as well as those of us seeking to remain healthy: **read this book carefully and buy a copy for everyone you love.**"
> — *Jane Heimlich, author,* What Your Doctor Won't Tell You

"Dr. Moss has written an invaluable guide for the cancer patient who understands that knowledge is his or her greatest ally. This book is a thoroughly researched collection of methods for cancer therapy; and **provides a "must read" guide for all cancer patients and clinicians.** For every patient who is told "There is nothing that can be done for you," read this book. For every skeptical clinician who claims that "There is no data supporting the use of nutrition for the cancer patient," read this book. *Cancer Therapy* is a major step in the right direction for the comprehensive and effective treatment of cancer patients." *—Patrick Quillin, Ph.D., R.D., author,* Healing Nutrients

"For nearly twenty years, Ralph W. Moss, Ph.D. has been in the forefront of those fighting for a fair evaluation of alternative cancer therapies. Through his books, films and newsletter, *The Cancer Chronicles,* he has championed the cause of medical freedom of choice...."His latest book, *Cancer Therapy: The Independent Consumer's Guide to Non-Toxic Treatments,* is **a must-have.** Its many references refute the notion that all non-toxic treatments are outside the realm of science. This astonishing book is destined to be **the Bible of alternative cancer therapy!**" *—Frank Wiewel, Exec. Director, People Against Cancer*

"This is an important book. A quarter of the world's population is fated to get cancer and probably die of it. But accurate information on how best to treat it is scattered and difficult to comprehend for most people. And the cancer 'establishment' is reluctant to accept beneficial modifications of conventional treatment or acknowledge new, superior approaches to defeating this malignancy. In fact, they are often hostile and repressive in their attitude....Since all people must accept for themselves a method of treatment or avoidance, it is important that they have in their hands as complete and as accurate information as possible. This is what Dr. Moss has done in **brilliant and lucid** fashion. The reader will learn the essence of every answer to every question that can be raised about cancer. Abundant references are provided for those who wish to dig more deeply." *—Alan C. Nixon, Past President, American Chemical Society*

"It is usual for medical establishment organizations to decry use of alternative treatments as being scientifically unproven. At the same time, they persist for years in using drugs that have little value and cause serious side reactions such as destruction of the immune system. In my own experience, a review of medical journals frequently proves that established methods have no proven scientific basis, but are retained due to habit or persistent backing by individuals at prestigious institutions. **Dr. Moss equitably provides the public with well-documented facts that enable people to judge** why an alternative or establishment cancer treatment may be suitable or unwarranted for their particular type of cancer." *—Henry J. Heimlich, M.D., Sc.D.*
President, Heimlich Institute

CANCER THERAPY

10/25/92

Best wishes,

[signature]

OTHER BOOKS BY RALPH W. MOSS, PhD

The Cancer Industry

Free Radical: Albert Szent-Gyorgyi
and the Battle Over Vitamin C

Caring
(with Annette Swackhamer, RN)

A Real Choice

An Alternative Approach to Allergies
(with Theron G. Randolph, MD)

The Cancer Syndrome

CANCER THERAPY:

THE INDEPENDENT CONSUMER'S GUIDE TO NON-TOXIC TREATMENT & PREVENTION

BY

RALPH W. MOSS, PHD

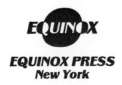

EQUINOX PRESS
New York

Designer: Martha Bunim
Typeface: 12/15 Century Expanded
Printer: BookCrafters

First Printing
99 98 97 96 95 94 93 92   5 4 3 2 1

Library of Congress Cataloging-in-Publication Data

Moss, Ralph W.
    Cancer therapy : the independent consumer's guide to non-toxic
treatment and prevention / Ralph W. Moss.
        p.   cm.
    Includes bibliographical references and index.
    ISBN 1-881025-06-3 (alk. paper) : $19.95
    1. Cancer—Popular works. 2. Cancer—Treatment.
    3. Cancer—Alternative treatment.   I. Title.
    RC263.M643   1992
    616.99'406—dc20   92-4076
                                                CIP

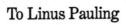

To Linus Pauling

To the Reader:

The information in this book is based on the journalistic research of the author and should be used only as a general guide. Each reader is urged to consult a qualified health professional before utilizing any of the treatments mentioned in this book. We do not advocate the use of any particular treatment for any medical condition, including cancer. Please understand that we cannot be responsible for any adverse effects resulting from the use of information in this book. We will be happy to refund the purchase price to anyone who cannot accept these conditions.

Acknowledgments

The author would like to thank the following people for their help in the preparation of this book:

At Equinox Press, I wish to thank the publisher Martha Bunim, as well as Jean Oschrin, Jennifer Sherman, Andrew Whitehead and Melissa Wolf, director of marketing. I also wish to give special thanks to Robert G. Houston and Patrick Quillin, PhD, RD, for the many detailed and helpful comments each made. Valuable suggestions were also contributed by the Hon. Berkley Bedell, Samuel S. Epstein, MD, Naomi Flack, George Klabin, Glenn McAnanama, Morton Walker, DPM, George Wald, PhD, and Frank Wiewel.

In addition, many scientists and health professionals have provided up-to-date information on their work. Needless to say, any errors are my responsibility alone.

TABLE OF CONTENTS

$\mathcal{P}$REFACE

I solemnly profess that I hate all pretences to secrets and I look upon the printed bills of quacks, who pretend to nostrums and private medicines, to be mere cheats and tricks to amuse the common people and to pick their pockets. But if any man can communicate a good medicine, he shows himself a lover of his country more than of himself, and deserves thanks of mankind.—Dr. William Simpson (1680 AD)

This book details nearly 100 non-toxic or less-toxic treatments for cancer. The effectiveness and safety of all of these methods are rigorously documented through nearly 1,000 references to the standard peer-reviewed scientific literature. In this way it is demonstrated once and for all that non-toxic therapies, far from being 'quackery,' are in fact a most promising avenue for cancer research.

This book would not be necessary if conventional cancer therapy were generally successful. Unfortunately, it is not. While great advances have been made in treating a minority of cancers, the majority of people who get cancer today still die of their disease. And although many billions of dollars have been spent on cancer research, we must conclude that little progress has actually been made in treating this tragic illness.

Such statements may be surprising, since for more than 40 years the public has been flooded with stories of dramatic breakthroughs and incredible cures. We do not mean to diminish the importance of real advances. But the 'cure mongering' surrounding two experimental treatments, interferon and interleukin, are still fresh enough for us to remain skeptical of all exaggerated claims. In fact, official records support this skeptical view: figures from the National Cancer Institute (NCI) reveal that there has been no substantial improvement in cancer cure rates over the last several decades (1).

Death rates for the major killers, such as lung, breast and colon, have remained essentially unchanged. The only substantial improvement has been for cancer of the cervix and for such relatively rare malignancies as choriocarcinoma, testicular cancer, lymphomas and childhood leukemias, when these are treated with radiation and/or toxic chemotherapy. However, even with such cures, there is a high incidence of delayed, or secondary, cancers due to the carcinogenic effects of the treatments themselves.

Cumulative figures from the US National Cancer Institute confirm the overall lack of progress. The five-year relative survival rates for cancer for all nationalities was 49 percent in 1974-75 and 50.7 percent in 1981-1986. This represents an improvement of only 1.7 percent in 13 years. The corresponding 'cure' rates for African-Americans in the same 13 year interval actually dropped from 38.6 percent to 38.2 percent (2). Furthermore, even the tiny improvement in the overall cancer 'cure' rate may be little more than a statistical artifact, reflecting recent trends toward earlier diagnosis (3).

At the same time, cancer incidence is rising throughout the industrialized world. These increases are real and cannot be explained away by improved diagnosis or increased longevity. From 1947 to 1984, for instance, the overall incidence of cancer in the general US population increased some 40 percent. For more common cancers, such as those of the breast, incidence rates have increased by over 30 percent; for prostate and male colon cancers by over 60 percent. Increases for some less common cancers, such as malignant melanoma, multiple myeloma, non-Hodgkin's lymphoma and male kidney cancer, are around 100 percent. Similar increases have been seen in other industrialized countries.

Behind these figures lurks a human tragedy of almost unimaginable proportions. Every one of those millions of deaths is a human life wasted and often a family ruined. The financial cost of this disaster is equally staggering. After years of underestimating the cost, in 1987 the US authorities admitted to a total annual expense of $71 billion for the nation as a whole. The figure today is probably well over $100 billion. Many individuals are bankrupted by the cost of such care and it contributes greatly to society's enormous medical burden. New high technology treatments, such as bone marrow transplantation, can cost well over $100,000 per procedure. One new drug called Neupogen, which is used only to counteract the toxic effects of chemotherapy, costs patients between $6,000 and $10,000 per year, according to the *Wall Street Journal* (2/22/91).

This is a situation calling out for radical alternatives.

For many years, however, the war on cancer has been dominated by powerful groups with closely interlocking professional financial interests (4). In the US, the principal components of this "cancer establishment" are the NCI; the American Cancer Society (ACS); the twenty-odd comprehensive cancer centers, such as New York's Memorial Sloan-Kettering and Boston's Dana-Farber Cancer Institute; an extensive network of NCI and ACS contractees and grantees at most major universities; the leading pharmaceutical houses; and the Food and Drug Administration (FDA), which regulates the marketplace on behalf of the very industries it is supposed to oversee.

Although most such organizations are non-profit, they generally follow the lead of the profit-driven industries. Thus, the hub of the cancer establishment is a highly profitable drug development system, led by chemical, pharmaceutical and biotechnology companies.

While it is in the interest of such companies to find patentable cancer treatments, there is no corresponding incentive to develop non-patentable natural methods. Since it currently costs around $200 million to develop a new drug in the US, mainly to comply with Byzantine FDA regulations, the drug companies claim they must seek enormous profits from each and every drug. And such profits are generally only available through patentable drugs, with their 17-year legal monopolies.

Yet most of the methods discussed in this book are not patented or patentable. Most are in fact readily-available natural substances, such as foods or food components. There are profits to be made selling such items, but these are obviously far less than those for purified, often toxic, pharmaceuticals. Thus there is a powerful economic rationale for favoring toxic treatments.

Another reason is that toxic treatments require the supervision and intervention of medical professionals skilled to the highest degree. Toxic or high-tech treatments keep the focus on high-paid cancer specialists and well-funded medical centers. Natural, non-toxic methods, on the other hand, enable primary care health givers, or sometimes even the patients themselves and their family members, to administer care.

Such non-toxic methods are thus more readily accepted by doctors, nurses and other professionals who are closer to the patients, while despised by those at the pinnacle of the medical elite. Interestingly, in a recent survey the American Cancer Society found that the greatest single source of referrals to such non-toxic "questionable" treatments were the front-line doctors themselves (4). As humble as they often are, these non-toxic treatments present a powerful competitive challenge to high profile toxic treatments, which happen to be hated and feared by most of their intended recipients.

The main argument used against non-toxic methods is that they are not supported by research in peer-reviewed scientific journals and do not conform to the rules of scientific evidence. Non-toxic methods are called questionable, unproven and unscientific. Only orthodox cancer treatments—surgery, radiation and chemotherapy—are "scientific," they say, and presumably not to be questioned.

I hope that this book will finally destroy the underpinnings of this fallacious argument. All the non-toxic and less-toxic methods in this book have been selected based on their appearance in the same selective journals that all doctors and scientists around the world depend upon. (In addition, I have added a small section of methods that are not yet documented in this way but bear further research.)

The obvious purpose of this book is to provide the person with cancer—and all of us who fear we might someday become one—with useful information on cancer alternatives. Its secondary purpose is to aid the patient to better exercise freedom of choice in medical care. Freedom of choice means that the major choices in cancer treatment belong to the patient, and no one else. The doctor is employed by the patient in what jurists call a "fiduciary" role. This means that the doctor's interests in the treatment is less immediate and compelling than those of the patient, who has to bear the full consequences of the treatment decisions (5).

This principle of medical freedom of choice is rooted in the Hippocratic tradition, in the US Declaration of Independence and the French Declaration of the Rights of Man and of the Citizen (1789). It was first explicitly formulated by the British philosopher John Stuart Mill more than a century ago, when he proclaimed that "over himself, over his own body and mind, the individual is sovereign" (*On Liberty*).

Judge Benjamin Cardozo enshrined this principle in US law when he wrote, in the landmark 1914 case of *Schloendorff v. Society of N.Y. Hospital,* "Every human being of adult years and sound mind has a right to determine what shall be done with his own body." This judgment was supported by the postwar Nuremberg Code which held that every patient "should be so situated so as to be able to exercise free power of choice..." And it was most recently reaffirmed by the Second Circuit US Court of Appeals, which wrote, in *Schneider v. Revici* (1987), that "we see no reason why a patient should not be allowed to make an informed decision to go outside currently approved medical methods in search of an unconventional treatment" (6).

The history of non-toxic therapies has been a sad one. There has been repression and neglect on one side, wild claims and paranoid fantasies on the other. With the formation of an office of unconventional medical practices at the National Institutes of Health there is now hope that such therapies can at last find acceptance by the medical profession. I hope this book can make a contribution toward that goal.

—Ralph W. Moss, PhD

⊕ References

1.   Cairns, J. The treatment of diseases and the war against cancer. Scientific American 253:51-9;Nov. 1985.

2.   National Cancer Institute, Cancer Statistics Review 1973-1987, NIH Publication No. 90-2789, Bethesda, MD, 1990.

3.   Bailar JC and Smith EM. Progress against cancer? New Eng J Med 314:1226-1232, 1986.

4.   Lerner IJ and Kennedy BJ. The prevalence of questionable methods of cancer treatment in the United States. Ca 42:181-191.

4.   Epstein, SS. The politics of cancer. San Francisco: Sierra Club Books, 1978 (Rev. ed. Garden City, NY: Anchor Press/Doubleday, 1979).

5.   Shultz MM. From informed consent to patient choice: a new protected interest. The Yale Law Journal 95:2, December 1985.

6.   817 Federal Reporter, 2nd Series: 987-996, 1987.

		BLADDER	BRAIN	BREAST	COLON/RECTUM	ESOPHAGUS	HEAD & NECK	HIV-RELATED	KIDNEY
1	Algae			✓					
2	Antineoplastons		✓					✓	
3	Arginine		✓						✓
4	Aspirin	✓			✓				
5	Astragalus								
6	Ayur-Veda			✓					
7	Azelaic Acid								
8	BCG	✓							
9	Benzaldehyde			✓					
10	Bestatin				✓			✓	
11	Beta-Carotene	✓		✓	✓		✓		
12	Bioflavonoids								
13	Bryostatins								✓
14	Butyric Acid								
15	B Vitamins	✓				✓			
16	Calcium			✓	✓				
17	Calorie Balance				✓				
18	Canthaxanthin			✓					
19	Cesium & Rubidium			✓	✓				
20	Chaparral		✓						
21	Chinese Herbs					✓			
22	Coley's Toxins			✓				✓	
23	CSF								
24	DMSO								
25	Electric Therapy			✓					
26	Ellagic Acid								
27	Enzymes								
28	Evening Primrose	✓							
29	Fiber			✓	✓				
30	Fish Oil			✓	✓				
31	Garlic			✓				✓	
32	Germanium							✓	
33	Gerson				✓				
34	Gossypol			✓					
35	Green Tea								
36	Heat Therapy		✓	✓			✓		
37	Hydrazine		✓	✓					
38	Indoles			✓	✓				
39	Inosine							✓	
40	Iscador			✓					
41	Kampo	✓							

	LEUKEMIA	LIVER	LUNG	LYMPHOMA	ORAL	PANCREAS	PROSTATE	SKIN	STOMACH	TESTICULAR	UTERUS (CERVIX)	GENERAL
1	✓											
2												
3		✓										
4												
5								✓				
6			✓									
7							✓					
8			✓				✓					
9								✓				
10	✓		✓	✓				✓				
11			✓		✓						✓	
12								✓				
13	✓											
14	✓											
15			✓					✓			✓	
16												
17												✓
18												
19		✓	✓	✓		✓	✓					
20	✓							✓				
21			✓									✓
22		✓		✓				✓			✓	✓
23	✓											
24	✓									✓		
25												
26			✓									
27	✓											
28		✓										
29												
30						✓						
31								✓				✓
32										✓		✓
33			✓									
34	✓					✓			✓	✓		
35		✓	✓					✓	✓			
36							✓	✓		✓		
37	✓		✓	✓				✓	✓			
38							✓		✓			
39								✓				
40			✓								✓	
41							✓	✓				✓

19

	BLADDER	BRAIN	BREAST	COLON/RECTUM	ESOPHAGUS	HEAD & NECK	HIV RELATED	KIDNEY
Krestin				✓				
Lactobacilli				✓				
Lentinan			✓	✓				
Levamisole				✓				
Linseed Oil			✓	✓				
Macrobiotics				✓				
Magnesium			✓					
Maruyama Vaccine								
Megace			✓				✓	
Methylene Blue	✓							
Molybdenum			✓		✓			
Monoclonals							✓	
MTH-68	✓		✓	✓				
Muroctasin								
Mushroom			✓				✓	
Onconase								✓
Pau d'Arco							✓	
Phototherapy				✓		✓	✓	
Psychotherapy			✓					
Seaweed			✓				✓	
Selenium	✓		✓	✓				
Shark Cartilage							✓	
SOD			✓					
Spices								
Splenopentin								
Staphage Lysate			✓					
Sulindac				✓				
Suramin			✓					✓
Tagamet							✓	
Tamoxifen			✓					✓
Thioproline			✓					
Thymic Factors							✓	
Urea					✓			
Vitamin A			✓		✓			
Vitamin C			✓	✓	✓		✓	✓
Vitamin D			✓	✓				
Vitamin E			✓					
Vitamin K	✓		✓	✓				✓
Zinc								

SUMMARY CHART

LEUKEMIA	LIVER	LUNG	LYMPHOMA	ORAL	PANCREAS	PROSTATE	SKIN	STOMACH	TESTICULAR	UTERUS (CERVIX)	GENERAL
✓								✓			
✓											
	✓							✓			
											✓
									✓		
									✓		
✓											
								✓			
✓							✓				
			✓								
✓			✓	✓		✓	✓	✓		✓	
											✓
✓	✓			✓		✓	✓	✓		✓	
		✓						✓		✓	
						✓	✓	✓			✓
			✓								
					✓						
	✓		✓					✓			
									✓		
			✓								
		✓						✓			
	✓					✓				✓	
	✓	✓	✓		✓	✓	✓		✓		
✓		✓		✓	✓	✓		✓	✓	✓	✓
✓						✓					
		✓						✓			✓
✓	✓	✓									
				✓							

How to Use This Book

By their very nature, most of the treatments in this book act on the immune system and therefore can apply to almost any kind of cancer. However, many readers are primarily interested in finding treatments for a single kind of cancer. And in fact much research has been done along those lines. The Summary Chart on pages 18-21 will help quickly locate treatments that have been shown to act on particular kinds of cancer. The chart will also guide people to treatments that have shown promise against HIV viral infections. References to less common kinds of cancer and a number of related conditions are found in the index.

Words in **bold face** are the subject of their own chapters elsewhere in the book. Please consult the table of contents or index to locate them.

In addition, there are three devices used throughout:

This handshaking symbol indicates that the substance under discussion works well in conjunction with conventional treatments, by either enhancing their cell-killing power or decreasing toxic side effects.

This lighthouse indicates a resource guide. These pages throw light on the practical aspects of therapy, such as how to obtain the treatments discussed. They are found at the end of each of the nine major sections of the book rather than after every particular chapter. In addition, there is a General Resources section at the end of the book.

This globe indicates a bibliographical reference section, which follows each chapter. The globe refers to the international nature of scientific research. Cancer is a worldwide problem and consequently we have attempted to scan and reflect the entire world's effort against this problem. It is our view that no one country's research is intrinsically better than any other's. We need to learn from the efforts of all nationalities and cultures if we are to overcome this disease.

The footnoted citations in these reference sections refer to articles in peer-reviewed scientific journals or occasionally to standard medical texts. Reference to some other works are embedded in the text of the book. The references are intended as a representative sample of the work in each field. The square brackets found in some of the references indicate that the article is written in a language other than English.

Actual citations from scientific or other texts are given in double quotes. Single quotes are used when alluding to unusual expressions or for the sake of emphasis.

This book summarizes many studies derived not just from human clinical trials but from test tube and animal experiments. How relevant are laboratory studies to the human situation? Most scientists believe that animal or test tube studies can predict anticancer activity. This is precisely why animals have been widely used in cancer research for over fifty years. In fact, the entire development of modern pharmaceuticals is inconceivable without them. Such studies are part of a very long process of testing that may end in human clinical trials.

Of course, research on people is even more valuable and we report on many such trials in this book. But clinical trials are expensive and difficult to arrange and are often inconclusive. As non-toxic therapies emerge into the mainstream, scientists will hopefully obtain more resources and more opportunities for clinical trials. However, people with cancer cannot wait, and deserve to be told whatever is currently known about such treatments.

*I*NTRODUCTION

This book provides crucial information for medical consumers who want to actively participate in making decisions about their health.

It is especially directed towards people who:

• **have been diagnosed with cancer** and need to make important decisions on what sort of treatments to choose.

• **have friends or family members with cancer.** They are in a difficult position, trying to act as adviser to their loved ones. This book will quickly bring them up to date on what is available around the world in cancer treatment.

• **do not have cancer, but are concerned** that someday they or someone close to them might face this situation. After all, two out of three families eventually will confront cancer. This book will prepare the reader in advance on how to deal with a situation we all fervently hope will never arise. It contains information on many simple and inexpensive ways of *preventing* cancer from ever attacking you or your loved ones. This information is based on scientific research from around the world.

• **have decided to follow the conventional route** and take surgery, radiation and chemotherapy. This book can also help them. It offers a discussion of many non-toxic substances that can reduce the side effects of chemotherapy while increasing its effectiveness.

This *Independent Consumer's Guide* is "independent" in two ways:

First, it is written for people who think for themselves. For example, these are the type of people who ask doctors for full explanations of procedures and who want to see their own medical records.

Second, the book itself is independent of vested interests in the cancer field. It offers positive and objective information, but also points out any negatives, drawbacks or side effects of the therapies, when they are scientifically-verified and relevant to the discussion. This pertains to both chemotherapy and to the less-conventional treatments discussed in the book.

The word consumer in the title recognizes the fact that there is a marketplace of cancer treatments and the cancer patient is a shopper in that market. Being a good consumer means understanding what your choices are and how they rate when stacked up against the competition. This information is being brought to the public for the first time in *Cancer Therapy: The Independent Consumer's Guide.*

The research cited comes from books and articles in the world's peer-reviewed scientific literature. These are the same reputable publications that scientists all over the world publish in and learn from. This means that other scientists in the same field have checked the work and found it sound enough to be published.

These references demonstrate that non-toxic treatments are now passing from the fringes of medicine into the mainstream. They are increasingly being adopted and verified by conventional scientists around the world. This is a heartening fulfillment of the World Health Organization's (WHO) call for a "New Medicine," which integrates the best of both scientific and traditional practices. The Office of Technology Assessment of the US Congress has called for a thorough investigation of these cancer therapies and a committee of the National Institutes of Health has now been established to do so.

Your doctor probably does not yet know about many of these treatments, for most of this information has been culled from specialized journals from around the world, which few practicing doctors have time to read.

We have tried to make this book a dependable 'guide for the perplexed' in cancer. We hope you will be helped by what you read about these treatments. But we can use *your* help, as well. Were any of these treatments beneficial to you? Were the resource sections helpful in obtaining the therapies under discussion? Do you have new phone numbers or addresses you could add? We would like to hear from you on your experiences—positive and negative—in using this consumer's guide. We will integrate such information into future editions and updates of this book. Please send your comments to: Equinox Press, 331 West 57th Street, Suite 268-B, New York, NY 10019.

US readers attempting to obtain these therapies will find that the Food and Drug Administration (FDA) has barred the marketing of some of the substances discussed in this book, such as IAT and the medicines of Dr. Hans Nieper. (For a full explanation of why this is so, the reader is referred to *The Cancer Industry*, chapter 17.)

In most cases, however, the FDA explicitly *allows* people with cancer (or AIDS) to obtain almost any substance for their *personal use.* In other countries, readers should contact their government's equivalent of the FDA.

The goal of *Cancer Therapy: The Independent Consumer's Guide to Non-Toxic Treatment and Prevention* is to empower you, the consumer, with the information you need to make intelligent choices in today's international medical marketplace.

$\mathcal{U}$ITAMINS

For years, many doctors looked down on nutrition. Even the great Hungarian-American biochemist Albert Szent-Gyorgyi (1893-1986) revealed this prejudice when he discovered a new chemical in adrenal glands in the 1920s. He suspected it was a vitamin, but put its study aside. Asked why he didn't pursue the lead, he answered, "I felt that vitamins were a problem for the cook!" Happily, Szent-Gyorgyi overcame his bias and won the 1936 Nobel Prize for isolating vitamin C from Hungarian paprika.

"Let your food be your medicine and your medicine be your food" was a dictum of the great physician, Hippocrates (fifth century BC). Most medical scientists are only now discovering that there are many powerful healing substances in food. And the ancient Greek's motto is being dramatically affirmed today by cancer research centers around the world.

As just one example, scientists in Germany tested various fruit and vegetable juices against mutation- and cancer-causing chemicals. About 80 percent of these juices displayed antimutation and anticancer activity. Juices from raw celery root, broccoli, red cabbage, carrots, green peppers, lettuce, asparagus, apricots, red-currants, gooseberries, raspberries and pineapple all showed more than 50 percent inhibition of these harmful chemicals (1).

This section assembles groundbreaking scientific work on food factors and cancer—work that has been steadily emerging from laboratories and clinics on six continents—and explains it to the non-scientist.

Some of this research has been well-publicized, but most

of it has never before been brought to the attention of the person who needs it most: the individual with cancer.

This science of using nutrition against cancer is still emerging, and some of the research is admittedly taking place only in test tubes or laboratory animals. Nevertheless, science's new emphasis on vitamins and other food factors represents an exciting departure, away from toxic drugs and towards more natural approaches.

⊕ References

1.   Edenharder R, et al. [Antimutagenic activities in vitro of vegetable and fruit extracts with respect to benzo(a)pyrene]. Z Gesamte Hyg Ihre Grenzgeb (GRD).1990;36:144-147.

⚘ VITAMIN A

Vitamin A was the first vitamin to be isolated and defined. It is a fat-soluble food factor that gives us the power of night vision. It also fortifies the mucous membranes, which serve as a barrier against poisons, microbial invaders and carcinogens (cancer-causing substances). It protects the thymus gland (crucial for immunity) and is essential for protein synthesis and normal growth. Like other powerful food factors, it is an antioxidant that destroys harmful chemicals called 'free radicals.' And it does much more.

Evidence for a link between vitamin A deficiency and cancer goes back over 60 years. It was first named in 1922. In 1926, a Japanese scientist found that laboratory animals deficient in vitamin A were more likely to develop cancer than those fed normal chow. Two years later, scientists found that a lack of vitamin A was an important factor in the development of human cancer, as well.

Around the same time, a Harvard researcher pointed out the similarity between vitamin A-deprived and cancer cells. After World War II, it was found that vitamin A enhanced the effectiveness of chemotherapy.

In 1963, vitamin A was first shown to cure and prevent a condition called leukoplakia—white, warty patches in the mouth that often precede cancer. Dr. Umberto Saffioti, dean of vitamin A studies, showed that mice could be protected against cancers of the lungs, stomach, gastrointestinal (GI) tract and uterus that were caused by carcinogens. Sometimes the protection was nearly 100 percent.

By 1981, there were more than 300 positive reports on vitamin A. In that year, a well-known British researcher suggested that a diet high in carrots and similar vegetables could reduce the risk of cancer.

"I believe there is now a light at the end of our tunnel in our fight against this disease," Dr. Richard Peto told a conference. He claimed there was a 40 percent lower risk of cancer among men who maintained above average consumption of vitamin A. Later, these studies were extended to A's non-toxic pro-vitamin, beta-carotene.

At Stockholm's Karolinska Hospital, scientists gave healthy subjects vitamin A pills. After a few years they found that vitamin A decreased the risk of cancer: the higher the dose, the less cancer developed. The Swedish scientists concluded that vitamin A may trap cell-damaging chemicals called free radicals and neutralize their cancer-causing effects. (They also found an increased risk of cancer in people who ate a lot of fried meat, fried potatoes or fat.) (1)

For ten years scientists at the NCI 'followed' (studied over time) nearly 2,500 men over the age of 50. Eighty-four of these men developed cancer of the prostate. Levels of vitamin A in their blood were found to be significantly lower than among men who did not develop this cancer. In fact, the lower their blood serum level of vitamin A, the greater their risk of developing prostate cancer. This was the first time that vitamin A and prostate cancer were subjected to a large 'prospective' study (in which scientists select a group of people and then check up periodically to see what diseases they have developed) (2).

In another NCI study, blood was obtained in 1974 from over 25,000 people. Over 100 of these developed prostate cancer during the next 13 years. Once again, the less vitamin A (retinol) they had in their blood, the greater their odds of developing prostate cancer (3).

Six hospitals in southwestern France provided 106 cases of lung cancer for a dietary study. As with prostate cancer, it was found that the lower the consumption of vitamin A and its pro-vitamin, beta-carotene, the greater the chances of developing lung cancer.

French scientists confirmed the protective value of beta-carotene and provided new evidence that vitamin A also has a protective effect. In experimental animals, cancer forms in two phases—initiation and promotion. This vitamin seemed to inhibit the tumor promotion phase, while beta-carotene complemented this action by inhibiting tumor initiation (4).

Dutch scientists have studied the blood levels of vitamin A in 86 patients with cancers of the head and neck. Some of these patients had tumors at other sites as well. Thirty-one percent of the patients with just head and neck cancers had low serum levels of vitamin A. But 60 percent of those with two kinds of cancer had low levels. About two-thirds of all these cancer patients had low beta-carotene levels.

The scientists concluded that it was possible that low vitamin A levels play a role in causing a second tumor of the head or neck. They recommended that patients with head and neck tumors be given vitamin supplements in order to prevent a second tumor from forming (5).

In early 1992, Italian scientists reported that a combination of vitamin A with vitamins C and E could correct abnormalities in the cells of the rectum in people who had had polyps removed. Such abnormalities are believed to eventually progress to cancer in many cases. They reported their finding in the *Journal of the National Cancer Institute (JNCI)*. The Bologna scientists found a decrease in the occurrence of malignant-type cells in patients who received the three vitamins, compared to controls. As an interesting side light, the patients in this study were given relatively high doses of vitamin A—25,000 to 50,000 IU per day for months. There were "no side effects" in the population studied, non-pregnant adults without liver problems (6).

Vitamin A is one of those few fat-based vitamins that is toxic in high doses (others are vitamins D, E and K).

A variant of vitamin A used in cancer therapy is the acne medication, Accutane® (13-cis-retinoic acid). This is not entirely non-toxic. Like vitamin A, when taken in excess, it can cause extremely dry skin, chapped lips, eye problems (conjunctivitis) and increased levels of fat in the blood.

Frank L. Meyskens, Jr., MD, is a prominent researcher at the University of California (UC), Irvine who has been studying vitamin A and its derivatives, called retinoids, for a dozen years. He has found them beneficial for some kinds of cancer.

"I think increasingly, we will find the retinoids in and of themselves will impact the prevention and treatment of cancer," he has said. For example, a rapidly growing kind of skin cancer (keratoacanthoma) responds to the retinoid-like Accutane.

In 1985, Dr. W.K. Hong of the Head, Neck and Thoracic Oncology Department at M.D. Anderson Cancer Center proposed the experimental use of Accutane in treating head and neck cancer (7). In the *New England Journal of Medicine* in 1990, he reported positive results using Accutane to treat tumors. M.D. Anderson scientists studied 103 patients who were disease-free after receiving standard treatment for cancers of the larynx, pharynx or the mouth. After receiving surgery or radiotherapy or both, they were assigned to receive either Accutane or a placebo (sugar pill), which they took daily for 12 months.

While there were no differences between the two groups in the number of recurrences of the primary cancers, the group receiving Accutane had "significantly fewer second primary tumors." After 32 months, only 2 patients (4 percent) in the Accutane group had second primary tumors, compared with 12 (24 percent) in the placebo group. Some of those in the placebo group had multiple cancers reappear. Of the 14 second cancers, 13 (or 93 percent) occurred in the head and neck, esophagus or lung, the Houston researchers said.

These scientists concluded that "daily treatment with high doses of Accutane is effective in preventing second primary tumors in patients who have been treated for squamous-cell carcinoma of the head and neck, although it does not prevent recurrences of the original tumor" (8).

Another variant on the vitamin (transretinoic acid) when topically applied benefitted a condition called dysplastic nevi syndrome, which can turn into the deadly skin disease, malignant melanoma. Some other advanced skin cancers and a kind of lymphoma of the skin have also shown benefit with this therapy. One patient had 30 skin cancer cell growths on his hands and was scheduled to have both hands amputated. He showed such tremendous improvement on Accutane that the surgery was called off and he has remained free of the disease for years.

By placing Accutane directly in cervical caps (a

barrier form of birth control) doctors have been able to get an 80 percent response to moderate cases of cervical dysplasia. (Beta-carotene and the B vitamin folate also benefit this condition.)

Negative: Scientists at the Evans Department of Clinical Research of University Hospital, Boston, MA studied the effect of Accutane on a wart-like condition called "respiratory papillomatosis." They used it as an adjuvant (helper) treatment to surgery with lasers. Four of the six patients experienced a recurrence while using the therapy, and so the study was discontinued (9).

Conclusion: Vitamin A and its derivatives are being proposed as "chemopreventive" agents. The biochemistry of vitamin A suggests a number of ways in which it could decrease the chance of cancer even getting started. Scientists are generally cautious about telling people to take supplements, especially since high doses of vitamin A can be toxic. But many concede that greater intake of beta-carotene and vitamin A-rich foods may be a 'prescription' worth following (10).

⊕ References

1.   Steineck G, et al. Vitamin A supplements, fried foods, fat and urothelial cancer, a case-referrent study in Stockholm in 1985-1987. International Journal of Cancer.1990; 45:1006-1011.

2.   Reichman M, et al. Serum vitamin A and subsequent development of prostate cancer in the first national health and nutrition examination survey epidemiologic follow-up study. Cancer Research. 1990; 50:2311-2315.

3.   Hsing A, et al. Serologic precursors of cancer. Retinol, carotenoids and tocopherol and the risk of prostate cancer. J Natl Cancer Inst.1990;82:941-946.

4.   Dartigues J, et al. Dietary vitamin A, beta-carotene and risk of epidermoid lung cancer in southwestern France. European Journal of Epidemiology.1990;6:261-265.

5.   De Vries N and Snow G. Relationship of vitamins A and E and

beta-carotene serum levels to head and neck cancer patients with and without second primary tumors. European Archives of Otorhino-laryngol.1990;247:368-370.

6. Paganelli G, et al. Effect of vitamin A, C, and E supplementation on rectal cell proliferation in patients with colorectal adenomas. J Natl Cancer Inst.1992;84:47-51.

7. Hong WK and Doos WG. Chemoprevention of head and neck cancer. Potential use of retinoids.Otolaryngol Clin North Am.1985; 18:543-9.

8. Hong WK, et al. Prevention of second primary tumors with isotretinoin in squamous-cell carcinoma of the head and neck [see comments]. N Engl J Med.1990;323:795-801.

9. Bell R, et al. The use of cis-retinoic acid in recurrent respiratory papillomatosis of the larynx: a randomized pilot study. Am J Oto-laryngol.1988;9:161-4.

10. Kummet T, et al. Vitamin A: evidence for its preventive role in human cancer. Nutr Cancer.1983;5:96-106.

☙ *B*ETA-*C*AROTENE

Beta-carotene is a natural chemical found in many fruits and vegetables, especially brightly colored ones like carrots, mangos, papayas and yams. It was discovered in 1928, as one of a family of about 500 colorful food pigments called carotenoids (ca-rót-en-oids). Beta-carotene is a pro-vitamin, converted into vitamin A in the human body. Recent research has indicated that in reducing the risk of cancer it also plays an important, independent role.

Beta-carotene slowly reaches more parts of the body for a longer time and gives more protection than plain vitamin A. It is considered one of the most promising natural anti-cancer agents. Studies have shown:

• Tumors took longer to develop in beta-carotene treated mice than in animals that did not get the pro-vitamin.

• Even when tumors were well-established, beta-carotene enabled the mice to live longer, with or without other treatments.

• All tumors disappeared for two months when mice were given radiation in addition to beta-carotene. Only one mouse showed a regrowth of tumor.

• Animals which continued to receive beta-carotene lived out their two-year life spans, but five out of six of those taken off beta-carotene died within 66 days.

The pioneering Western Electric study of beta-carotene's health effects was conducted by scientists at Chicago's Rush Presbyterian-St. Luke's Hospital and Northwestern University School of Medicine. These scientists set out to study people's diets and correlate them with death rates. They gained access to blood samples and histories of employees of Western Electric, a large manufacturer of telephone equipment, first in 1957; after one year; and then again 19 years later. They followed up on nearly 2,000 middle aged men and were able to show that a below-average intake of beta-carotene often preceded the development of cancer.

One surprising finding was that cigarette smokers who had relatively high levels of beta-carotene in their diet had a risk of lung cancer about the same as men who had never smoked but had lower levels of beta-carotene in the diet. This meant that not eating carrots and other beta-carotene-rich foods was a dangerous practice, analogous (as far as lung cancer was concerned) to regular cigarette smoking. The more beta-carotene the men got, the less lung cancer they developed.

Oddly, the intake of pre-formed vitamin A in food such as liver, or through vitamin A supplement pills, did not significantly reduce the risk of lung cancer. Nor, in this study, did beta-carotene significantly decrease the risk of cancer taken as a whole. But men who developed cancers of the head and neck also tended to have lower beta-carotene levels. While the study seemed to support the view that smokers could decrease their risk of cancer by getting abundant beta-carotene, the authors cautioned that "cigarette smoking also increases the risk of serious diseases other than lung cancer," and there was no evidence that beta-carotene affects these other risks in any way (1).

The discovery that beta-carotene (but not vitamin A) prevented the development of lung cancer took many researchers by surprise. Until that time, scientists had thought that beta-carotene did not have any independent qualities (2). How then does a pro-vitamin do things that its vitamin counterpart cannot do? One theory is that cigarette smoke instantly destroys vitamin A, but when the body has an abundance of beta-carotene this remains available in the bloodstream to instantly replenish the supply and protect the lungs and other organs. (There is probably more to it than that, since carotenoids which are not precursors of vitamin A also have anticancer effects.)

In addition, scientists at Albert Einstein College of Medicine in the Bronx, NY measured the tissues of women with a kind of uterine growth called leiomyomas. They found that beta-carotene levels were significantly lower in fibroid tissue than in the normal tissue. Beta-carotene levels in cancers of the cervix, endometrium, ovary, breast, colon, lung, liver and rectum were also all found to be lower than in the adjacent normal tissues. This suggests that beta-carotene deficiency might play a role in the origin of many other kinds of cancer, as well (3).

Similarly, in a 1990 NCI study, doctors examined 83 breast cancer patients and compared them to 113 people without cancer. They looked at the dietary and blood concentrations of carotene and various vitamin A look-alikes.

BETA-CAROTENE

On average, the breast cancer patients also had lower concentrations of beta-carotene in their blood. But doctors could not say whether such low carotene levels were a cause of the illness, or simply the result, of the disease process (4).

Unfortunately, there have been few studies that have tested high doses of beta-carotene as a treatment against human cancer. One not-quite-cancerous condition that has been clinically studied is leukoplakia ("white patches"), which is often associated with an increased risk of mouth cancer.

Vitamin A-like substances, particularly the acne medication Accutane® (13-cis-retinoic acid) can often reverse leukoplakia. However, this drug is fairly toxic and is considered unsuitable for large-scale use in the prevention of oral cancer. Beta-carotene, on the other hand, is naturally-occurring and non-toxic. In 1986, scientists designed a study of a toxic drug versus non-toxic beta-carotene (30 milligrams per day) as a treatment of leukoplakia.

However, they faced a patient rebellion: 11 out of the first 16 patients refused to even participate unless they were guaranteed to receive beta-carotene. Therefore, the scientists had to change their design and furnish just beta-carotene for three months. Patients who had a positive response to the treatment were continued on it for another three months. Cells from their oral lesions were examined under the microscope at the beginning of the study. Eventually, 24 patients were treated: 17 had major responses (2 complete, 15 partial), with an overall response rate of 71 percent. There was no significant toxicity.

These results indicated, scientists said, that beta-carotene was a very useful drug for such pre-malignant conditions of the mouth. And because of its general lack of toxicity, "it is an excellent candidate for a preventive agent for oral cancer" (5).

37

Scientists are also examining whether beta-carotene can be used to treat certain other conditions that often turn into cancer such as the very common, localized form of uterine cancer called 'carcinoma in situ.' Although definitive evidence is not in, many people are already using both vitamin A or beta-carotene as part of their treatment program.

When mice which had been given a cancer-causing virus were also given beta-carotene they developed fewer tumors; lived a longer time before cancers occurred; and had a higher rate of tumor regression. When beta-carotene supplements were given after tumors had already developed, it greatly increased the rate at which the tumors regressed. Beta-carotene also decreased damage to the thymus gland caused by the virus. Such protective action on the thymus gland is "believed to underlie part of beta-carotene's antitumor activity" (6).

Cytokines are powerful substances, such as interferon, interleukin and **tumor necrosis factor** (TNF), produced by the body itself to boost immunity and fight cancer. Like other immune boosters, beta-carotene increased the levels of cytokines.

Blood that had been pretreated with beta-carotene was able to kill four out of the six different kinds of human cancer cells in the test tube. This tumor-killing activity, triggered by beta-carotene, was due to cytokines. But it was found to be distinct from the activity of any known cytokine, according to scientists at the University of Arizona in Tucson. This has led them to believe that beta-carotene stimulates the production of some still unidentified cytokine (7).

The colorful pro-vitamin may also prevent a second tumor in patients who have been cured of an initial cancer but now stand at an increased risk of developing new cancers in the upper part of the digestive tract (8, 9).

At the University of Pavia in Italy, 15 patients were given beta-carotene supplements (along with another food constituent) to prevent recurrences after lung, breast, colon, urinary bladder, and head and neck surgery. They had a "longer than expected disease-free interval" (10).

To find out what causes the high rate of liver cancer in parts of China, scientists studied the connection between diet and liver cancer deaths in 65 Chinese counties. Death rates were definitely linked to previous hepatitis-B virus infections. Rates were also higher in counties where people had high cholesterol levels and consumed much liquor, rapeseed oil or moldy corn. Wheat may have conferred a protective effect. But no significant connection with liver cancer deaths was found for consumption of beta-carotene or other vitamins and minerals (11).

People who had had a previous non-melanoma skin cancer showed no decrease in the re-occurrence rate after being given beta-carotene over a five year period (12).

Toxicity: While vitamin A in high doses is toxic, beta-carotene can be taken in large amounts without any appreciable harm, besides turning the palms and soles orange.

⊕ References

1. Shekelle RB, et al. Dietary vitamin A and risk of cancer in the Western Electric study. Lancet.1981;2:1186-90.
2. Peto R, et al. Can dietary beta-carotene materially reduce human cancer rates? Nature.1981;290:201-8.
3. Palan PR. Decreased b-carotene tissue levels in uterine leiomyomas and cancers of the reproductive and nonreproductive organs. American Journal of Obstetrics and Gynecology.1989;161:1649-1652.
4. Potischman N, et al. Breast cancer and dietary plasma concentrations of carotenoids and vitamin A. American Journal of Clinical Nutrition.1990;52:909-15.
5. Garewal HS, et al. Response of oral leukoplakia to beta-carotene. J Clin Oncol.1990;8:1715-20.
6. Seifter E, et al. Moloney murine sarcoma virus tumors in CBA/J

mice: chemopreventive and chemotherapeutic actions of supplemental beta-carotene. J Natl Cancer Inst.1982;68:835-40.

7. Abril ER, et al. Beta-carotene stimulates human leukocytes to secrete a novel cytokine. J Leukoc Biol.1989;45:255-61.

8. Garewal HS. Potential role of beta-carotene in prevention of oral cancer. Am J Clin Nutr.1991;53:294S-297S.

9. Malone WF. Studies evaluating antioxidants and beta-carotene as chemopreventives. Am J Clin Nutr.1991; 305S-313S.

10. Santamaria LA and Santamaria AB. Cancer chemoprevention by supplemental carotenoids and synergism with retinol in mastodynia treatment. Med Oncol Tumor Pharmacother.1990;7:153-67.

11. Hsing AW, et al. Correlates of liver cancer mortality in China. Int J Epidemiol.1991;20:54-9.

12. Greenberg ER, et al. A clinical trial of beta carotene to prevent basal-cell and squamous-cell cancers of the skin. The Skin Cancer Prevention Study Group [see comments]. N Engl J Med.1990;323:789-95.

ᵠ ℬ 𝒰ITAMINS

The B vitamins are extremely important for the general maintenance of health. They enhance immune function; restore the nutritional status of cancer patients, especially those receiving conventional treatment; and enhance the effects while diminishing the side effects of chemotherapy.

Both cancer and its treatment with chemotherapy can lead to serious nutritional deficiencies. In particular, toxic drugs called antimetabolites —by their very design—interfere with the synthesis of essential nutrients, such as vitamins.

"Deficiencies of vitamins B_1, B_2, and K and of niacin, folic acid, and thiamine also may result from chemotherapy," scientists at the University of Texas Health Science Center in Houston stated (1).

B vitamin supplementation may be a logical way to counteract some of these serious side effects.

Vitamin B_6 (pyridoxine) bolsters the immune system, according to researchers at Loma Linda University in Riverside, CA. They note that whole grains, lean meats, liver, kidney, halibut and vegetables are all good sources of this vitamin. At the Nassau Hospital Cancer Center in Mineola, NY, and at Temple University's Fels Research Institute in Philadelphia, PA, doctors have been using a concentrated topical application of vitamin B_6 to treat melanoma. Dr. Gerald Litwack of Fels says that B_6 triggers the production of another substance, which stops the cancer's growth.

Litwack and his colleagues showed that vitamin B_6 could retard and eventually kill rat liver cancer cells in the test tube. However, the B_6-supplemented growth medium had little effect on human breast cancer cells. The resistance of these breast cancer cells suggested that B_6 must first be altered in the body by another substance, before it can act as a growth inhibitor. "These findings suggest the potential use of vitamin B_6 as an antineoplastic agent," the Fels scientists concluded (2).

A lack of B_6 also interferes with the formation of DNA (genetic material) and cuts down on the formation of disease-fighting antibodies. It interferes with other kinds of immune function as well (3). A 1989 Russian study showed that injections of B_6 stopped the formation of lung cancers in experimental animals that had previously received a carcinogen (4).

Riboflavin: In 1983, a large-scale experiment was undertaken in China to see if vitamins could stop the formation of esophageal (gullet) cancer, which is common in parts of that country. In one such area, Heshun Village in Linxian County, nearly 7,000 people ranging in age from 40 to 65 were examined. Remarkably, over half at least showed the first signs of cancer of the gullet: 1,729 with "marked dysplasia," i.e., misshapen, precancerous cells, and another 2,411 with mild dysplasia.

Those with mild dysplasia were given either riboflavin (vitamin B_2) or a placebo ('sugar pill'). Those who had marked dysplasia were put into one of three groups to receive either "antitumor B," a Chinese herbal preparation, a vitamin A-type substance (retinamide) or a placebo.

After three years, these people were re-examined. The incidence of esophageal cancer in the group that received Chinese herbs was reduced by 53 percent compared to the placebo group. Esophageal cancer in the retinamide and the riboflavin groups was reduced by 33.7 and 19 percent, respectively. Taking such herbs and vitamins is therefore "effective in the prevention of esophageal cancer," according to scientists at the Cancer Institute of the Chinese Academy of Medical Sciences, Beijing (5).

Folic Acid: This is another member of the vitamin B family, found in abundance in liver, kidney, mushrooms, spinach, yeast and green leafy vegetables. It has been used for decades to prevent and treat certain forms of anemia. But folic acid also increases the production of white blood cells crucial in the defense against cancer. In the late 1980s, scientists at the University of Alabama Medical Center found that the folic acid in dark leafy vegetables, oranges and liver could act together with vitamin B_{12} to prevent injuries to lung tissue and retard the development of cancer among cigarette smokers.

These researchers found that smokers whose lung cells were injured had low levels of both folic acid and vitamin B_{12}. Since these nutrients are necessary to synthesize DNA, a deficiency of one or both of these vitamins could make cells more susceptible to the effects of carcinogens. These vitamins also offered protection against birth defects and cancerous changes in cervical cells.

Folate (a salt of folic acid) also showed protective effects against lung cancer. Smokers form a thick mucous in their lungs called sputum, which often contains premalignant cells. To test whether folate and vitamin B_{12} could modify premalignant growths found in sputum, University of Alabama scientists conducted a study of smokers who exhibited such cancer-like changes in their lungs.

Seventy-three men who smoked 20 or more packs of cigarettes a year were given either a placebo or ten milligrams of folate as well as 500 micrograms of vitamin B_{12}. After four months the Birmingham nutritionists saw a reduction of such cancer-like changes in the lungs of smokers who received these two B vitamins. This provided evidence that such precancerous changes "may be reduced by supplementation with folate and vitamin B_{12}."

However, writing in the *Journal of the American Medical Association* (*JAMA*), the scientists cautioned that "the results should not be construed as pointing to a potential way of preventing lung cancer in individuals who continue to smoke or as supporting self-medication with large doses of folate or B_{12} by smokers" (6).

Cervical cancer is the ninth most common cause of death among women in the US. It is also "by far the commonest" cancer among women in the developing world, where rates are sometimes six times US levels. This kind of cancer is usually preceded by suspicious readings on Pap smears, a condition called "cervical dysplasia."

Although little is done to prevent this widespread disease, a 1992 study in *JAMA* showed that dietary intervention might be possible. University of Alabama Comprehensive Cancer Center scientists demonstrated that a folate deficiency was often associated with cervical dysplasia. Such deficiency was said to "enhance the effect of other risk factors" and particularly that of the human papillomavirus (HPV), a known cause of cervical cancer (7). Thus, although a lack of folate may not be cancer-causing in itself, deficient cells are more susceptible to the effects of carcinogens (8). Chinese scientists noted that dysplastic changes in women's cervical cells cleared up after they were given folate supplements (9).

Nicotinamide: A large single dose of another B vitamin, nicotinamide, enhanced the cancer cell-killing ability of the conventional drug, L-PAM. This enhancement was at its maximum when nicotinamide was given one hour before L-PAM injections. In fact, it more than doubled the effectiveness of the drug. It also more than tripled the time that the chemotherapy stayed in the bloodstream. As the dose of nicotinamide was decreased, the enhancement of L-PAM was also reduced, British scientists reported (10).

Nicotinamide also increased the antitumor activity of another conventional anticancer drug, cisplatin. Survival time of mice more than doubled in a group receiving both substances. Yet nicotinamide by itself showed no antitumor activity. Pathological changes in cells were partially prevented "by a single protective dose" of the vitamin. Toxicity of the drug was also "partially reversed" by the vitamin. Scientists at Sun Yat-sen University of Medical Sciences in Guangzhou, China suggested that the combination of chemotherapy and nicotinamide "might be used clinically in the future" (11).

People with advanced bladder cancer who had been operated on were given nicotinic acid or aspirin at commonly used doses before and after receiving gamma-ray radiation therapy. Another group of patients did not receive the vitamins or drugs. The results were dramatic: there were 76.3 percent relapses in the group that received standard therapy, but only 33.3 percent

relapses in the nicotinic acid/aspirin group. Five-year
survival in the vitamin-treated group was 72.5 percent
but only 27.4 percent in the controls. Administration of
nicotinic acid and aspirin to patients during radiation therapy was shown to raise the body's antitumor resistance,
Russian scientists reported (12).

⊕ References

1. Dreizen S, et al. Nutritional deficiencies in patients receiving cancer chemotherapy. Postgraduate Medicine.1990;87:163-168.

2. DiSorbo DM and Litwack G. Vitamin B6 kills hepatoma cells in culture. Nutr Cancer.1982;3:216-22.

3. De Simone C, et al. Vitamins and immunity: II. Influence of L-carnitine on the immune system. Acta Vitaminol Enzymol. 1982;4:135-40.

4. Draudin-Krylenko V, et al. [Anticarcinogenic action of vitamins PP and B6 in the natural initiation of malignant growth in mice]. Vopr Onkol.1989;35:34-8.

5. Lin PZ, et al. [Secondary prevention of esophageal cancer—intervention on precancerous lesions of the esophagus]. Chung Hua Chung Liu Tsa Chih. 1988;10:161-6.

6. Heimburger DC, et al. Improvement in bronchial squamous metaplasia in smokers treated with folate and vitamin B12. Report of a preliminary randomized, double-blind intervention trial [published erratum appears in JAMA 1988;259:3410]. JAMA 1988;259:1525-30.

7. Butterworth C, et al. Folate deficiency and cervical dysplasia. JAMA.1992;267:528-533.

8. Eto I and Krumdieck C. Role of vitamin B12 and folate deficiencies and carcinogenesis. Adv Exp Med Biol.1986;206:313-330.

9. Ran J, et al. Selective folate deficiency in one but not another cell line. Blood. 1990;76S:114A.

10. Horsman MR, et al. Changes in the response of the RIF-1 tumour to melphalan in vivo induced by inhibitors of nuclear ADP-ribosyl transferase. Br J Cancer.1986;53:247-54.

11. Chen G and Pan QC. Potentiation of the antitumor activity of cisplatin in mice by 3-aminobenzamide and nicotinamide. Cancer Chemother Pharmacol.1988;22:303-7.

12. Popov AI. [Effect of the nonspecific prevention of thrombogenic complications on late results in the combined treatment of bladder cancer]. Med Radiol (Mosk).1987;32:42-5.

ᵀ CARNITINE

....

Carnitine is a little-known B vitamin, vitamin Bᴛ (tau). It is found in meat but also can be manufactured by the liver from two amino acids (lysine and methionine), provided that adequate amounts of other co-factors such as vitamin C, iron, nicotinic acid and vitamin B_6 are present. There has been a long debate over whether carnitine is truly a vitamin. A recent review concluded that it is indeed an essential nutrient, especially in infancy, fasting, pregnancy and breast feeding, even though technically carnitine can be manufactured by the human body (1).

For many years, scientists knew that carnitine was present in animal tissue, but they did not know precisely what it did. Then it was discovered that carnitine was an essential nutrient for one animal, the mealworm (a beetle larva commonly used in experiments). This suggested that it might be necessary for some important function in people as well. (It may be ego-deflating, but metabolically we are not all that different from our creeping cousins.) And indeed, it was eventually shown that carnitine was essential for the transport or oxidation of fatty acids within the energy centers of human cells (mitochondria).

Carnitine deficiencies, while rare, can occur in people with certain genetic disorders. They can also result from unusual liver diseases or from dialysis (the medical filtration of the blood) in cases of severe kidney failure. The symptoms of a carnitine deficiency are low blood sugar and skeletal muscle weakness.

Recent research indicates that carnitine may also influence the course of cancer. This is because of its influence on mitochondria. It is known that responses of T (thymus mediated) white blood cells slow as people get older. Scientists studied the effects of two forms of carnitine on the ability of cells to proliferate (reduplicate themselves). They found that white blood cell proliferation was "markedly increased" in the blood samples that were exposed to carnitine. This effect was especially notable in older people's blood. Cells from such people "considerably improved their defective proliferative capability" under the influence of this vitamin. Carnitine also protected seniors' white blood cells, when these were exposed to free radicals (harmful chemicals that can cause cancer and other damage) (2).

Other studies show that carnitine, even in small amounts, can counteract the damage that certain fats do to the immune system (3, 4).

In another survey, scientists looked at carnitine blood levels in 54 people with cancer and 81 hospital patients who did not have the disease. They found that the concentration of one kind of carnitine, called acid-soluble acylcarnitine, was significantly lower. In fact, the levels were half of those found in people without the disease. Large variations were also found among people with different types of cancer. The scientists were uncertain whether the lower levels of this kind of carnitine in people with cancer could be explained as an effect of the disease itself or of their therapy (5).

Two years later, in 1989, scientists tentatively concluded that chemotherapy destroys carnitine in the body. They took blood serum and urine samples from 21 cancer patients with metastatic (distantly spread) disease who were receiving toxic drugs. They compared them to 13 healthy people, looking at carnitine levels. Serum concentrations of carnitine were "significantly lower" in the female cancer patients than in women without cancer. Cancer patients also were expelling more carnitine in their urine than people without the disease. This increased

CANCER THERAPY

excretion of carnitine-type substances was thought to be a "response to chemotherapy" and represented "a loss of energy to the cancer patient" (6).

Azelaic acid is an experimental substance that kills melanoma cells in the test tube. It is believed to interfere with cancer cells' mitochondria. By adding carnitine, scientists increased the transport of azelaic acid into these energy centers and thereby increased that drug's cell-killing effect. The addition of carnitine had no effect by itself or with low concentrations of azelaic acid.

Scientists concluded that "carnitine may reduce the time or concentration needed for azelaic acid to have a toxic effect" on melanoma cells (7). It may, therefore, be a useful agent in improving the effects of other anticancer drugs.

Negative? Carnitine actually protected some tumor cells from damage to their mitochondria by the experimental anticancer drug, MGBG. But carnitine also protected experimental animals from acute toxicity and death caused by MGBG (8).

⊕ References

1. Giovannini M. Is carnitine essential in children? Journal of International Medical Research.1991;19:88-102.
2. Franceschi C, et al. Immunological parameters in aging: studies on natural immunomodulatory and immunoprotective substances. Int J Clin Pharmacol Res.1990;10:53-7.
3. De Simone C, et al. Vitamins and immunity: II. Influence of L-carnitine on the immune system. Acta Vitaminol Enzymol. 1982;4:135-40.
4. De Simone C, et al. [Reversibility by L-carnitine of immunosuppression induced by an emulsion of soya bean oil, glycerol and egg lecithin.] Arzneimittelforschung.1982;32:1485-8.
5. Sachan DS and Dodson WL. The serum carnitine status of cancer patients. J Am Coll Nutr.1987;6:145-50.

6.   Dodson WL, et al. Alterations of serum and urinary carnitine profiles in cancer patients: hypothesis of possible significance. J Am Coll Nutr. 1989;8:133-42.

7.   Ward BJ, et al. Effect of L-carnitine on cultured murine melanoma cells exposed to azelaic acid. J Invest Dermatol. 1986;86:438-41.

8.   Janne J, et al. S-adenosylmethionine decarboxylase as target of chemotherapy. Adv Enzyme Regul.1985;24:125-39.

❦ VITAMIN C

Vitamin C is a powerful antioxidant found in many foods, including lemons, oranges and green peppers. It is also one of the most promising items in the anticancer arsenal. Also known as ascorbic acid, this vitamin was discovered in the adrenal gland in the 1920s by the Hungarian scientist Albert Szent-Gyorgyi, who later isolated it from paprika. He won the Nobel Prize for his discovery in 1936 and continued to study the relationship between vitamin C and diseases such as cancer into his nineties (1).

The existence of a food substance that prevents scurvy had been suspected for centuries. Brews of a pine tree called *arborvitae* had been given to explorer Jacques Cartier by North American Indians to cure the scurvy rampant among his crew. We now know the reason why this treatment was effective: the tree's leaves and bark contained vitamin C.

In the eighteenth century, Dr. James Lind performed a landmark experiment in which sailors who received citrus fruit were dramatically cured of scurvy, while seafarers who did not receive such fruit in their diets died. After decades of hesitation, this treatment was officially adopted by the British navy. Vitamin C thus help Britain's 'limeys' rule the waves for over a century.

Researchers have hardly exhausted the wonders of

vitamin C. It not only prevents scurvy but is required for tissue growth and repair, the functioning of the adrenal glands and healthy gums. It is a prime fighter against free radicals in the body. Prof. Linus Pauling, the only person to win two solo Nobel prizes (Chemistry, 1954; Peace, 1962), has argued eloquently that large doses of vitamin C can affect the occurrence, severity and length of colds. It has also been shown to affect the toxicity and cancer-causing ability of more than 50 common pollutants (2). It is vital in maintaining the health of the liver, for the absorption of iron and for the efficiency of the immune system (3).

As early as 1933, Szent-Gyorgyi suggested in a letter that "a partial lack of this vitamin manifests itself in a decreased resistance of the body." (See the author's *Free Radical: Albert Szent-Gyorgyi and the Discovery of Vitamin C*, NY: Paragon House, 1988.) He thought that large doses of the vitamin might have an influence on colds and other diseases. This theory was elaborated in the 1960s by Dr. Irwin Stone and later popularized and developed by Pauling, who wrote a popular book, *Cancer and Vitamin C*, on the subject with Scottish surgeon Ewan Cameron. According to these authors, "vitamin C is closely related to both scurvy and cancer." They believed that "vitamin C may turn out to be the most important of all nutrients in the control of cancer."

The US government's Recommended Daily Allowance (RDA) of vitamin C is between 35 milligrams (for infants) and 60 milligrams (for most adults). It is suggested that pregnant and lactating women get 20 and 40 milligrams more. For heavy smokers, after operations or traumas or during bouts of infections, doctors may recommend between 100 to 200 milligrams a day. And in the treatment of frank scurvy doctors might give as much as 1,000 milligrams (one gram), according to the *Merck Manual* (15th Ed.). But the conventional view is that for most people more than this amount a day is worthless. At doses over two grams a day, there is even said to be a decrease in the scavenging ability of the white blood cells (3).

Pauling and the 'orthomolecular' physicians who follow him believe that all adults, at least, should take several grams a day of the vitamin to stay well, and that cancer and other patients can profitably take 10, 20 or even more grams per day of the vitamin—many thousand times the amount needed to prevent frank scurvy. Pauling claims that such large amounts of vitamin C extend life, inhibit the growth of cancer and improve one's general well-being. Vitamin C, he says, inhibits cancer "at each stage of its development" (4).

Is this an unnatural amount? Pauling says no. Humans are nearly unique in the animal kingdom for not producing our own supply of the vitamin. Other animals produce the human equivalent not of mere milligrams but of full grams of this crucial nutrient.

Physicians have generally reacted to Pauling's proposals with skepticism and scorn. In the 1970s, he and Cameron published several scientific reports on their treatment for cancer. The first two appeared, amid great controversy, in the Proceedings of the National Academy of Sciences of the USA (PNAS), a prestigious scientific body of which Pauling is a member (5, 6). All clinical experiments were carried out in Scotland, under Cameron's direction.

One hundred terminally ill cancer patients were given vitamin C and then compared to 1,000 similar patients not receiving the vitamin. Survival time, they concluded, was more than four times greater in the vitamin C subjects (more than 210 days) compared to the controls (50 days).

"The results clearly indicate that this simple and safe form of medication is of definite value in the treatment of patients with advanced cancer," they wrote (5).

51

A further study revealed that the vitamin C group lived on average about 300 days more than those who did not receive vitamin C. Many of these patients lived on for years after being declared terminal, while those who did not receive the vitamin died (6).

They also compared patients with lung cancer who received vitamin C to other cases taken from the medical records. In their study, the average increase in survival time (after the date of their first admission to hospital) was about 101 days in one study, and 119 in the second one. The scientists concluded that this increase in survival time "together with the previously reported symptomatic relief and improved sense of well-being" justified the use of vitamin C in cases of lung cancer (7).

Pauling's cause was injured, however, by two Mayo Clinic studies which claimed that high doses of vitamin C had no effect as a cancer treatment. The first study was announced in September, 1979 and claimed that large amounts of vitamin C were ineffective in curing cancer or alleviating the pain of patients with advanced disease (8).

Pauling complained that this test was invalid because the Mayo patients had previously received chemotherapy, which undermines the body's ability to fight disease. And so, the Mayo scientists performed the study again, this time on patients who had not received prior chemotherapy. Once again, they claimed that vitamin C had no effect on the outcome of cancer (9).

This was a public relations disaster for Pauling, accompanied by negative editorials and television appearances by vitamin C's prominent detractors. Their sweeping conclusion was that "high-dose vitamin C therapy is not effective against any advanced malignant disease regardless of whether the patient has had any prior chemotherapy."

Pauling pointed to serious deficiencies in the Mayo study. Upon analysis, he said, it was clear that the vitamin had been discontinued at any sign of worsening, even in subjective symptoms or in performance status of the patients. Thus, if patients merely said they felt worse, they could be yanked off vitamin C. The result was that patients received vitamin C for a median time of only ten weeks, which represented a significant departure from the Cameron protocol that supposedly had been followed to the letter.

In fact, no Mayo patient died while receiving vitamin C. They only died when the vitamin was taken away from them. And suddenly stopping vitamin C could bring on the well-known "rebound effect," a downturn that follows sudden removal of the vitamin (10).

In addition, there was evidence that some of the people in the control group were surreptitiously taking vitamin C. (Patients in controlled studies often eliminate the possibility of not getting the experimental drug by sneaking that substance on their own.)

"Some of the controls were clearly taking vitamin C independently of the trial," a sociologist concluded in the British journal, *New Scientist.*

Finally, after being yanked off the vitamin C, about half the patients were given the toxic drug 5-FU, despite the fact that Mayo scientists themselves had once written that this drug was useless for this type of advanced cancer. Pauling concluded that the Mayo studies are "so flawed as to be themselves of no value" (10).

Since that time, evidence has continued to accumulate about the beneficial effects of vitamin C in cancer. Some of this is taking place, surprisingly, at institutions affiliated with the National Cancer Institute.

The formation of cancer-causing compounds "is inhibited by vitamin C, vitamin E, and certain antioxidants. This fact can be used to decrease deliberately the risk of gastric cancer" (11). For example, stomach cancer is more common in areas where nitrite in the food is not balanced by the presence of vitamin C as well as other antioxidants.

When leukemic mice were given a combination of vitamin C (sodium ascorbate) and vitamin B_{12} for ten days, there was a 70 percent increase in their survival (12).

Chinese scientists, seeking the cause of high rates of esophageal cancer in Linxian County isolated a carcinogenic chemical in pickled vegetables called RRME. This caused 63 percent tumors in experimental animals. But massive doses of vitamin C and a form of vitamin A "showed an obviously inhibitory effect on promoting action" of this carcinogen (13).

In 1980, vitamin C was shown to kill cancer cells preferentially in the test tube. It is "selectively toxic to at least one type of malignant cell—a melanoma—at concentrations that might be attained in humans," according to an article in *Nature* (14). A decade later, it was shown that a modified form of vitamin C (called 6-Br-AA) had a "highly pronounced inhibiting effect" on the growth and normal functioning of melanoma cells, according to scientists in Zagreb, Yugoslavia. These tumor-suppressing effects on melanoma were attained with just nine milligrams of the substance, given three times a day for 16 days. Yugoslav scientists suggested that this substance "could serve as a potential antitumor agent" (15).

NCI scientists found that they could greatly extend the lifespans of mice which had melanoma by:

• giving them a form of the drug levodopa (routinely used to treat Parkinsonism);

• restricting their intake of two amino acids, phenylalanine and tyrosine; and

• administering vitamin C in the drinking water.

In mice fed a diet deficient in these two amino acids, the combination of vitamin C and levodopa "retarded tumor

growth and increased survival dramatically by 123 percent." This could "become an important strategy for treating malignant melanoma," NCI scientists suggested (16).

In 1990, Pauling teamed up with Abram Hoffer, MD,
PhD, a well-known Canadian biochemist and psychiatrist,
who had been treating schizophrenic patients with megadoses of vitamin B₃ for decades. Together, they published
a study of women with cancer who received high dose
vitamin C (17).

The paper used a statistical analysis developed by Pauling in 1989 based on the "Hardin Jones principle" (10, 18).
This principle was formulated by the late Prof. Hardin
Jones of the UC Berkeley in 1956 (19). It implies a set of
criteria for showing the validity of a clinical test for cancer
patients who have survived for different lengths of time.

This study was not planned. Its inception was Hoffer's
observation that cancer patients referred to him by other
doctors survived much longer when they followed a nutritional supplement program that included beta-carotene
and about ten grams a day of vitamin C.

The mean survival time of patients who did not follow
the megavitamin program was 5.7 months. Those who
received vitamin C fell into two groups. The poor responders, constituting about 20 percent of the entire group,
lived an average of ten months, almost twice as long. But
the other 80 percent who received vitamin C responded
much better. In fact, these good responders, as they were
called, lived 16 times as long as those who did not get the
treatment. Many of them were still alive at the time the
paper was written in 1990 (17).

The results were particularly impressive for women
with cancers of the ovary, breast and fallopian tubes. Of 11
such women who did not take vitamin C, all but one had
died, and the one survivor was very ill. But, after a comparable period of time, 21 of forty women who received the

vitamins were alive and all but two of these were well.

Hoffer and Pauling strongly recommended "that patients with cancer follow the regimen described in this paper, as an adjunct to appropriate conventional therapy."

In addition, they recommend that "physicians consider administering a large amount of sodium ascorbate by intravenous infusion to patients with advanced cancer." Such treatment is already being practiced by a number of orthomolecular physicians (20).

In September 1990, NCI sponsored a symposium on "Ascorbic Acid: Biological Functions and Relation to Cancer." The meeting was held at the Lister Hill Auditorium of the National Institutes of Health (NIH), NCI's parent body. Forty papers were presented, with 130 scientists in attendance from all over the world.

At this historic meeting, Dr. Balz Frei of UC Berkeley said he considered vitamin C "the most effective antioxidant in human blood plasma." Frei showed that some of the chemical reactions that cause cancer simply could not take place as long as vitamin C was present. But oxygen damage to body fats would occur as soon as the vitamin C supplementation was discontinued (21-23). Dr. E. Niki from the University of Tokyo stated that harmful free radicals are destroyed faster by vitamin C than by any other antioxidant (24-27). He has also shown that vitamin C interacts particularly well with vitamin E. Pauling showed that most animals manufacture the bodily equivalent of ten grams per day of vitamin C.

Two researchers from the Linus Pauling Institute of Science and Medicine, Palo Alto, CA, Drs. Raxit J. Jariwalla and Constance S. Tsao, reported on the benefits of vitamin C on AIDS and in mammary tumor fragments in mice. For example, they showed that vitamin C had an "anti-HIV effect," by diminishing the production of protein by viruses in infected cells. It also decreased the stability of certain proteins crucial to the virus when it is outside the cell (28).

Dr. Joachim Liehr from the University of Texas at Galveston reported that vitamin C inhibits the incidence of kidney tumors induced by female sex hormones. But pretreatment of hamsters with vitamin C protected them against the effects of DES (a cancer-causing synthetic hormone) injections. Dr. M.E. Poydock of the Mercyhurst College Cancer Research Center, Eire, PA, told of a patient who showed a significant reduction in tumor after just three injections of vitamin C and B_{12} (29-31).

Dr. Okunieff showed that when vitamin C was administered to animals with cancer, they needed only half the usual amount of radiation therapy. And Dr. Gary Meadows of Washington State University showed that vitamin C added to drinking water inhibited the growth of cancer in mice, while increasing the cell-killing activity of chemotherapy. In men who had very low levels of vitamin C in their blood, Dr. Jacob of San Francisco found increased levels of mutagens in their stool; such mutagens are suspected of causing or promoting colorectal cancer.

The symposium was concluded by Dr. Gladys Block of NCI who reviewed the evidence in the scientific literature on the value of vitamin C. Of the 46 studies in which the intake of vitamin C in people's food was calculated, 33 demonstrated a protective effect. In fact, people with high levels of vitamin C in their diet had half the chance of contracting cancer as those who had a low intake.

Since vitamin C is commonly found in fruits, scientists have also tried to estimate the overall protective value of eating fruit and drinking fruit juice. Of 29 additional studies that simply looked at fruit intake, 21 found "significant protection" from cancer. For cancers of the esophagus, larynx, oral cavity and pancreas, evidence for a protective effect of vitamin C or some other component in fruit is "strong and consistent." For cancers of the stomach, rectum, breast, and cervix there is also good evidence, she said.

In a 1991 article, Block added, "It is likely that ascorbic acid, carotenoids, and other factors in fruits and vegetables act jointly. Increased consumption of fruits and vegetables in general should be encouraged" (32).

A second conference on vitamin C was held at NIH in September, 1991. By this time it had become apparent to all that vitamin C was beginning to get "a little respect," in the words of *Science* (10/18/91). According to this magazine, vitamin C may have had a "checkered past" because of the "fringe group" associated with its use, but the scientific tide was turning in its favor.

Dr. Block, who had moved from NCI to the School of Public Health at UC Berkeley, said "there is no question that the status of vitamin C has changed in a lot of researchers' minds." Her own studies continue to show that the "protective effect of vitamin C for non-hormone-dependent cancers is strong."

Hiroshi Kan Shimpo, of Fujita Health University in Japan, reported that vitamin C can block the damage to heart muscles that often occurs when doctors treat cancer patients with highly toxic drugs like adriamycin and interleukin-2 (IL-2), a form of immunotherapy whose promise has been limited by its great toxicity. (The side effects of IL-2 include fever, chills, rapid heartbeat, low blood pressure, vomiting, diarrhea and fluid retention.) Peter Wiernick of the Montefiore Medical Center, NY found that people undergoing IL-2 treatment suffered an 80 percent drop in vitamin C, to levels low enough to cause scurvy. Such levels became "undetectable" in 8 of 11 patients. Not surprisingly, those with the lowest levels tended to do worst on IL-2, contributing to the notorious toxicity of that treatment (33).

However, many researchers still dismiss Pauling and his vitamin C crusade out of hand. "We're talking about speculations that have nothing to do with public health," nutritionist Robert Olson of the State University of New York (SUNY) at Stony Brook told *Science*.

There have been numerous media reports of vitamin C's alleged toxicity, and even a flurry of reports that it promotes cancer. In 1979, Scottish doctors described three patients (two with Hodgkin's disease and one with lung cancer) in whom high doses of vitamin C appeared associated with the development of potentially harmful symptoms. They suggested that vitamin C therapy "should be given with caution in malignant disease, with a slow buildup over several days to high levels of dosage" (39). According to another 1988 study, vitamin C administration to rats seemed to accelerate the formation of liver cancer when a carcinogen was put in the animals' drinking water (40).

Dr. S. Fukushima of Nagoya City University Medical School has also shown that an extremely high dose of sodium L-ascorbate, as five percent of the diet, amplified the effects of bladder carcinogens under experimental conditions, "while a high dose [one percent] does not" (34).

But that was with the sodium salt of the vitamin. What about the more common ascorbic acid, which contains no sodium? In 1985, Fukushima reported that administration of five percent ascorbic acid did not cause or promote bladder cancer (35). It turns out to be the sodium (salt) version of the molecule that promotes cancer, not vitamin C per se. In 1991, scientists at the University of Nebraska Medical Center, Omaha affirmed that "ascorbic acid showed no tumor-promoting activity," but that salts of many compounds did so (36). This appears to be another example of the cancer-promoting effects of high-sodium diets that are deficient in potassium.

There have also been claims that vitamin C promotes the formation of oxalate crystals (the salt of oxalic acid, which is damaging to the kidneys) and kidney stones. In 1977, South African scientists studied the formation of oxalate crystals in baboons given high doses of vitamin C over a long period of time. Microscopic inspection "did not reveal oxalate crystals in any of the soft tissues obtained from 16 baboons fed very high doses of ascorbic acid for a period of 20 months," they reported (37).

Indian biochemists also studied this question and found "neither stone nor calcium oxalate crystal deposition" in the kidneys of rats which were fed 60 milligrams of vitamin C daily for three months. They attributed the lack of such stones to the acidity of the mice's urine after receiving the vitamin as well as to their reduced calcium excretion (38).

This is not to say that vitamin C cannot be toxic under certain circumstances. Some patients report stomach upset, rectal itching and diarrhea after very high doses. Such symptoms can be relieved by cutting back the dose or changing to the calcium ascorbate form of the vitamin. By and large, vitamin C appears to be a very non-toxic substance, which most people can take in large amounts for long periods of time without harm.

⊕ References

1. Fodor G, et al. The search for new cancerostatic agents. Ciba Found Symp.1978;67:165-74.
2. Calabrese EJ. Does exposure to environmental pollutants increase the need for vitamin C? J Environ Pathol Toxicol Oncol. 1985;5:81-90.
3. Kolb E. [Recent knowledge concerning the biochemistry and

significance of ascorbic acid]. Z Gesamte Inn Med.1984;39:21-7.

4.   McCarty MF. An antithrombotic role for nutritional antioxidants: implications for tumor metastasis and other pathologies. Med Hypotheses.1986;19:345-57.

5.   Cameron E and Pauling L. Supplemental ascorbate in the supportive treatment of cancer: Prolongation of survival times in terminal human cancer. Proc Natl Acad Sci USA.1976;73:3685-3689.

6.   Cameron E and Pauling L. Supplemental ascorbate in the supportive treatment of cancer: Reevaluation of prolongation of survival times in terminal human cancer. Proc Natl Acad Sci USA.1978;75:4538-4542.

7.   Cameron E and Pauling L. Survival times of terminal lung cancer patients treated with ascorbate. J Int Acad Prev Med. 1979;6:21-27.

8.   Creagan E, et al. Failure of high-dose vitamin C (ascorbic acid) therapy to benefit patients with advanced cancer. New England Journal of Medicine.1979;301:687-690.

9.   Moertel C, et al. High-dose vitamin C versus placebo in the treatment of patients with advanced cancer who have had no prior chemotherapy. New England Journal of Medicine.1985;312:137-141.

10.   Pauling L and Herman Z. Criteria for the validity of clinical trials of treatments of cohorts of cancer patients based on the Hardin Jones principle. Proc Nat Acad Sci USA.1989;86:6835-6837.

11.   Weisburger JH and Horn CL. Human and laboratory studies on the causes and prevention of gastrointestinal cancer. Scand J Gastroenterol Suppl. 1984;104:15-26.

12.   Pierson HF, et al. Depletion of extracellular cysteine with hydroxocobalamin and ascorbate in experimental murine cancer chemotherapy. Cancer Res.1985;45:4727-31.

13.   Lin PZ, et al. [Carcinogenic and promoting effects of Roussin red methyl ester (RRME) on the forestomach epithelium of mice and esophageal epithelium of rats, and its inhibition by retinamide and vitamin C]. Chung Hua Chung Liu Tsa Chih.1986;8:405-8.

14.   Bram S, et al. Vitamin C preferential toxicity for malignant melanoma cells. Nature.1980;284:629-31.

15.   Osmak M, et al. 6-Deoxy-6-bromo-ascorbic acid inhibits growth of mouse melanoma cells. Res Exp Med (Berl).1990;190:443-9.

16.   Pierson HF and Meadows GG. Sodium ascorbate enhancement of carbidopa-levodopa methyl ester antitumor activity against pigmented B16 melanoma. Cancer Res.1983;43:2047-51.

17.   Hoffer A and Pauling L. Hardin Jones biostatistical analysis of mortality data for cohorts of cancer patients with a large fraction surviving at the termination of the study and a comparison of survival times of cancer patients receiving large regular oral doses of vitamin C and other nutrients with similar patients not receiving those doses. Journal of Orthomolecular Medicine.1990;5:143-154.

18. Pauling L. Biostatistical analysis of mortality data for cohorts of cancer patients. Proc Nat Acad Sci USA.1989;86:3466-3488.

19. Jones H. Demographic consideration of the cancer problem. Trans NY Acad Sci.1956;18:298-333.

20. Riordan H, et al. High-dose intravenous vitamin C in the treatment of a patient with adenocarcinoma of the kidney. J Orthomol Med. 1990; 5:5-7.

21. Frei B, et al. Ascorbate is an outstanding antioxidant in human blood plasma. Proc Natl Acad Sci U S A.1989;86:6377-81.

22. Frei B, et al. Ascorbate: the most effective antioxidant in human blood plasma. Adv Exp Med Biol. 1990;264:155-63.

23. Frei B, et al. Gas phase oxidants of cigarette smoke induce lipid peroxidation and changes in lipoprotein properties in human blood plasma. Protective effects of ascorbic acid. Biochem J. 1991;277:133-8.

24. Niki E, et al. Inhibition of oxidation of methyl linoleate in solution by vitamin E and vitamin C. J Biol Chem.1984;259:4177-82.

25. Niki E. Lipid antioxidants: how they may act in biological systems. Br J Cancer Suppl.1987;8:153-7.

26. Niki E. Interaction of ascorbate and alpha-tocopherol. Ann NY Acad Sci.1987;498:186-99.

27. Niki E. Antioxidants in relation to lipid peroxidation. Chem Phys Lipids.1987;44:227-53.

28. Harakeh S, et al. Suppression of human immunodeficiency virus replication by ascorbate in chronically and acutely infected cells. Proc Natl Acad Sci U S A.1990;87:7245-9.

29. Poydock ME, et al. Inhibiting effect of vitamins C and B12 on the mitotic activity of ascites tumors. Exp Cell Biol.1979;47:210-7.

30. Poydock ME, et al. Inhibiting effect of dehydroascorbic acid on cell division in ascites tumors in mice. Exp Cell Biol.1982;50:34-8.

31. Poydock ME, et al. Mitogenic inhibition and effect on survival of mice bearing L1210 leukemia using a combination of dehydroascorbic acid and hydroxycobalamin. Am J Clin Oncol.1985;8:266-9.

32. Block G. Vitamin C and cancer prevention: the epidemiologic evidence. Am J Clin Nutr.1991;53:270S-282S.

33. Marcus SL, et al. Severe hypovitaminosis C occurring as the result of adoptive immunotherapy with high-dose interleukin 2 and lymphokine-activated killer cells. Cancer Res.1987;47:4208-12.

34. Fukushima S, et al. Promoting effects of sodium L-ascorbate on two-stage urinary bladder carcinogenesis in rats. Cancer Res. 1983;43:4454-7.

35. Fukushima S, et al. Significance of L-ascorbic acid and urinary electrolytes in promotion of rat bladder carcinogenesis. Int Symp Princess Takamatsu Cancer Res Fund.1985;16:159-68.

36. Cohen SM, et al. Comparative bladder tumor promoting activity of

62

sodium saccharin, sodium ascorbate, related acids, and calcium salts in
rats. Cancer Res.1991;51:1766-77.

37. du Bruyn D, et al. High dietary ascorbic acid levels and oxalate crys-
tallization in soft tissues of baboons. S Afr Med J.1977;52:861-2.

38. Singh PP, et al. An investigation into the role of ascorbic acid in renal
calculogenesis in albino rats. J Urol.1988;139:156-7.

39. Campbell A and Jack T. Acute reactions to mega ascorbic acid therapy in malignant disease. Scott Med J.1979;24:151-3.

40. Birk RV, et al. [Effect of ascorbic acid on the hepatocarcinogenic action of N- nitrosodiethylamine in rats]. Eksp Onkol.1988;10:66-8.

ᕥ ᗷIOFLAVONOIDS

Bioflavonoids are brightly colored substances commonly found alongside vitamin C, in nature as in the health food store. Both substances were discovered by Albert Szent-Gyorgyi and isolated from paprika in the 1930s. Szent-Gyorgyi himself called bioflavonoids "vitamin P," and suggested they were crucial for the integrity of the small blood vessels and as a treatment for a skin disease called purpura. Influential nutritionists refused to acknowledge this designation, however. Bioflavonoids have existed in a kind of nutritional limbo ever since then.

Some of the best-known bioflavonoids are citrin, hesperidin and rutin. Bioflavonoids are abundantly found in the white pulp of citrus fruits and in grapes, plums, black currants, apricots, buckwheat, cherries, blackberries and rose hips. They remove toxic copper from the body and protect vitamin C from the destructive action of some copper-containing enzymes. In reasonable amounts they are believed to be non-toxic. They thus may have a role to play in promoting vitamin C's anticancer effects.

Bioflavonoids are being evaluated, by themselves and together with other substances, in the treatment of cancer.

The general consensus is that a synthetic relative of bioflavonoids, flavone acetic acid, or FAA, is an immune booster, although not a very useful drug by itself (1). FAA increases natural killer (NK) cell activity in mice (2). In Italian laboratory tests, FAA produced mixed results. Some transplanted human tumors were unaffected, but those grown under the skin and in the liver of test animals were significantly inhibited. This test demonstrated, Italian scientists said, the "great importance of the site of tumour growth for FAA efficacy" (3).

FAA was also clinically evaluated in cancer. Fifty-four patients were given large infusions for up to six hours. No objective responses were seen in this trial, however (4). Scientists are puzzling over why this drug works much better in mice than in people. Some have concluded that there is "a clear immunological component in the mechanism of action of FAA" (5).

However, FAA seems to have one powerful effect. Combined with interleukin-2 (IL-2) the two become very powerful together. As an added plus, IL-2 taken with FAA does not have its usual severe toxicity. In mice, kidney cancer treated with FAA and IL-2 resulted "in up to 80 percent long term survival" whereas either substance alone was "unable to induce any long term survivors." The two substances appeared to work by stimulating natural killer (NK) cells (6) as well as the production of natural **tumor necrosis factor** (7). Used together in people, there were nearly 60 percent more long-term survivors than when either drug was used alone (2).

Another flavonoid, quercetin, derived from the common horse chestnut, is also found in many plants, including edible fruits and vegetables. It is an enzyme inhibitor. Japanese scientists found that it markedly inhibited the growth of human stomach cancer cells (8).

FAA's side effects: Doctors saw uncomfortable warmth and flushes, nausea, diarrhea and visual complaints. Low blood pressure was also seen in some patients (4, 9).

⊕ References

1. Kerr DJ, et al. Phase II trials of flavone acetic acid in advanced malignant melanoma and colorectal carcinoma. Br J Cancer. 1989;60:104-6.

2. Hornung RL, et al. Augmentation of natural killer activity, induction of IFN and development of tumor immunity during the successful treatment of established murine renal cancer using flavone acetic acid and IL-2. J Immunol.1988;141:3671-9.

3. Pratesi G, et al. Differential efficacy of flavone acetic against liver versus lung metastases in a human tumour xenograft. Br J Cancer. 1991;63:71-4.

4. Kerr DJ, et al. Phase I and pharmacokinetic study of flavone acetic acid. Cancer Res.1987;277:6776-81.

5. Bibby MC, et al. Antitumour activity of flavone acetic acid (NSC 347512) in mice— influence of immune status. Br J Cancer.1991;63:57-62.

6. Wiltrout RH, et al. Flavone-8-acetic acid augments systemic natural killer cell activity and synergizes with IL-2 for treatment of murine renal cancer. J Immunol.1988;140:3261-5.

7. Pratesi G, et al. Role of T cells and tumour necrosis factor in antitumour activity and toxicity of flavone acetic acid. Eur J Cancer. 1990; 26:1079-83.

8. Yoshida M, et al. The effect of quercetin on cell cycle progression and growth of human gastric cancer cells. Febs Lett. 1990;260:10-3.

9. Kaye SB, et al. Phase II trials with flavone acetic acid (NCS. 347512, LM975) in patients with advanced carcinoma of the breast, colon, head and neck and melanoma. Invest New Drugs.1990;8:S95-9.

☙ VITAMIN D

. . . .

Unlike any other nutrient, vitamin D is manufactured in the body by exposure to sunlight. Together with the mineral calcium, it may play an important role in preventing colon and other kinds of cancer.

Much of the work establishing the relationship between vitamin D and cancer in various populations has been done by two San Diego brothers, Cedric and Frank Garland. They began their investigations at the Johns Hopkins University School of Hygiene and Public Health. They then moved to Southern California, where Cedric became director of the epidemiology program at the UC San Diego Cancer Center. His younger brother Frank is associate professor and head of occupational medicine at the Naval Health Research Center.

In 1974, the Garlands took blood samples from over 25,000 people in Washington County, MD to investigate the relationship between this vitamin and the risk of colon cancer. Between 1975 and 1983, 34 cases of colon cancer developed in this group. The chances of getting colon cancer were 80 percent less in the subjects who had the highest levels of vitamin D. The Garlands concluded that vitamin D exerts a protective effect against colon cancer (1).

They then studied colon cancer in a variety of locales which received differing amounts of exposure to sunlight. Death rates from this type of cancer were highest precisely in those places where people received the least amount of sunlight, including smoggy cities (2).

A few years later, the Garlands made the startling and iconoclastic proposal that sunlight might actually *protect* against malignant melanoma. Sunlight is commonly thought of as a major cause or promoter of this deadly form of skin disease. Their argument ran as follows:

Melanoma is the second most common malignancy among US sailors (after cancer of the testicles). Between 1974 and 1984, active duty sailors came down with a total of 176 cases of melanoma. But surprisingly it was not outdoors sailors but Naval personnel working indoors who exhibited the highest rates. Sailors whose jobs required spending time indoors and outdoors had the lowest rate.

Melanomas on the trunk of the body were more common than on the sunlit areas of the head and arms. What could this mean? That brief, regular *exposure* to sunlight was probably beneficial in preventing melanoma, while either too little or too much exposure was potentially harmful. This finding fit in with laboratory studies showing that vitamin D suppressed the growth of melanoma cells in the test tube. Vitamin D also seemed to inhibit very small melanomas from developing into clinical cases of cancer (3).

The annual death rate from breast cancer varies considerably from region to region, practically doubling from the US South and Southwest to the high-risk Northeast. In addition, the risk of fatal breast cancer in the major cities is "inversely proportional to intensity of local sunlight." It increased in low sunlight areas and decreased in sunnier climes. Vitamin D, created in the course of exposure to sunlight, is thus associated with a low risk of fatal breast cancer. The Garlands concluded that differences in the amount of ultraviolet light reaching the population may account for the striking regional differences in breast cancer deaths (5). The same was true in the Soviet Union (6).

Now, sulfur dioxide (a main ingredient in smog) absorbs ultraviolet light in the very part of the spectrum that triggers the production of vitamin D in the skin. 'Acid haze' (a high concentration of sulfur dioxide in the air) may thus lead to vitamin D deficiencies and therefore breast and colon cancer. In 20 Canadian cities, there was a positive association between air pollution and the death rate from colon cancer in both women and men, as well as breast cancer in women (7).

It is generally believed that a high fat diet by itself promotes breast cancer. But biochemists at the University of Western Ontario in London, Canada, suspected that vitamin D and calcium might also play a crucial role. To test this idea, 40 rats were fed a diet supplemented with sunflower seed oil (for fat), calcium and vitamin D. After one week, each rat was given a carcinogen. A week later, these same animals were switched to diets varying in fat, calcium and vitamin D content. In the animals fed the high-fat diet, a concurrent reduction of calcium and vitamin D increased the total number of breast tumors from four to sixteen. The Canadian scientists suggested that lowering the amounts of calcium and vitamin D "increase the promoting effects of a high-fat diet" on the development of breast cancer in rats (8).

In colon cancer, a 19-year study of nearly 2,000 men in Chicago found that a high dietary intake of vitamin D per day was associated with a 50 percent reduction in the incidence of cancer of the colon and rectum. An intake of 1.2 grams or more calcium per day was associated with a 75 percent reduction. Clinical and laboratory studies further support these findings. In addition, a study of over 25,000 people showed that even moderately larger amounts of vitamin D were associated with "large reductions in the incidence of colorectal cancer" (9).

But how does vitamin D actually work? For many years that was a mystery. The "revolution of information" on vitamin D began in 1968, when J.W. Blunt and colleagues discovered the form of vitamin D that actually circulates in the blood (25-OH-D3) (10). This hormonal form of the vitamin, created in the kidneys, is ultimately responsible for the classical action of the vitamin. At the molecular level, some cancer cells appear to have receptors on their surfaces that are capable of receiving the vitamin D molecule. Scientists studied cancer cells from 136 patients with breast cancer. Those whose cancers had such vitamin D receptors "had significantly longer disease-free survival" periods than those whose tumors did not.

Vitamin D also stopped the growth of several kind of human breast cancer cells in the test tube. Treatment of mice with breast cancer "produced significant inhibition of tumor progression," according to pathologists at St George's Hospital Medical School in London, UK. Taken together, these studies suggest vitamin D may inhibit the growth of cancers that have receptors for the vitamin (4).

In the early 1980s it was shown that high doses of vitamin D suppressed growth and changed cancer cells into a different type (11). This stimulated interest in using vitamin D in treatment. However, even small amounts of the hormonal form of the vitamin will cause an early stage of leukemic cells to mature into healthy blood cells (13). This raised the possibility that the vitamin D-hormone could be used to suppress the growth of leukemia and render malignant cells benign. In mice it was shown that injections of the vitamin D-hormone three times a week greatly increased their survival time (14).

But vitamin D also happens to be toxic in doses of more than 50,000 units a day. Its hormonal form is similarly toxic, except that the amounts needed to produce damage are much smaller (12). In fact, the problem with using vitamin D as therapy is that at effective doses it causes an excess of calcium in the blood (hypercalcemia) that is great enough to kill the patient.

Scientists at the University of Wisconsin, Madison are therefore trying to find other forms of the vitamin D-hormone that are more active but less toxic (10).

Russian scientists have also shown that a diet rich in

vitamin D is not particularly beneficial unless vitamin C is also present. The levels of calcium and vitamin D in the blood both decreased by as much as 50 percent in the face of vitamin C deficiencies. This study demonstrated "a critical role for ascorbic acid in vitamin D metabolism," according to scientists at the Academy of Medical Sciences in Moscow (15).

The Garlands recommend that people try to get ten to fifteen minutes of sunlight per day, without using the popular PABA type of sunscreen during that period. They also think that people should generally try to limit exposure to sunlight using clothing and shade rather than sunscreen: these lotions, they say, may actually block the very kind of light necessary to produce vitamin D, while ironically allowing exposure to precisely the kind of light that promotes skin cancer. The Garlands feel that most PABA sunblockers actually promote the occurrence of three out of four of the most common kinds of cancers. Such exposure is all the more important in northern climes and during winter months.

There is also a fascinating theory, first proposed by innovative researcher John Ott, that light itself performs a dual physiological function: to see by, of course, but also to stimulate the hypothalamus gland and maintain one's general physical and mental health (16). Ott has similarly suggested that people need exposure to whole spectrum solar radiation and that most indoor lighting is lacking in the beneficial effects of whole spectrum light. He too suggests that people try to get outside every day, take off their eyeglasses, and absorb full-spectrum light through the eyes (without of course staring directly into the sun) (17-19). Such 'sunworshiping' ideas are now being given powerful support in laboratories around the world.

⊕ References

1. Garland CF, et al. Serum 25-hydroxyvitamin D and colon cancer: eight-year prospective study [see comments]. Lancet.1989;2:1176-8.

2. Garland CF and Garland FC. Do sunlight and vitamin D reduce the likelihood of colon cancer? Int J Epidemiol.1980;9:227-31.

3. Garland FC, et al. Occupational sunlight exposure and melanoma in the U.S. Navy. Arch Environ Health.1990;45:261-7.

4. Colston KW, et al. Possible role for vitamin D in controlling breast cancer cell proliferation. Lancet.1989;1:188-91.

5. Garland FC, et al. Geographic variation in breast cancer mortality in the United States: a hypothesis involving exposure to solar radiation. Prev Med.1990;19:614-22.

6. Gorham ED, et al. Sunlight and breast cancer incidence in the USSR. Int J Epidemiol.1990;19:820-4.

7. Gorham ED, et al. Acid haze air pollution and breast and colon cancer mortality in 20 Canadian cities. Can J Public Health.1989;80:96-100.

8. Jacobson EA, et al. Effects of dietary fat, calcium, and vitamin D on growth and mammary tumorigenesis induced by 7,12-dimethylbenz(a)anthracene in female Sprague-Dawley rats. Cancer Res.1989;49:6300-3.

9. Garland CF, et al. Can colon cancer incidence and death rates be reduced with calcium and vitamin D? Am J Clin Nutr.1991;54:193S-201S.

10. DeLuca H and Ostrem V. Analogs of the hormonal form of vitamin D and their possible use in leukemia. In: Tryfiates G and Prasad K (Eds). Nutrition, Growth, and Cancer. NY: Alan R. Liss, 1988.

11. Frampton R, et al. Inhibition of human cancer cell growth by 1,25-dihydroxyvitamin D3 metabolites. Cancer Res.1983;43:4443-4447.

12. Tanaka Y, et al. Biological activity of 1,25-dihydroxyvitamin D3 in the rat. Endocrinology.1973;92:417-422.

13. Tanaka H, et al. 1(alpha),25-dihydroxycholecalciferol and a human myeloid leukaemia cell line (HL-60). The presence of a cytosal receptor and induction of differentiation. Biochem J.1982;204:713-719.

14. Honma Y, et al. 1(alpha),25-dihydroxyvitamin D3 and 1 (α)-hydroxyvitamin D3 prolong survival time of mice inoculated with myeloid leukemia cells. Proc Natl Acad Sci USA.1983;80:201-204.

15. Sergeev IN, et al. Ascorbic acid effects on vitamin D hormone metabolism and binding in guinea pigs. J Nutr.1990;120:1185-90.

16. Ott J. The influence of light on the retinal hypothalamic endocrine system. Ann Dent. 1968;27:10-6.

17-19. Ott J. The eyes' dual function. I., II, III, Eye Ear Nose Throat Mon. 1974;53:276-7; 309-16; 465-69.

℣ VITAMIN E

Vitamin E is an essential nutrient found abundantly in wheat germ, cottonseed and palm oils as well as in whole grains, lettuce and liver. A deficiency of vitamin E (or more specifically, the crucial portion known as alpha-tocopherol) produces sterility in rats. For this reason, E became known as the 'antisterility' vitamin and even gained an undeserved reputation as an aphrodisiac. There is indeed evidence that it benefits the heart and circulatory system, but there have been numerous, if less publicized, studies showing that it has a protective effect against cancer, as well.

For example, 17 women with a form of premalignant breast disease called 'mammary dysplasia' as well as six controls were treated with 600 International Units (IUs) of vitamin E per day. Scientists studied their blood levels of the vitamin, as well as of the hormones estradiol, estriol and progesterone. Eighty-eight percent of the patients showed a "clinical response" to vitamin E therapy.

To protect against breast cancer, the amount of the hormone progesterone should be high compared to estradiol. It is dangerously low in women who have mammary dysplasia. But the ratio between these two substances improved after women received vitamin E therapy. According to doctors at North Charles General Hospital in Baltimore, MD the "results of this study indicate that vitamin E therapy may correct an abnormal progesterone/estradiol ratio in patients with mammary dysplasia, with implications on reducing future risk for malignant breast disease" (1). The same Baltimore scientists have reported that "vitamin E supplementation may be of value in women with severe PMS symptoms" (2-4).

Kedar N. Prasad, PhD is a leading vitamin researcher at the University of Colorado. He has also written a thoughtful book on *Vitamins Against Cancer* for the layperson (Rochester, VT: Healing Arts Press, 1989). Dr. Prasad has found that one form of vitamin E stops the growth of melanoma cells. His data show that this form of vitamin E "may be a potentially useful tumor therapeutic agent" (5).

Vitamin E has been shown to reduce the toxicity of chemotherapy. When standard drugs such as 5-FU, methotrexate, cyclophosphamide or vincristine were given to rats, they produced harmful free radicals in internal organs. But rats that received vitamin E at the same time had free radical levels that were significantly lower (7).

Polish scientists exposed human blood in the test tube to seven standard drugs known to harm white blood cells. A high blood level of vitamin E protected the white blood cells against the toxicity of all the drugs, except nitrogen mustard (8). (**Aspirin** also protected the cells against four of the drugs.)

Bone Marrow Transplantation (BMT) is an experimental procedure, being used with increasing frequency in an attempt to treat advanced cancer. Before bone marrow transplantation is started, doctors give "conditioning therapy" of high-dose chemotherapy, combined with total body irradiation. Patients who received such "conditioning therapy" were found to have lower levels of vitamin E and beta carotene. The loss of these antioxidants, doctors at Tubigen University, Germany concluded, is possibly the cause of the toxicity seen with BMT.

CANCER THERAPY

"We suggest high-dose supplementation of essential antioxidants for patients undergoing BMT," the German doctors wrote in 1989 (9).

Scientists at Louisiana State University studied patients with lung cancer. Vitamin E was significantly lower in patients hospitalized for lung cancer. They concluded that low serum vitamin E levels may well be associated with an increased risk of lung cancer (10, 11).

Vitamin E versus Carcinogens: In a 1989 study, Russian scientists gave rats a powerful carcinogen. This compound caused tumors of the digestive tract in more than 90 percent of the cases, on average five tumors per rat. When they gave these rats vitamin E, however, there was a 37 percent decrease in the incidence of such tumors (12).

Selenium is a mineral with anticancer activity. But the anticancer effects of selenium are greatly reduced when there is an insufficient intake of vitamin E. Rats who receive a normal amount of vitamin E in their diets showed a 45 percent decrease in tumors when they were given selenium. But they only had a 25 percent decrease if their diet was low in vitamin E. In fact, vitamin E was considered more important than selenium in decreasing "oxidant stress" to the fat of the breast (13).

Finland has been a center of vitamin E research. Between 1968 and 1971, over 15,000 women took part in a large-scale study of vitamin E and cancer by that country's national health insurance agency. At the start, all were free of cancer. During the next eight years, cancer was diagnosed in 313 of these women. Vitamin E levels were then measured from frozen blood samples. The more vitamin E in the blood, the less cancer, scientists concluded. Women with the lowest levels of vitamin E in their blood had a more than one-and-a-half times greater chance of developing cancer than women with the highest levels of the vitamin. Low level of vitamin E strongly predicted major kinds of cancer (14). For example, a small number of melanoma patients had significantly lower levels of vitamin E and **beta-carotene** in their blood (6).

Finnish scientists concluded that "low vitamin E intake is a risk factor for cancer in many, but not all, organs" (14).

The association between vitamin E and cancer was also studied in more than 21,000 Finnish men. The first examination was conducted between 1968 and 1972. By 1982, over 450 cases of cancer had been found in these men.

The risk of cancer in men with higher amounts of vitamin E in their blood was one-third less than those with the lower amounts. This association was strongest for cancers not related to smoking. Scientists again concluded that a high vitamin E level was associated with a reduced risk of cancer. "These findings agree with the hypothesis that high vitamin E intake protects against cancer," said the Finnish researchers (15, 16).

Over 36,000 Finnish men and women were also studied for cancers of the gastrointestinal (GI) tract. There were 150 cases of GI cancer during the next ten years. Again, it was found that people with lower levels of vitamin E or selenium had a higher risk of cancer of the stomach and esophagus. The risk of cancer among men with the lowest amounts of selenium in their bloodstream was several times as great as among those with relative high amounts. The scientists concluded that selenium, and possibly vitamin E, may protect against GI tract cancer, especially among men (17).

Although few doctors are reporting on the use of vitamin E as a cancer treatment, some therapy studies have been published on animals. South African scientists reported in a veterinary journal that they used gamma linolenic acid (GLA) and other essential fatty acid (EFA) metabolites in malignant cancer treatment. Two dogs with

75

lymphoma were given daily doses of GLA, linoleic acid and vitamin E. After about one week, the veterinarians saw a "slight to marked reduction in size" of the enlarged lymph nodes, spleen, skin nodules and tonsils. Both animals continued to improve, but then later deteriorated "due to complications, apparently unrelated to therapy" (18).

Nitrosamines are powerful carcinogens that can form in the stomach. Vitamin E was effective in preventing their formation, however, especially when used in conjunction with **vitamin C.** German nutritionists suggest that vitamin E, when taken together with food, may reduce human exposure to cancer-causing nitrosamines (19).

A Cautious Man: Despite the fact that his own studies provide the strongest support for the cancer-vitamin E link, in 1991 a leader of the Finnish studies cautioned that "no definite conclusions about a causal connection between vitamin E and the occurrence of cancer can be drawn until the final results of current large-scale intervention trials are published" (20).

In addition, it should be noted that one Dutch study showed a protective value for beta-carotene and **vitamin A,** but no conclusive benefit for vitamins C or E (11).

⊕ References

1.   London RS, et al. Endocrine parameters and alpha-tocopherol therapy of patients with mammary dysplasia. Cancer Res.1981;41:3811-3.

2.   London RS, et al. The effect of alpha-tocopherol on premenstrual symptomatology: a double-blind study. J Am Coll Nutr.1983;2:115-22.

3.   London RS, et al. The effect of alpha-tocopherol on premenstrual symptomatology: a double-blind study. II. Endocrine correlates. J Am Coll Nutr.1984;3:351-6.

4.   London RS, et al. Efficacy of alpha-tocopherol in the treatment of the premenstrual syndrome. J Reprod Med.1987;32:400-4.

5.   Prasad KN and Edwards PJ. Effects of tocopherol (vitamin E) acid succinate on morphological alterations and growth inhibition in melanoma

cells in culture. Cancer Res.1982;42:550-5.

6.   Knekt P, et al. Serum micronutrients and risk of cancers of low incidence in Finland. Am J Epidemiol.1991;134:356-61.

7.   Capel ID, et al. Vitamin E retards the lipoperoxidation resulting from anticancer drug administration. Anticancer Res. 1983;3:59-62.

8.   Szczepanska I, et al. Inhibition of leucocyte migration by cancer chemotherapeutic agents and its prevention by free radical scavengers and thiols. Eur J Haematol.1988;40:69-74.

9.   Clemens MR, et al. Decreased essential antioxidants and increased lipid hydroperoxides following high-dose radiochemotherapy. Free Radic Res Commun.1989;7:227-32.

10.   LeGardeur B, et al. A case-controlled study of serum vitamins A, E and C in lung cancer patients. Nutrition and Cancer.1990;14:133-140.

11.   Stam J. Vitamins and lung cancer. Lung.1990;Suppl:1075-1081.

12.   Bespalov VG, et al. [The effect of tocopherol and ascorbic acid on the development of experimental esophageal tumors].Vopr Onkol. 1989;35:1332-6.

13.   Ip C. Attenuation of the anticarcinogenic action of selenium by vitamin E deficiency. Cancer Lett.1985;25:325-31.

14.   Knekt P. Serum vitamin E level and risk of female cancers. Int J Epidemiol.1988;17:281-6.

15.   Knekt P, et al. Serum cholesterol and risk of cancer in a cohort of 39,000 men and women. J Clin Epidemiol.1988;41:519-30.

16.   Knekt P, et al. Determinants of serum alpha-tocopherol in Finnish adults. Prev Med.1988;17:725-35.

17.   Knekt P, et al. Serum vitamin E, serum selenium and the risk of gastrointestinal cancer. Int J Cancer.1988;42:846-50.

18.   Williams JH. The use of gamma linolenic acid, linoleic acid and natural vitamin E for the treatment of multicentric lymphoma in two dogs. J S Afr Vet Assoc.1988;59:141-4.

19.   Lathia D and Blum A. Role of vitamin E as nitrite scavenger and N-nitrosamine inhibitor: a review. Int J Vitam Nutr Res.1989;59:430-8.

20.   Knekt P. Role of vitamin E in the prophylaxis of cancer. Ann Med.1991;23:3-12.

❧ VITAMIN K

Vitamin K is a little known, but essential nutrient, necessary for both blood clot formation and liver function. There are three main kinds of this vitamin. The first two are fat-soluble and are generally manufactured in the intestines in the presence of bacteria. Vitamin K_3, also known as mena-dione, is a synthetic bright yellow crystal that is given to people who cannot manufacture their own vitamin K. Several experiments suggest that vitamin K, with or without other drugs, may be an effective anticancer agent.

Vitamin K_3 was first synthesized in 1940 and by the 1970s was being tested as an anticancer and antimicrobial product (1). Dr. Kedar Prasad of Colorado found that it inhibited the growth of mammalian tumor cells in culture (2). In 1985, Dr. Rowan Chlebowski of UCLA-Harbor Medical Center published a definitive review of the evidence for the use of this vitamin (3).

He also studied the effects of vitamin K_3 on human tumor colony formation in 34 tumor samples (4). There was also complete inhibition of the mouse leukemia L1210 using vitamin K_3 as well as vitamin K_1 (the natural form of the vitamin). The **anticoagulant** warfarin also killed cancer cells. Somewhat surprisingly (since their actions seem contradictory) vitamin K and warfarin enhanced cell-killing ability. Small amounts of K_3 together with warfarin "resulted in nearly complete inhibition of L1210 growth."

There was a more than 70 percent inhibition in colony formation in some kinds of leukemia and hepatoma (liver cancer) cells. Some other tumor types that responded to this treatment were breast, ovary, colon, stomach, kidney, lung, melanoma and bladder (4).

A 1991 report from Taiwan similarly found that vitamin

K_3 was effective against liver cancer cells (5).

The activity of the vitamin may be due to its ability to cut down on the cancer cell's energy centers. Cells treated with K_3 caused a more than 90 percent decrease in ATP, the energy packets that normally fuel the cell. This resulted in irreversible damage, according to scientists at the Academy of Medical Sciences of the former USSR (6). This conclusion was more recently disputed, however (7).

In a wide-ranging 1991 review, scientists in Taiwan found that 4 out of 15 standard anti-cancer drugs were enhanced by the addition of vitamin K_3. The vitamin was found to possess "a broad spectrum of anticancer activity." The researchers called for further clinical trials of the vitamin (7).

This vitamin was also found to increase the effectiveness and reduce the toxicity of toxic anticancer drugs. While the drug NMF increased the life span of mice with cancer by 82 percent, giving NMF with a form of vitamin K_3 lead to a 126 percent increase of life span (8). Mice with liver cancer were given combined vitamin K_3 as well as vitamin C before or after receiving a single injection of six different standard drugs commonly used in human cancer therapy.

The vitamins "produced a distinct chemotherapy-potentiating effect for all drugs examined, especially when injected before chemotherapy," scientists at Catholic University of Louvain in Brussels, Belgium wrote in 1987 (9).

Negative: In a study of quail in the journal *Poultry Science*, Ohio State University scientists reported that "a high dietary level of vitamin K_3 had no influence on tumor development" (10).

⊕ References

1.   Mohsen A, et al. Some novel phthiocol and menadione thiosemicarbozone derivatives as potential anticancer and antimicrobial agents. Pharmazie.1978;33:81-2.

2.   Prasad KN, et al. Vitamin K3 (menadione) inhibits the growth of mammalian tumor cells in culture. Life Sci.1981;29:1387-92.

3.   Chlebowski RT, et al. Vitamin K in the treatment of cancer. Cancer Treat Rev.1985;12:49-63.

4.   Chlebowski RT, et al. Vitamin K3 inhibition of malignant murine cell growth and human tumor colony formation. Cancer Treat Rep.1985; 69:527-32.

5.   Su WC, et al. The in vitro and in vivo cytotoxicity of menadione (vitamin K3) against rat transplantable hepatoma induced by 3'-methyl-4-dimethyl-aminoazobenzene. Kao Hsiung I Hsueh Ko Hsueh Tsa Chih.1991;7:454-9.

6.   Gabai VL, et al. Oxidative stress, disturbance of energy balance, and death of ascites tumour cells under menadione (vitamin K3) action. Biomed Sci.1990;1:407-13.

7.   Nutter LM, et al. Menadione: spectrum of anticancer activity and effects on nucleotide metabolism in human neoplastic cell lines. Biochem Pharmacol.1991;41:1283-92.

8.   Osswald H, et al. The influence of sodium ascorbate, menadione sodium bisulfite or pyridoxal hydrochloride on the toxic and antineoplastic action of N-methylformamide in P 388 leukemia or M 5076 sarcoma in mice. Toxicology.1987;43:183-91.

9.   Taper HS, et al. Non-toxic potentiation of cancer chemotherapy by combined C and K3 vitamin pre-treatment. Int J Cancer.1987;40:575-9.

10. Nestor KJ, et al. Research note: lack of an effect of high levels of menadione on tumor development in Japanese quail females. Poult Sci.1991;70:2382-5.

⌖ Resources

Food sources of vitamins:

Vitamin A: Preformed vitamin A is only present in animals that have digested the carotene contained in its vegetable food. One of the richest sources of preformed A is fish-liver oil. Cream and butter also contain both vitamin A and its precursor, beta-carotene.

Beta-carotene: Green leafy vegetables, such as beet greens, spinach, broccoli and carrots.

The B-complex vitamins include thiamine, riboflavin, niacin, pantothenic acid, pyridoxine, cyanocobalamin, biotin, choline, folic acid, inositol, PABA and probably carnitine as well. Good natural sources of B vitamins include brewer's yeast, liver and whole-grain cereals. B vitamins are also manufactured by intestinal bacteria, which grow well in the presence of milk sugar and small amounts of fat. Milk-free diets or the intake of sulfonamides and other antibiotics may destroy these bacteria.

Vitamin C: Red and green peppers of all kinds, paprika, parsley, black currants, broccoli, kale, mustard greens, cauliflower, cabbage, chives, lemons, oranges and grapefruits.

Vitamin D is created when the ultraviolet rays of the sun activate a form of cholesterol in the skin. Dietary sources include fish-liver oil and fortified milk. Vitamin D is found in milk and milk products. The RDA of vitamin D is 400 IU, which is what the Balches recommend. One cup of milk contains 30 percent of one's recommended daily allowance (RDA) of calcium and 25 of one's vitamin D requirement. Pauling recommends 800 IU per day. Weil claims you do not need extra vitamin D "unless you live in a basement or are a total shut-in."

Food sources of vitamin E include cold-pressed vegetable oils, dark leafy vegetables, nuts and seeds, legumes and whole grains. It is also found in dry beans, brown rice, cornmeal, eggs, dessicated liver, milk, oatmeal, organ meats, sweet potatoes and wheat germ. Do not take iron at the same time as vitamin E. Also, people who have diabetes, rheumatic heart disease or an overactive thyroid should not use high doses. It is advisable for those with high blood pressure to start with a small amount and gradually increase the dose.

Vitamin K is generally produced in the body by bacteria in the intestines. Some natural sources of vitamin K are alfalfa, green leafy vegetables and kelp. Other sources are milk, egg yolks, molasses, safflower and other polyunsaturated oils. Some reports say that eating yogurt helps the body manufacture vitamin K.

Bioflavonoids (Vitamin P): Apricots, blackberries, black currants, buckwheat, grapefruit, grapes, lemons, plums and rose hips.

Vitamin Supplements:

For most people it is impractical to get all their vitamins from food. Cancer patients may have very high requirements for nutrients, because of the cancer as well as the effects of therapy. In addition, normal requirements for many people are probably far higher than government estimates.

Vitamins are of course widely available in supermarkets, pharmacies and health food stores. There is a debate over whether it is worthwhile to pay more for "natural" vitamins. Pauling, for example, believes that synthetic vitamin C is just as good as (in fact, identical to) the natural product. Others are convinced that there are subtle differences to natural products. One not so subtle difference is the price: natural is usually more expensive.

The most economical way to buy supplements is by mail. There are many excellent sources that will ship vitamins within a few days of purchase. Several recommended sources:

• Bronson Pharmaceuticals, Inc., 4526 Rinetti Lane, La Canada, CA 91011. Phone: 800-235-3200. Ask for attractive catalog. They accept credit cards. Deliveries usually come within a week to ten days.

• L&H Vitamins, 37-10 Crescent Street, Long Island City, New York 11101. Phone: 800-221-1152 (includes entire USA and Canada). Fax: 718-361-1437. They publish a tabloid style newsletter, *Health Newsline*. They are open Saturdays and take credit cards.

• Eclectic Institute, although primarily an herb maker, also offers vitamins and vitamin-botanical combinations. Interesting educational materials with purchase. 11231 S.E. Market Street, Portland, OR 97216. Phone: 800-332-HERB (-4372).

Folate is available through the L&H vitamin catalogue. The product is called Intrinsic B12 Folate Tablets. The dose is two tablets daily or as directed by a doctor. The price is $7.96 for 60 tablets.

Bioflavonoids: Citrin, hesperidin, rutin and quercetin are available in combinations from L&H or General Nutrition Centers (GNC) for $10.76 for 100 capsules.

Flavone Acetic Acid (FAA) is available through L&H and manufactured by Freeda Vitamins. Cost is $12.60 for 250 tablets.

How much to take?

There is clearly no one answer for everyone to this difficult question. Recommendations are usually given for well people, and even so differ widely. Many doctors will tell you not to take supplements, since you get enough vitamins through your normal "balanced" diet to suffice. Thus, they would say all you need are the government's recommended daily allowances (RDAs). Others might say that taking a vitamin pill or two will "do no harm," with the implication that it will do no good, either. Others may prescribe doses hundreds, or even thousands, times greater than the government's suggestions. The reader will obviously have to make up his or her own mind, based on the information given in the book and other sources. Consult Dr. Kedar N. Prasad,*Vitamins Against Cancer* and Prof. Linus Pauling, *How to Live Longer and Feel Better* (New York: W.H. Freeman, 1986).

Bear in mind that the fat-based vitamins are not readily excreted and so can become toxic. These include vitamins A, D, E and K. It is best to consult with a knowledgeable medical professional.

Medical Centers Using Vitamins

NCI's "chemoprevention program" is sponsoring over 20 human efficacy studies. These trials are testing beta-carotene, other vitamin A-like substances, as well as folic acid, vitamins C and E, and minerals as inhibitors of colon, lung, esophagus, cervix, bladder and skin cancer. They are looking at the overall incidence of cancer, the incidence of specific cancers, the rate of regression or progression of precancerous changes, as well as changes in cells and blood. Participants in these studies include volunteers from the general population; people at high risk for cancer; people who have previously been treated for cancer; as well as people who have precancerous conditions. To find out about such trials call the government's Cancer Information Service at 800-4-CANCER. (It may take 15-20 minutes to get through.)

In addition, scientists at various medical centers are giving various types of vitamin treatments, often in a research setting. (One often stands the risk in such studies of only receiving a placebo instead of the substance under study.) Cancer Treatment Centers of America, for example, is currently giving as "usual care" for most patients: 12 grams of vitamin C; 100,000 IU of beta-carotene; Immuno Max (their custom-designed broad spectrum vitamin and mineral supplement); 400 IU of vitamin E; 400 mcg of selenium (for a total of 800 mcg when coupled with Immuno Max); and 2 grams daily of eicosapentaenoic acid (EPA). They are also beginning to use more enzymes (Wobenzym 30 caps/day on empty stomach). They claim that this is probably higher dosages and a greater range of nutrients than other medical centers.

Some of those who have conducted vitamin or vitamin-related research:

Dr. Gary E. Goodman, Fred Hutchinson Cancer Research Center
1124 Columbia, Seattle, WA 98104 USA
Phone: 206-667-4672 Fax: 206-667-5530
Trial (the CARET study) focused on the prevention of lung cancer by using beta-carotene and vitamin A. The study is still open to new people and is randomized. Groups are mostly made up of smokers and workers who have been exposed to asbestos.

Dr. Nicholas J. Lowe, Skin Research Foundation of California
2001 Santa Monica Blvd., Suite 490 West
Santa Monica, CA 90403. Phone: 310-828-8887. Fax: 310-828-8504
Treatment of skin cancers using retinoids. Dr. Lowe is Clinical Professor of Dermatology at UCLA. He is also in private practice:

Dr. Nicholas Lowe, 2001 Santa Monica Bldg., Suite 490 West
Santa Monica, CA 90403. Phone: 310-828-2282. Fax: 310-828-8504.
An initial consultation fee is $110. Fees vary depending on the course of the treatment.

Dr. William A. Robinson, Professor of Medicine, University of Colorado
Health Science Center, 4200 East 9th Avenue, Denver, CO 80262
Phone: 303-399-1211 Fax: 303-270-8825
Treatment of cancer using vitamin A.

CANCER THERAPY

Dr. G.J.S. Rustin, Department of Medical Oncology
Charing Cross Hospital, London, W68RF, England
Phone: 081-846-1421 Fax: 081-846-1443

Dr. W.J. Uphouse, Cancer Center of Hawaii
1236 Lauhala Street, Rm 301, Honolulu, Hawaii 96813
Phone: 808-433-5394

Dr. Linus Pauling, Linus Pauling Institute of Science and Medicine
440 Page Mill Road, Palo Alto, CA 94306
Phone: 415-327-4064, Fax: 415-327-8564
Does not provide advice on treatment but information on cancer.

Dr. F. Morishige, Tachiarai Hospital,
842-1, Yamaguma Miwa-machi, Asa-kura-gun, Fukuoka, 838, Japan
Treatment of human cancer with vitamin C.

Dr. A. Hanck, Unit of Social and Preventive Medicine
University of Basel, Switzerland
Treatment of human cancer with vitamin C.

Voula Kodoyianni, University of Wisconsin, Madison
Molecular Biology Building, 1525 Linden Drive
Madison, WI 53706. Phone: 608-262-3026
Information on vitamin D analogues.

Dr. Joel Schwartz, Beth Israel Hospital, 330 Brookline Avenue
Boston, MA 02215. Phone: 617-732-3349
Treatment for Kaposi's sarcoma with vitamin E and beta-carotene.

Dr. Joel Schwartz, Brigham and Women's Hospital, 75 Francais St.
Boston, MA 02115. Phone: 617-732-3349
Treatment for advanced cancer with vitamin E and beta-carotene. Study
will begin as soon as sufficient numbers of patients enroll.

Dr. Charles Leonard, University of Colorado, 4200 East 9th Street
Denver, CO 80262. Phone: 303-270-7819. Fax: 303-270-8074
Treatment of mucositis with beta-carotene. Phase 3 study.

John M. Fink's very useful directory of alternative clinics, *Third Opinion*,
(Garden City Park, NY: Avery, 1992, $14.95) mentions many practition-
ers using vitamins as part of an overall therapy. One well-known German
clinic offering emulsified vitamin A is:

Robert Janker Clinic, Fachklinik für Tumorerkrankungen
Baumschulallee 12-14, 5300 Bonn 1 Germany
Wolfgang Scheef, MD, medical director
Phone: 011-49-228-7291-101 (secretary), Fax: 011-49-228-631832

Accutane® (13-cis-retinoic acid) is a well-known acne drug available by prescription. It also has uses in cancer therapy. A number of clinical trials are underway on Accutane and cancer.

Study of Accutane for reducing risk of second primary tumors in patients who have had head and neck cancer controlled by surgery and/or radiotherapy. For information:
Waun Ki Hong, University of Texas, M.D. Anderson Cancer Center
Division of Medicine, 1515 Holcombe Boulevard,
Houston, TX 77030. Phone: 713-792-63634

Accutane is also being tested in head and neck cancer patients by:
Robert Wells Carlson, Stanford University Medical Center
Division of Medical Oncology, M-2111, 300 Pasteur Drive
Stanford, CA 94305. Phone: 415-723-7621

Another Accutane study to establish usefulness of treatment with Accutane on chronic smokers (at least 15 years), excluding women of childbearing age (under 50). Patients may have had a prior malignancy provided they are currently free of disease.
Contact: Waun Ki Hong, University of Texas, M.D. Anderson Cancer Center, Division of Medicine, 1515 Holcombe Boulevard, Houston, TX 77030. Phone: 713-792-63634

Yet another study of Accutane for the prevention of skin cancer in patients with xeroderma pigmentosum or nevoid basal cell carcinoma syndrome, and to determine lowest effective dose orally.
Contact: John J. DiGiovanna, Dermatology Branch, IRP, DCBDC, National Cancer Institute, National Institutes of Health, Building 10, Room 12N238, 9000 Rockville Pike, Bethesda, MD 20892. Phone: 301-496-6421

Vitamin A testing in patients treated for laryngeal, oral cavity, and non-small cell lung carcinoma, concerning development of second primary cancers.
Contact: Ugo Pastorio, Istituto Nazionale per lo Studio e la Cura dei Tumori, Department of Thoracic Surgery, Via Venezian 1, 20133 Milano, Italy. Phone: 39-2-2390-601

Beta-carotene and vitamin E study:
On preventing lung cancer in a high-risk group. For men 50 to 69 years old who smoke at least 5 cigarettes a day.
Contact: Demetrius Albanes, Cancer Prevention Studies Branch, CPRP, DCPC, National Cancer Institute, National Institutes of Health, Executive Plaza North, Room 211, Bethesda, MD 20892 Phone: 301-496-8559

Another trial of beta-carotene and vitamin E:
To determine benefit for patients with stage I/II head and neck cancer (two year study).
Contact: Omer Kucuk, Cancer Research Center of Hawaii, 1236 Lauhala Street, Honolulu, HI 96813. Phone: 808-586-2975

Vitamin E study:
To determine usefulness of Vitamin E therapy in Community Clinical Oncology Programs (CCOPs), using Vitamin E to treat oral leukoplakia. Contact: Rodger J. Winn, Univ. of Texas, M.D.Anderson Cancer Center Box 501, 1515 Holcombe Boulevard, Houston, TX 77030.
Phone: 713-792-8515

More tests on vitamin E and beta-carotene at Harvard School of Dental Medicine:
Purpose is to find out the effectiveness of beta-carotene and/or vitamin E as either a preventative for cancer or as a way of enhancing therapy.
For more information, contact: Joel Schwartz, DMD, DMSc, Department of Oral Pathology, Harvard School of Dental Medicine, 188 Longwood Avenue, Boston, MA 02115.
Phone: 617-732-3349

ℳINERALS

As life evolved it incorporated various mineral elements into organic forms. In human beings, some minerals are required in abundance, like calcium. Others, such as copper and iodine, so-called trace minerals, are required in minute amounts. Yet others, like mercury or cadmium, are toxic. And sometimes the trace minerals become toxic when they are oversupplied. Research into the biological effects of minerals shows that some of them can have a profound effect in preventing and possibly treating the disease. This field is wide open for further investigation.

ℭALCIUM

Calcium is the most abundant mineral in the human body. About 99 percent goes to build and maintain healthy teeth and bones. The remaining percent helps nerves and muscles, the parathyroid gland and the blood-clotting mechanisms function properly. One of calcium's most important uses is to aid in the metabolism of vitamin D.

Calcium itself needs other minerals such as magnesium and phosphorus, as well as vitamins A, C, D and possibly E to carry out its many jobs.

How much calcium do we need? Probably more than we get. Scientists now speculate that most people in industrialized countries need higher levels of this mineral. The reasons for this are historical. As a race, we grew up receiving abundant calcium in our diet. The agricultural revolution, several thousand years ago, resulted in a "substantial decrease in human calcium intake," according to scientists at the Oregon Health Sciences University. Therefore, "calcium intakes typical of contemporary humans may well be inadequate for many individuals."

A number of slowly developing chronic diseases such as osteoporosis (the progressive loss of calcium from the bones), high cholesterol and high blood pressure now are thought to be either caused or exacerbated by the low levels of calcium typical of Western diets. Not only is the amount of calcium deficient, but the body must make a constant, debilitating effort to adapt to the consequences of this loss (1). Colon cancer, for example, may be among the disastrous effects of low calcium intake.

As early as 1980, it was proposed that calcium, together with its partner, **vitamin D**, could reduce the risk of colon cancer in humans. As our discussion of vitamin D has shown, this suggestion was based on the fact that deaths from colon cancer decreased as one travelled from north to south. Southern climes are rich in sunlight, which triggers the production of vitamin D in the skin. But what is vitamin D's role? One function is the proper metabolism of calcium.

A study of nearly 2,000 Chicago men found that a dietary intake of greater than 3.75 micrograms of vitamin D per day was associated with a 50 percent reduction in the incidence of cancer of the colon or rectum. Even more startlingly, an intake of 1200 milligrams of calcium a day was associated with a 75 percent reduction, according to scientists at UC San Diego. Clinical and laboratory studies support these findings. Blood serum drawn from over 25,000 people showed that moderately elevated concentrations of vitamin D was associated with large reductions in the incidence of cancer of the colon and rectum (2).

A diet in which total fat makes up only 20 percent of calories and in which cereal fibers are high (about 30 grams per day) is widely believed to help prevent colon cancer. Scientists say that such a diet most likely would also reduce the risk of colon cancer recurrences "in patients who have been treated successfully by conventional means."

Scientists at the American Health Foundation of Valhalla, New York add that regular intake of yellow and green vegetables, foods containing calcium, as well as selenium and other micro-nutrients further lowers the risk (3).

High-fat diets are known to cause breast cancer in rats. Scientists also gave rats receiving such high-fat, cancer-causing diets, supplements of calcium and vitamin D. In one experiment, 40 female rats were divided into 5 groups and fed differing amounts of fat, vitamin D, phosphorus and calcium. By reducing the amount of calcium and vitamin D, scientists increased the incidence of breast cancer in these animals from 37 to 75 percent. The total number of tumors jumped from 4 to 16. In addition, the tumors in the low-supplement group were larger.

Next, 126 rats were tested in a similar way. As in the first experiment, animals fed a high-fat, low-calcium and low-vitamin D diet had nearly twice as many breast tumors, with bigger tumors as well. Biochemists at the University of Western Ontario, Canada concluded that the less calcium and vitamin D these animals got, the greater their risks of breast cancer (4).

Scientists at Memorial Sloan-Kettering Cancer Center, NY studied the growth and spread of cancer in the colons of ten people who had a high hereditary risk of colon cancer. Some of these test subjects were given supplements of 1250 milligrams of calcium carbonate daily.

"Two to three months after supplementation had been started," they stated, "proliferation [of cancer-like cells] was significantly reduced...."

In fact, their colon cells now resembled those of people who were at low risk for this type of cancer (5, 6).

Scientists at the Free University of Brussels also gave nine patients at high risk of colon cancer 1,500 milligrams of calcium for four to eight weeks. After this period, colon cells in six of these patients came to resemble those of patients at low risk of developing colon cancer. Biopsy specimens from such high-risk patients showed a decrease in proliferation when they were grown in the test tube (7).

Certain types of fats are known to damage the colon and lead to cancerous changes. The Belgian scientists also showed that calcium could block the toxicity of such fats when the supplement was given at the same time as the injurious agents (8).

Negative? In one animal study using a cancer-causing chemical, University of Chicago scientists saw no significant reduction of colon cancer incidence through the use of calcium supplements. However, they found that calcium did "decrease the number of rats with multiple tumors and reduced tumor size." A vitamin D deficiency seemed to wipe out any protective effects of the calcium (9).

⊕ References

1.   McCarron DA, et al. Dietary calcium and chronic diseases. Med Hypotheses.1990;31:265-73.

2.   Garland CF, et al. Can colon cancer incidence and death rates be reduced with calcium and vitamin D? Am J Clin Nutr.1991;54:193S-201S.

3.   Weisburger JH and Horn CL. Human and laboratory studies on the causes and prevention of gastrointestinal cancer. Scand J Gastroenterol Suppl.1984;104:15-26.

4.   Jacobson EA, et al. Effects of dietary fat, calcium, and vitamin D on growth and mammary tumorigenesis induced by 7,12-dimethylbenz(a)anthracene in female Sprague-Dawley rats. Cancer Res.1989;49:6300-3.

5.   Lipkin M and Newmark H. Effect of added dietary calcium on colonic epithelial-cell proliferation in subjects at high risk for familial colonic cancer. N Engl J Med.1985;313:1381-4.

6.   Lipkin M, et al. Colonic epithelial cell proliferation in responders and nonresponders to supplemental dietary calcium. Cancer Res.1989; 49:248-54.

7.   Buset M, et al. Inhibition of human colonic epithelial cell proliferation in vivo and in vitro by calcium. Cancer Res.1986;46:5426-30.

8.   Buset M, et al. Injury induced by fatty acids or bile acid in isolated human colonocytes prevented by calcium. Cancer Lett.1990;50:221-6.

9.   Llor X, et al. K-ras mutations in 1,2-dimethylhydrazine-induced colonic tumors: effects of supplemental dietary calcium and vitamin D deficiency. Cancer Res.1991;51:4305-9.

❦ CESIUM & RUBIDIUM

Cesium and rubidium are rare alkali metals widely distributed in tiny amounts throughout the earth's crust (1). Like that better-known mineral salt, lithium carbonate, rubidium chloride has a conventional medical use as an antidepressant (2). In 1860, cesium was the first element discovered through the use of the spectroscope. It produced blue lines in that optical instrument, hence its name ('sky blue' in Latin). Rubidium (Latin for 'ruby red') was discovered in the same way in the following year.

The long-lived radioactive isotopes of cesium have been used in cancer therapy for many years as radioactive 'seeds' implanted in cancer patients. It has even been suggested that "large cesium doses can protect against radiation toxicity by blocking sites on red blood cells and thereby result in increased excretion and clearance of the radioactive forms of cesium," according to scientists at the

Princeton Brain Bio Center (3).

The non-radioactive form of cesium has also been used with rubidium, selenium and other minerals and vitamins as a relatively non-toxic treatment for advanced cancer.

This 'high pH therapy' for cancer was arrived at theoretically by scientists. (pH is the standard measurement of alkalinity/acidity. A pH of 7 is neutral.) First, they evaluated diets in areas with a low incidence of cancer and found relatively high amounts of alkali metals in the soil of such regions. These findings suggested that similar alkali metals might be useful as chemotherapeutic agents.

The rationale for such high pH therapy lies in changing the acidic pH of the cancer cell towards "weak alkalinity" (a pH of 8 or so). At that pH, they said, "the survival of the cancer cell is endangered." In addition, toxic and acidic materials, normally formed in the cancer cells, could be "neutralized and eliminated" (4).

In the late 1970s, scientists tested this theory in mice by feeding them the mineral rubidium carbonate. Tumors were transplanted into the abdomen of mice and allowed to grow for eight days. The mice were then divided into two groups. The control group was fed conventional mouse chow. But the test group, in addition to their mouse chow, got 1.11 mg of rubidium carbonate in distilled water. At the end of 13 more days, tumors in the controls had grown to a large size, which were then removed and weighed.

"The tumors in the test animals weighed essentially one-eleventh of those in the controls," they wrote. "In addition the test animals were showing no adverse effects from the cancers" (5).

Chloride salts of lithium and cesium were studied for their ability to influence the growth of sarcomas in mice. Daily doses of either cesium to these mice "reduced the incidence and size of tumor implants," scientists wrote in the *Journal of Surgical Oncology*. This effect was not seen in animals receiving small doses of the same drug. Lithium had no beneficial effect. Cesium is very similar to potassium, and so the scientists suspected that cesium was taken up preferentially by cancer cells where it interfered with those cells' metabolism (6).

Mice were also given cesium chloride for 14 days before sarcomas were implanted. There was an initial reduction in the number of mice who died from their cancers. Potassium built up inside the tumors of the mice that received cesium. These results were somewhat surprising and suggested that "a critical balance between these two alkali metals may be required" in order for cesium to exert its anticancer effects (7).

In another experiment, rats were given cesium chloride for 12 consecutive days. They then were injected with liver cancer cells. Rats that got the cesium treatment had lower death rates. When the rats were given potassium chloride as well, their death rate decreased even further. But this effect was only seen when the potassium was given alone, not when it was combined with cesium chloride. The scientists called this a "paradoxical effect" and again suggested that there was a "critical intercellular balance" between cesium and potassium that was responsible for the destruction of tumors (8).

Predetermined amounts of cesium chloride, cesium carbonate, **zinc** gluconate and **vitamin A** were administered together to alter growth of colon cancer in mice. The use of these compounds in a treatment protocol was responsible for repression of tumor growth (9).

Potassium, rubidium, and especially cesium are thus all said to be taken up very efficiently by cancer cells. Such uptake is enhanced by **vitamin C**, as well as vitamin A, zinc and **selenium.**

"The amount of cesium taken up was sufficient to raise the cell to the 8 pH range," the scientists said. At this pH, all cell division stopped and the life of the cell was abruptly terminated. Mice fed cesium and rubidium "showed marked shrinkage in the tumor masses within two weeks."

Tests have also been carried out on over 30 humans, the report continued.

"In each case the tumor masses disappeared."
Also all pains and side effects associated with cancer
disappeared within 12 to 36 hours.

The more morphine the patient had taken, however, the longer the withdrawal period (10).

By the mid 1980s, a total of 50 patients had been treated over a three-year period with cesium chloride. Most of them no longer responded to conventional therapy and were considered 'terminal.' Their experimental high pH therapy consisted of cesium chloride together with vitamins, minerals, chelating agents and the salts of magnesium, potassium and selenium. In addition, they were given a special diet.

There was said to be an "impressive 50 percent recovery of various cancers," including cancers of the breast, colon, prostate, pancreas, lung, liver, lymphoma, Ewing's sarcoma of the pelvis and an adenocarcinoma of the gallbladder, according to this report.

Twenty-six percent of the patients died within the first two weeks, and another 24 percent died within the first year. A "consistent finding in these patients was the disappearance of pain within the initial three days of cesium treatment," scientists at the Life Science Universal Medical Center said. A small number of autopsies of patients who died of other causes was performed. They "showed the absence of cancer cells in most cases." Doctors at the

Washington, DC medical facility called this "a remarkably successful outcome of treatment" (11).

Cesium is considered "moderately toxic" (12). In one case, a man in upstate New York "volunteered to experience on himself the effect of short-term, i.e., 36 consecutive days, oral administration of cesium chloride." The subject was given six grams per day into two equally divided doses. The drug was dissolved in a glass of liquid and taken immediately after breakfast and dinner.

For the first three weeks, his meals consisted solely of wheat bran and other grain products, in order to attain approximately one percent potassium intake. "There was an initial general feeling of well-being and heightened sense perception," the man reported. "At first there was a gradual decrease in appetite, which later stabilized. There was also some nausea and diarrhea, which was decreased by the use of foods with high amounts of potassium.

The man also experienced a tingling sensation in his lips and cheeks 15 minutes after taking the cesium chloride. These same sensations occurred with "moderate intensity in hands and feet" by the end of the one-man experiment. The author noted no adverse effects in performance of math problems or driving skill. He concluded that cesium chloride was devoid of toxicity, as long as adequate diet and supplements were administered (13).

In one experiment, however, cesium appeared very toxic to rats with liver cancer. About two-thirds died after just sixteen days. But when the mice were given alcohol (ethanol) at the same time the alcohol exerted a "protective action" that cut the death rate in half (14).

⊕ References

1. Messiha F. Cesium: A bibliography update. Pharmacol Biochem Behav.1984;21:113-129.

2. Loo H and Cuche H. [Biochemical prospects in treatment of depressive illness]. Ann Biol Clin (Paris).1979;37:65-72.

3. Braverman E, et al. Cesium chloride: Preventive medicine for radioactive cesium exposure? Med Hypotheses.1988;26:93-95.

4. Sartori HE. Nutrients and cancer: an introduction to cesium therapy. Pharmacol Biochem Behav.1984;1:7-10.

5. Brewer AK, et al. The effects of rubidium on mammary tumour growth in C57 blk/6J mice. Cytobios.1979;24:99-101.

6. El Domeiri A, et al. Effect of alkali metal salts on Sarcoma I in A/J mice. J Surg Oncol.1981;18:423-9.

7. Messiha FS. Biochemical aspects of cesium administration in tumor-bearing mice. Pharmacol Biochem Behav.1984;1:27-30.

8. Messiha FS and Stocco DM. Effect of cesium and potassium salts on survival of rats bearing Novikoff hepatoma. Pharmacol Biochem Behav.1984;1:31-4.

9. Tufte MJ, et al. The response of colon carcinoma in mice to cesium, zinc and vitamin A. Pharmacol Biochem Behav.1984;25:25-6.

10. Brewer A. The high pH therapy for cancer tests on mice and humans. Pharmacol Biochem Behav.1984;21/suppl 1:1-5.

11. Sartori HE. Cesium therapy in cancer patients. Pharmacol Biochem Behav.1984;1:11-3.

12. Pinsky C and Bose R. Pharmacological and toxicological investigations of cesium. Pharmacol Biochem Behav.1984;21:17-23.

13. Neulieb R. Effects of oral intake of cesium chloride: a single case report. Pharmacol Biochem Behav.1984;21:15-16.

14. Messiha F. Effect of cesium and ethanol on tumor bearing rats. Pharmacol Biochem Behav.1984;21:35-50.

☙ GERMANIUM

Germanium is a mineral widely used in the electronics industry as a semiconductor. It is also found in minute amounts in almost all food (1). Germanium has a limited use in conventional medicine (as an intestinal astringent in animals and an antibiotic) (2). In 1976, Japanese scientists announced the synthesis of an organic form of the mineral, called Ge-132 (3). Several studies have since reported that Ge-132 has anticancer effects (4, 5).

Germanium has also been reported to be an effective immune enhancer (6). This discovery led to widespread advocacy of germanium as a 'miracle cure.' One advocate even literally attributed the 'miracles' of Lourdes to the presence of germanium in the water at that French shrine. In Japan, germanium preparations have been extremely popular since the 1970s, where they are regarded as a kind of tonic. Popularity in the UK, the US and Germany followed, starting in 1987, when advocates claimed that germanium would "rebuild your compromised immune system." This appeal, an article in the *Lancet* asserted, was clearly directed at people with AIDS (7). In the late 1980s there were about 15 different brands of germanium on the market in the UK.

In 1979, scientists at the Sasaki Institute, Tokyo, tested Ge-132 against several different strains of liver cancer in rats. They reported "remarkable life prolongation" in animals with transplanted tumors. Such antitumor activities were entirely due to the activation of the animals' immune system. "Ge-132," they concluded, "has no cytotoxicity," or ability to directly kill cancer cells. They called Ge-132 "the first germanium compound in which antitumor activity has been proven" (8).

Other Effects: Mice with burns produce less of the beneficial cytokine interferon-gamma than uninjured mice. But when these same mice were given Ge-132 they once again produced the same amount of this immune protein as normal mice, according to doctors at the Shriners Burn Institute of Galveston, TX. Researchers also found that Ge-132 lowered blood pressure and slowed the heart beat, while according to others germanium is able to restore "to some extent the impaired immunoresponses in aged mice" (9).

The Asai Germanium Research Institute in Japan is a center of research on this mineral. Scientists there studied the effects of combinations of germanium and other anti-cancer agents. Mice with lung cancer were given oral doses of Ge-132, with chemotherapeutic drugs such as 5-FU. They found that this combination inhibited tumor growth, decreased the spread of metastases, prolonged survival time, and prevented the loss of body weight.

Such antitumor effects could also be transferred from germanium-treated mice to mice which had just received the antimetabolite 5-FU through the injection of spleen cells. Ge-132 also increased the anti-tumor activity of the standard drug bleomycin (10).
Japanese scientists also found that Ge-132 stimulated natural killer (NK) cells to produce interferon. The largest amount was produced after about three days. A major portion of the interferon was of the gamma type. These results suggested that organic germanium might have a special affinity to NK cells, causing them to create a potentially valuable form of cancer-fighting interferon (11).

According to scientists at the University of Texas Medical Branch, in Galveston, TX, Ge-132 is "an immuno-potentiating agent with low toxicities" in animals. It stimulates macrophages in mice (12).

In another experiment, Ge-132 had varying effects on metastases. Depending on the dose schedule, it either reduced or promoted the number of metastases. Scientists at Tohoku University, Sendai called this a "preferential antimetastatic effect" but only under "strictly defined conditions."

In addition, when mice had small tumors, a single dose of germanium on the first day delayed the appearance of metastatic tumor (13).

Korean scientists studied the effects of **garlic, indoles** (from cabbage) and germanium on cancer. Liver cancer in rats "was significantly inhibited by treatment with all three compounds," scientists from the Korea Cancer Center Hospital in Seoul reported. Administration of germanium also significantly slowed the development of cancer of the lung and thyroid (14).

At Hungary's Semmelweis University researchers found that Ge-132 controls white blood cell activity. Ge-132 by itself was not found to be a destroyer of harmful free radicals. But at higher concentrations Ge-132 did seem to have the ability to stabilize cell membranes, which are often attacked by such free radicals (15).

Dangers? Despite all these positive reports, germanium remains a controversial substance, even among alternative physicians. The reason is a well-justified fear of toxicity. Several studies, including a 1991 report in the journal *Renal Failure*, have demonstrated that kidney damage can be caused by the wrong kind of germanium (16). Japanese scientists have also reported several cases of kidney damage from the use of germanium (17, 18).

Rats were given a nonorganic form of the mineral, germanium oxide (GeO_2) until it accumulated in their kidneys. The same kinds of changes were seen in their kidneys as in humans exposed to germanium. This included degeneration in the mitochondria (energy centers) of some cells.

Almost all the damage is done by germanium oxide, not organic Ge-132. For example, a 1991 study by scientists at Tokyo Medical and Dental University, found serious and long-lasting kidney damage from germanium dioxide but not from Ge-132 (19). Unfortunately, most scare stories do not differentiate between the various forms of germanium. With one exception (20), all cases have been connected only to non-organic forms of the mineral.

But nervousness over germanium runs high. Dr. Jonathan Collin, editor of the alternative *Townsend Letter for Doctors*, has advised his colleagues against routine use of germanium in their practice. "Given the malpractice concerns of alternative practitioners," he has written, "germanium supplementation should not play a role in the general practice of medicine, without firm documentation of need and careful monitoring of kidney function."

The major problem with Ge-132 is that it can be contaminated with germanium dioxide in the production process. At present, there is no reliable testing procedure for monitoring the purity and safety of germanium products.

⊕ References

1. Schroeder H and Balassa J. Abnormal trace metals in man: germanium. J Chronic Dis.1967;20:211-244.
2. Sijpesteijn A, et al. Antimicrobial activity of organogermanium derivatives. Nature.1964;201:736.
3. Tsutsui M, et al. Crystal structure of "carboxyethylgermanium sesquioxide". J Am Chem Soc.1976;98:8287-8289.
4. Suzuki F, et al. Ability of sera from mice treated with Ge-132, an organic germanium compound, to inhibit experimental murine ascites tumours. Br J Cancer.1985;52:757-763.
5. Suzuki F, et al. Importance of T-cells and macrophages in the antitumour activity of carboxyethylgermanium sesquioxide (Ge-132). Anticancer Res.1985;5:479-484.
6. Aso H, et al. Induction of interferon and activation of NK cells and macrophages in mice by oral administration of Ge-132, an organic germa-

nium compound. Microbiol Immunol.1985;29:65-74.

7. Anonymous. Germanium dangerous. Lancet.1989;2

8. Satoh H and Iwaguchi T. Antitumor activity of new organogermanium compound, GE-132. Gan To Kagaku Ryoho.1979;6:79-83.

9. Mizushima Y, et al. Restoration of impaired immunoresponse by germanium in mice. Int Arch Allergy Appl Immunol;.1980;63:338-339.

10. Kobayashi H, et al. [Effect of combination immunochemotherapy with an organogermanium compound, Ge-132, and antitumor agents on C57BL/6 mice bearing Lewis lung carcinoma (3LL)]. Gan To Kagaku Ryoho.1986;13:2588-93.

11. Munakata T, et al. Induction of interferon production by natural killer cells by organogermanium compound, Ge132. J Interferon Res.1987; 7:69-76.

12. Suzuki F, et al. Macrophage involvement in the protective effect of carboxyethylgermanium sesquioxide (Ge-132) against murine ascites tumours. Int J Immunotherapy.1986;2:239-45.

13. Kumano N, et al. Antitumor effect of the organogermanium compound Ge-132 on the Lewis lung carcinoma (3LL) in C57BL/6 (B6) mice. Tohoku J Exp Med.1985;146:97-104.

14. Jang JJ, et al. Modifying responses of allyl sulfide, indole-3-carbinol and germanium in a rat multi-organ carcinogenesis model. Carcinogenesis. 1991;12:691-5.

15. Pronai L and Arimori S. Protective effect of carboxyethylgermanium sesquioxide (Ge-132) on superoxide generation by 60C0-irradiated leukocytes. Biotherapy.1991;3:273-9.

16. Schauss A. Nephrotoxicitry in humans by the ultratrace element germanium. Renal Failure.1991;13:1-4.

17. Nakano T, et al. An ultrastructural study of rats treated with germanium. J Clin Elect Microscopy.1987;20:850-851.

18. Matsusaka T, et al. Germanium-induced nephropathy: report of two cases and review of the literature. Clin Nephrology. 1988;30:341-345.

19. Sanai T, et al. Chronic tubulointestinal changes induced by germanium dioxide in comparison with carboxyethylgermanium sesquioxide. Kidney International.1991;40:882-890.

20. Okuda S, et al. Persistent renal dysfunction induced by chronic intake of germanium-containing compounds. Current Therapeutic Research.1987;41:265-275.

❦𝐿ITHIUM

....

Lithium is a naturally-occurring alkali metal widely used in the treatment of mental illness. Fierce controversy surrounded the early use of lithium in psychiatry, but it has now become a standard treatment for manic-depressive disease, despite the fact that its mechanism of action remains unknown (1). Lithium treatment, while remarkably effective in many cases, can result in acute and chronic toxicity and must be carefully administered and monitored by a physician.

Lithium's use is also being extended into cancer. Hans Nieper, MD, an unconventional German physician, has long used lithium orotate, which he claims is less toxic, at doses of around 450 milligram per day. He claims there is no need to even check blood serum levels of patients using this compound, in contrast to therapy with lithium carbonate (2).

Lithium has also been found to counteract "the infectious complications that accompany systemic chemotherapy" (3). Twenty out of 45 people with lung cancer who were receiving both combination chemotherapy and radiation therapy, also received lithium carbonate. The people with cancer who received lithium suffered about one-tenth as many days with neutropenia (lack of neutrophils, a kind of white blood cell) as the people who did not receive this mineral supplement.

Only one patient who received lithium ran a fever, compared to seven in the other group. Lithium patients were also hospitalized for about one-tenth the number of days. And none died of infections, compared to five who so died in the untreated group. Several different kinds of white

LITHIUM

blood cells "were significantly higher in the lithium group"—in this case considered a good sign. The scientists concluded: "We believe that lithium carbonate shows promise as a means of lowering the risk of infection among patients receiving cytotoxic therapy" (4).

Doctors have began to use lithium carbonate along with chemotherapy. For example, a 61-year-old man with a disease called Felty's syndrome (a kind of rheumatoid arthritis with leukopenia and enlargement of the spleen), had previously had his spleen removed. By giving him lithium first they were able to raise his white blood cell level to that of normal individuals and begin chemotherapy (5).

An analysis carried out in Italy demonstrated that "lithium carbonate performs a protective action" against the toxic effects of chemotherapy on the blood; most importantly, "the action is long term" (6).

In a Hungarian study, lithium made "a great number of cells" mature in the marrow of people which had previously been depleted (7).

In a 1983 Israeli study, lithium chloride with two standard anticancer drugs, bleomycin and vinblastine, caused "a significant delay in the first appearance of the tumors, a higher degree of tumor kill, and a longer survival rate" in animals, Tel Aviv University hematologists said (8).

Scientists at the State University of Ghent, Belgium also reported that lithium chloride increases the activity of **tumor necrosis factor** (TNF) in both test tube and animals. An injection of TNF plus lithium caused acute inflammation in a mouse's skin. After two hours this stirred up the neutrophils, and other white blood cells were activated within 24 hours. This beneficial effect "remained present for several days," they said. Lithium helped white blood cells penetrate into the area around the tumor. However, the treatment did not destroy tumors, nor did lithium by itself seem to have much positive effect (9).

Negative: French doctors have reported on eight people who contracted leukemia after receiving lithium therapy. "Our findings suggest that lithium may initiate or promote leukemia," they wrote (10). An equally disturbing report came from the University of South Florida College of Medicine in Tampa. Although lithium carbonate reduced the incidence and severity of infections caused by chemotherapy, it did not actually improve patient survival.

In addition, 14 out of 100 lung cancer patients receiving lithium died suddenly of heart disease. These deaths occurred among patients with previous heart conditions.

For such patients, "lithium administration was associated with a greater risk of sudden death and shorter survival," the Florida oncologists wrote. A particular risk was posed for patients who also used bronchodilators to help them breathe. The scientists concluded: "Lithium treatment is a major risk factor for sudden death in cancer patients" (11).

Lithium carbonate is available only by prescription, under a number of brand names. The drug's label generally carries the warning that "lithium toxicity is closely related to serum lithium levels and can occur at doses close to therapeutic levels."

⊕ References

1. Berkow R. The Merck manual of diagnosis and therapy (15th ed.) Rahway, NJ: Merck & Co., 1987:2696.

2. Nieper HA. The clinical applications of lithium orotate. A two years study. Agressologie.1973;14:407-11.

3. Lyman GH, et al. The use of lithium carbonate to reduce infection and leukopenia during systemic chemotherapy. N Engl J Med.1980; 302:257-60.

4. Steinherz PG, et al. The effect of lithium carbonate on leukopenia after chemotherapy. J Pediatr.1980;96:923-7.

5. Pazdur R and Rossof AH. Cytotoxic chemotherapy for cancer in

Felty's syndrome: role of lithium carbonate. Blood.1981;58:440-3.

6. Spina MP, et al. [Protective effect of lithium carbonate in neutropenia induced by antiblastic agents and evaluation of its long-term efficacy]. Minerva Med.1981;72:3323-8.

7. Molnar S and Kajtar P. Effect of lithium carbonate on the bone marrow of patients treated for haematological malignancies. Acta Paediatr Hung.1983;24:211-6.

8. Ballin A, et al. The effect of lithium chloride on tumour appearance and survival of melanoma-bearing mice. British J Cancer.1983;48:83-87.

9. Beyaert R, et al. Induction of inflammatory cell infiltration and necrosis in normal mouse skin by the combined treatment of tumor necrosis factor and lithium chloride. Am J Pathol.1991;138:727-39.

10. Witz F, et al. [Lithium and acute myeloid leukemia]. Sem Hop Paris.1983;59:559-60.

11. Lyman GH;, et al. Sudden death in cancer patients receiving lithium. J Clin Oncol (USA).1984;2:1270-1276.

℞ $\mathcal{M}$AGNESIUM

Magnesium is a mineral with many beneficial effects in the human body. There is also some data that it may have a beneficial effect in cases of cancer, as well.

For example, Indian scientists showed that four common food supplements could have a marked impact on the occurrence of breast cancer in rats. They first gave rats a common carcinogen, DMBA, which produced malignant breast tumors in all the animals. They then gave the same rats four minerals or vitamins, either alone or in combination: **selenium** (in the form of sodium selenite), magnesium chloride, **vitamin C** or **vitamin A** (retinyl acetate). Each item given singly reduced the breast cancer rate approximately in half. When these substances were given in combinations of twos they all reduced tumors to about a third of the no-supplement rate. When they were given in combinations of three, the rate went down to about a quarter. Finally, "when all four modulators were given concurrently the tumor incidence was only 12 percent," the scientists reported in the *Japanese Journal of Cancer Research*.

Supplement given	% of rats with tumors
Vitamin C	57
Selenium	52
Vitamin A	48
Magnesium	46
All supplements	12

In addition, the number of tumors per animal also declined as the number of agents increased (1).

Little other work has been done on the anticancer effects of magnesium. However, animal studies have reported increased cancer in rodents which received magnesium deficient diets. There has also been a preventive effect in animals fed high levels of the mineral. There is also evidence from studies of human populations that the less magnesium in their environment, the greater the number of deaths. Several theories have been propounded for why this is so. One is that magnesium "may enhance the fidelity" of the way genetic material is copied in the cell; or magnesium in cell membranes may prevent those changes that trigger the beginning of cancer (2).

⊕ References

1. Ramesha A, et al. Chemoprevention of 7,12-dimethylbenz[a]anthracene-induced mammary carcinogenesis in rats by the combined actions of selenium, magnesium, ascorbic acid and retinyl acetate. Jpn J Cancer Res.1990;81:1239-46.

2. Blondell JM. The anticarcinogenic effect of magnesium. Med Hypotheses.1980;6:863-71.

‽c𝓜OLYBDENUM
....

Molybdenum is another trace mineral found in almost all plant and animal tissues. It is essential for the synthesis of two enzymes, one of which aids in the mobilization of iron from the liver, the other in the oxidation of fats. Good food sources of molybdenum are meats, grains, legumes and some green leafy vegetables.

Molybdenum in the food supply is dependent on its abundance in the soil. Lack of molybdenum may figure in some large-scale occurrences of cancer.

For example, cancer of the esophagus is very common in the Taihang Mountain range in northern China. More than coincidentally, chickens in that high incidence area also have unusually high rates of cancer of the gullet (a structure analogous to the human esophagus). This fact has led scientists to look for cancer-causing substances in the physical environment.

"Massive epidemiological studies" have shown that both people and animals were eating moldy food and pickled vegetables that contained potent carcinogens, such as nitrosamines. But Chinese scientists have suggested that there are other pieces to this puzzle. These include a lack of certain trace elements in the soil (1).

A prime suspect is molybdenum. By fortifying the soil with this mineral and adding it, along with vitamin C, to the food supply, they have been able to decrease the incidence of esophageal cancer in that part of their country.

Molybdenum is a free radical scavenger and provides protection against chemical carcinogens in the laboratory. Just two parts per million of molybdenum in the drinking water "significantly inhibited" the formation of either esophageal or stomach cancer (2).

In addition, molybdenum might be useful for treating breast cancer. Female rats were given molybdenum in their drinking water. Some others were given tungsten, molybdenum's harmful antagonist. After 15 days, all animals received an injection of a carcinogen. After almost 200 days, the breast cancer incidence in the group receiving molybdenum was 50 percent, but it was 90 percent in the group receiving just the carcinogen. In the tungsten group the results were even worse—over 95 percent tumors.

In addition, the first palpable breast tumor was found in the tungsten-supplemented group just 56 days after the injection, whereas in the molybdenum group the first tumor was not felt until 85 days. This study shows for the first time the inhibitory effect of molybdenum on the formation of breast cancer and the tumor-promoting effect of its antagonist, tungsten (3).

A derivative of molybdenum, called molybdocene dichloride, has been tested against Ehrlich ascites tumor in mice. By giving this chemical 24 hours after transplantation of the tumor cells, scientists got "100 percent tumor inhibition until day 30" (4).

⊕ References

1.   Yang CS. Research on esophageal cancer in China: a review. Cancer Res.1980;40:2633-44.

2.   Luo XM, et al. Inhibitory effects of molybdenum on esophageal and forestomach carcinogenesis in rats. J Natl Cancer Inst.1983;71:75-80.

3.   Wei HJ, et al. [Effect of molybdenum and tungsten on mammary carcinogenesis in Sprague-Dawley (SD) rats]. Chung Hua Chung Liu Tsa Chih.1987;9:204-7.

4.   Kopf MP, et al. [Molybdocene dichloride as an antitumor agent]. Z Naturforsch [c].1979;34:1174-6.

♀ SELENIUM

Selenium (from *selene*, Greek for moon) is a nonmetallic grey mineral of the sulfur family. While toxic in high doses, a relatively high intake of selenium in the diet has repeatedly been linked to lower-than-usual incidences of cancer. Since the 1940s, some organic forms of selenium have been used in cancer therapy by alternative physicians, most prominently Emanuel Revici, MD of New York.

It is needed in small amounts to maintain health and there are harmful effects in animals and people from getting too little, as well as too much, selenium. Deficiencies are mainly seen in regions where the supply of selenium in the soil or water is limited; in cases of protein-calorie deprivation; and in patients who are on medically-controlled "parenteral" nutrition, from which selenium supplements have been omitted. Some scientists still do not accept the need for selenium supplements and argue against its protective effect against cancer and other diseases (1). Others endorse the value of moderate amounts of selenium added to the diet.

In the laboratory, selenium has shown a wide range of anticancer effects.

• It inhibits chemical substances and viruses that cause cancer in many cells and animals.

• It protects against ultraviolet light.

• It fights against the harmful effects of several cancer-promoting minerals.

• It slows cancer growth, causing a reduction in tumor volume, prolonging survival and reducing the "take rate" of transplanted tumors.

Harold Ladas, Ph.D., a Hunter College professor, gathered references to dozens of such studies in a comprehensive review article on the subject (2).

The mechanism of selenium's anticancer action is not known, although several explanations have been suggested. For example, selenium might:

• Stop carcinogens from corrupting the genetic material of the cell. Selenium repairs DNA and keeps chemicals from harming the genetic "blueprint." Selenium is found in an enzyme that plays a crucial role in eliminating harmful free radicals.

• Slow the spread of cancer cells. A study at Georgia Tech showed that selenium and other trace minerals were present in significantly higher concentrations in cancerous than in normal tissues. They concluded that this is "possibly an effort of the body to inhibit the growth of tumors" using this anticancer element (2).

• Enhance the body's normal anticancer immunity. Scientists at the University of Nebraska Medical Center found that natural killer (NK) cells were greatly enhanced by even small amounts of the mineral. NK cells are relatively inactive in cancer patients. But the Nebraska scientists found that animals receiving selenium supplements had elevated activity of these natural killers (3).

Scientists believe this may explain why people who have a relatively abundant supply of selenium in their diets experience less cancer (3). The statistics for breast cancer are particularly striking. "The higher the selenium, the lower the breast cancer," said Prof. Ladas (2). Similar associations have been found with leukemia, as well as cancers of the intestines, rectum, ovary, prostate, lung, pancreas, skin and bladder (4, 5).

In Yugoslavia, scientists studied 33 patients with breast cancer. These women had selenium levels in their bloodstream only half those of healthy volunteers. The doctors suggested that examining blood for low serum selenium levels could be used as a non-invasive way of discovering if a woman was developing breast cancer (6).

In a study of almost 40,000 Finnish men and women from 1968-1972, with ten-year follow up, over 1,000 new cases of cancer were detected. Selenium levels in the blood of men with cancer were significantly lower than for men who did not have cancer. (Among women, there was no such correlation, however.) Low selenium levels were particularly associated with cancers of the stomach and the lung (7).

At the Yunnan Tin Corporation in China there is a very high rate of lung cancer among the miners. Forty healthy miners were given selenium supplements for a year. The selenium, which increased in their blood, boosted a key detoxifying enzyme system while simultaneously decreasing dangerous lipid peroxide levels by nearly 75 percent. It also protected against cancer-causing substances and ultraviolet radiation. Doctors at the Chinese Academy of Medical Sciences concluded that selenium supplements were a safe and effective food supplement for people (8).

There have also been a number of reports of selenium's toxicity or even its alleged ability to cause cancer. There is no question that excess selenium in the soil (in the form of its compounds, selenite or selenate) can kill grazing animals and could probably in sufficiently large doses kill humans as well. The symptoms of selenium poisoning are readily apparent without a doctor's assistance, according to Dr. Gerhard Schrauzer, a world expert on the topic. These symptoms include a heavy garlic odor, pallor, nervousness, depression, a metallic taste, skin eruptions, irritability, discolored teeth and hair loss (9).

There is some doubt about the carcinogenicity studies. For instance, one study showed toxic effects for inorganic, but not organic, forms of the mineral. Schrauzer says that the World Health Organization (WHO) has discredited earlier findings on the mineral's toxicity. Nor does this necessarily pertain to Revici's (and others') organic forms of the mineral used as a part of cancer treatment.

As a preventative, selenium is generally ineffective unless there is also a high level of **vitamin E** in the blood. One study of breast cancer in rats showed that selenium was largely ineffective as an anticancer element, if the intake of vitamin E was deficient. Selenium in the diet reduced the total amount of tumor by 45 percent. This dropped to 25 percent when the mice were given less vitamin E. A low vitamin E intake significantly increased the peroxidation of fats, which may contribute to cancer (10).

Aside from Revici's work, little has been done to investigate the use of this mineral as a cancer treatment. In 1911, Prof. August von Wasserrman achieved growth inhibition, shrinkage and eventually the disappearance of tumors by injecting selenium directly into mouse tumors. Four years later, two doctors caused the shrinkage and the eventual disappearance of small tumors in cancer patients, although larger tumors failed to respond (11).

The National Academy of Sciences advises that no more than 150 micrograms of selenium be taken orally daily. But Revici's "bivalent negative selenium"— a combination of the mineral with various organic substances, such as the fatty acids of sesame oil—is said to be so non-toxic that huge amounts, up to one million micrograms, have been injected (in the treatment of drug addiction), apparently without any ill effects. In the treatment of cancer the dosage is generally about 10,000 micrograms, still nearly one hundred times the National Academy of Science's recommended dose.

Revici's treatment is more complicated than just organic selenium. He only uses selenium in patients whom he deems to be in a "catabolic," as opposed to an "anabolic," state. He has devised a number of urine tests to find whether a patient is in one condition or the other. Selenium is given when the urine has a low specific gravity, a high surface tension and a pH above 6.0. The alkalinity of the urine is supposed to reflect the state of the body's defenses against tumors.

In an unpublished study of Revici in 1955, Robert Ravitch, MD evaluated 1,047 patients with advanced cancer. He is said to have found good results in some of the patients treated with amyl selenide, a Revici compound (12). Prof. Joseph Maisin, a former president of the International Union Against Cancer, is also said to have used Revici's compounds and reported good results. Amyl selenide was tested by NCI in the P388 test system and was found to act against tumors in mice (2). Doctors at the University of Milan are also said to have used another Revici compound (Rel) in the treatment of cancer and "reported dramatic life extension" (2). Two doctors unconnected to Revici reproduced parts of his work. They found that organic selenium compounds had strong antitumor activity and low toxicity in animal studies (13).

Scientists sometimes have short memories. In a 1980 review, for example, one doctor seriously stated that no human experiments with selenium had ever been performed. Yet at that time, Dr. Revici had been using organic selenium in his practice for about four decades and had published a medical textbook describing such work (*Research in Physiopathology as Basis of Guided Chemotherapy, with Special Application to Cancer.* Princeton: D. Van Nostrand and Company, Inc., 1961). Prof. Ladas concluded, "The time is long overdue to merge these two lines of research" on cancer prevention and treatment using selenium (2).

⊕ References

1. Neve J, et al. Selenium deficiency. Clin Endocrinol Metab.1985; 14:629-56.

2. Ladas HS. The potential of selenium in the treatment of cancer. Holistic Medicine.1989;4:145-156.

3. Petrie HT. Differential regulation of lymphocyte functional activities by Selenium. [Ph.D. dissertation.] University of Nebraska Medical Center, 1988.

4. Schrauzer G. Selenium and cancer. A review. Bioinorganic Chemistry.1975;5:275-81.

5. Schrauzer GN, et al. Cancer mortality correlation studies. III. Statistical associations with dietary selenium intakes. Bioinorganic Chemistry.1977;7:23-24.

6. Ksrnjavi H and Beker D. Selenium in serum as a possible parameter for assessment of breast disease. Breast Cancer Research and Treatment. 1990;16:57-61.

7. Knekt P, et al. Serum selenium and subsequent risk of cancer among Finnish men and women. Journal of the National Cancer Institute.1990;82:864-868.

8. Yu S-Y, et al. Intervention trial in selenium for the prevention of lung cancer among tin miners in Yunnan, China. Biological Trace Element Research.1990;24:105-108.

9. Budavari S, et al. (Eds.). The Merck index: an encyclopedia of chemicals, drugs, and biologicals. Rahway, NJ: Merck & Co., Inc., 1989:1606.

10. Ip C. Attenuation of the anticarcinogenic action of selenium by vitamin E deficiency. Cancer Lett.1985;25:325-31.

11. Schrauzer G. Selenium and cancer: historical developments and perspectives. In: Spallholz M and Spallholz G, (Ed.) Westport: Avi Publishing Co., 1981.

12. Ravich RA. Revici method of cancer control: evaluation of 1047 patients with advanced malignancies treated from 1946-1955. In: Unpublished manuscript prepared for John Heller, former director of NCI and Sloan-Kettering. Cited in Ladas, 1989, 1955.

13. Schwartz K and Pathak K. The biological essentiality of selenium, and the development of biologically active organoselenium compounds of minimum toxicity. Chemica Scripta.1975;8A:85-95.

❧ *T*ELLURIUM

Tellurium is another mineral of the sulfur family which is useful against cancer. Tellurium is rarely found in its native state but is fairly common in combination with other minerals. And in fact it was discovered in the late eighteenth century in Transylvanian gold. Scientists were confused about its nature and so called it the "metallum problematicum." It was not until 1832 that its chemistry was finally elucidated.

Tellurium can be combined with certain organic compounds to create organotelluriums, much as germanium and selenium can also be so combined. Tellurium's organic forms are said to have germicidal properties. Eating as little a one micromole (a very small amount) can give one's breath the penetrating odor of garlic, which appears within half an hour of ingestion. Some sources claim that as little as two grams of sodium tellurite can be lethal.

In 1972, organotelluriums were the subject of a symposium at the New York Academy of Sciences (1). However, it wasn't until the late 1980s that one particular organotellurium began to be used in the treatment of chronic diseases.

AS-101 is that new synthetic organic tellurium compound. It was found to boost the immune system by increasing cytokine production in both the test tube and in humans. Toxicity and early efficacy clinical trials (Phase I/II) were conducted in Israel on AIDS and cancer patients. Patients treated with AS-101 showed significant increases in various kinds of white blood cells and their anticancer "cytokines," without significant toxicity.

Together with another substance called PMA, AS-101 increased the production of interleukin-2 (IL-2) and colony-stimulating factor (CSF) by human and mouse cells. Scientists at Bar Ilan University in Ramat Gan also found a synergistic effect between AS-101 and **bryostatins,** new compounds derived from sea invertebrates.

By working together, these compounds greatly enhanced the production of IL-2, as well as **tumor necrosis factor** and interferon-gamma. Israeli scientists called bryostatins "particularly good candidates, in combination with AS-101, for immunomodulation" of patients whose immune systems had been devastated by conventional cancer treatments (2, 3).

They concluded that "AS-101 is an active biological response modifier..." that could be useful in cancer and AIDS (4).

In Mexico, 15 patients with systemic lupus erythematosus (SLE) were tested. AS-101 was found to be non-toxic and to increase the production of IL-2. It also enhanced suppressor cells in lupus patients. Since such cells are known to be defective in these patients, and since AS-101 seems to be a safe drug, "this immunoregulatory compound holds promise for a novel and effective treatment of SLE," doctors at the Instituto Nacional de la Nutricion Salvador Zubiran in Mexico City said (5).

The ability of "spleen cells of mice with SLE to produce IL-2 was restored after administration of AS-101," Israeli scientists concluded. But despite its beneficial effect on IL-2 production, AS-101 exerted no influence on harmful auto-antibodies in the blood of mice. It also had no effect on the clinical course of the disease itself. Doctors at the Sheba Medical Centre in Tel Hashomer concluded that "defective IL-2 production in SLE is probably secondary to other disease processes" and does not account for the production of auto-antibodies in this disorder (6).

This mineral was toxic in some studies. Rats were injected for four weeks with AS-101 in small amounts and there were few deaths at this level. "A garlic odor pervaded the room," Israeli scientists reported. As the dose went up, the animals' body weight and food consumption decreased. There were harmful effects on the blood-forming system and signs of liver damage. On examination "organs were found to have a grayish-blue discoloration." Other changes were seen in the bone marrow, eyes, heart, kidney, liver and thymus. The toxicity was similar to that seen with other tellurium-containing compounds. Scientists at Life Science Research Israel in Ness Ziona raised the "possibility that some of the effects may have been elicited due to selenium-vitamin E deficiency" (7).

⊕ References

1. Wynne KJ. Some donor and acceptor complexes of organoselenium and organotellurium halides. Ann NY Acad Sci.1972;192:107-14.

2. Sredni B, et al. A new immunomodulating compound (AS-101). with potential therapeutic application. Nature.1987;330:173-6.

3. Sredni B, et al. Cytokine secretion effected by synergism of the immunomodulator AS-101 and the protein kinase C inducer bryostatin. Immunology.1990;70:473-7.

4. Sredni B, et al. The biological activity and immunotherapeutic properties of AS-101, a synthetic organotellurium compound. Nat Immun Cell Growth Regul.1988;7:163-8.

5. Alcocer VJ, et al. Effect of the new immunoregulator AS-101 on in vitro functions of mononuclear cells from patients with systemic lupus erythematosus. Clin Exp Immunol.1989;77:319-23.

6. Blank M, et al. The effect of the immunomodulator agent AS-101 on interleukin-2 production in systemic lupus erythematosus (SLE) induced in mice by a pathogenic anti-DNA antibody. Clin Exp Immunol.1990; 79:443-7.

7. Nyska A, et al. Toxicity study in rats of a tellurium based immunomodulating drug, AS-101: a potential drug for AIDS and cancer patients. Arch Toxicol.1989;63:386-93.

⚕ 𝐙INC

··

Zinc is another mineral essential for health. Many studies have shown that the amount of this mineral naturally present in epithelial cells of the prostate is high: it is a "zinc-rich gland" (1). It has become a popular supplement, especially for treatment of enlarged or infected prostates.

Studies have consequently been performed all over the world, attempting to show a correlation between zinc intake and prostate cancer. The studies so far have shown an association, but no clear cause-and-effect relationship.

The most positive association came from a 1989 NCI report. Cadmium is another mineral, one which can cause cancer. Scientists studied the ability of zinc to modify cadmium's carcinogenic effects over a two-year period. After a single cadmium injection in laboratory animals, zinc was given in three separate doses or in the drinking water. It was no surprise when cadmium caused cancer at the injection site, as well as in the testes.

But tumor incidence at the injection site "was markedly reduced" (by 50 percent) by high dose injections of zinc. And it "was almost abolished" by zinc supplements in the water (92 percent reduction). Testicular tumors were also reduced by zinc injections: the more zinc, the less cancer.

"These results indicate that zinc inhibition of cadmium carcinogenesis is a complex phenomenon, depending not only on dose and route but also on the target site in question," the NCI scientists reported (2).

In a study of the tissues of men with prostate cancer there were "significant decreases not only of the zinc but also of the potassium concentration, in the cancerous tissue." Nitrogen, phosphorus and magnesium concentrations, however, remained normal. The composition of

ZINC

benign, but enlarged, prostates was similar to normal (3). In a 1984 Danish study, zinc concentrations were lower in a part of the cancerous tissue, when compared to enlarged but benign specimens (4).

African-Americans have a very high rate of prostate cancer, but African black men have one-tenth that amount. Scientists therefore measured zinc levels in both the blood serum and in the prostate of healthy Nigerian men, those with benign enlargement of the prostate (BPH), and prostate cancer. Unfortunately, there was little difference in these levels, or those of another metal, cadmium, between African and African-American men.

"This suggests that these metals do not primarily play any significant role in the reported low incidence rate of prostatic cancer in our community," surgeons at the Lagos University Teaching Hospital reported (5).

Norwegian doctors studied tissue taken from needle biopsies of ten patients. Seven had enlargement of the prostate, while three had cancer. These samples were then contrasted with normal prostate tissue. The amount of calcium in all the prostates was far higher than either magnesium or zinc. And they found a zinc deficiency in some of these patients' prostates (6).

In Utah, scientists studied 358 cases with prostate cancer and 679 controls. Dietary fat was the strongest risk factor. There was "little association between prostate cancer and dietary intake of zinc, cadmium, selenium, vitamin C, and beta-carotene." Total vitamin A intake had a "slight positive association with all prostate cancer" but not with aggressive tumors. Similar results had been seen in a study of African-American men in the Washington, DC area (7). These findings suggest that dietary intake, especially fats, may increase the risk of aggressive prostate tumors in older men (8).

⊕ References

1. Larue JP, et al. [Zinc in the human prostate]. J Urol (Paris).1985; 91:463-8.

2. Waalkes MP, et al. Cadmium carcinogenesis in male Wistar [Crl:(WI)BR] rats: dose-response analysis of effects of zinc on tumor induction in the prostate, in the testes, and at the injection site. Cancer Res.1989;49:4282-8.

3. Marczynska A, et al. The concentration of zinc in relation to fundamental elements in the diseased human prostate. Int Urol Nephrol.1983; 15:257-65.

4. Leake A, et al. Subcellular distribution of zinc in the benign and malignant human prostate: evidence for a direct zinc androgen interaction. Acta Endocrinol (Copenh).1984;105:281-8.

5. Ogunlewe JO and Osegbe DN. Zinc and cadmium concentrations in indigenous blacks with normal, hypertrophic, and malignant prostate. Cancer.1989;63:1388-92.

6. Tvedt KE, et al. Intracellular distribution of calcium and zinc in normal, hyperplastic, and neoplastic human prostate: x-ray microanalysis of freeze-dried cryosections. Prostate.1989;15:41-51.

7. Heshmat MY, et al. Nutrition and prostate cancer: a case-control study. Prostate.1985;6:7-17.

8. West DW, et al. Adult dietary intake and prostate cancer risk in Utah: a case-control study with special emphasis on aggressive tumors. Cancer Causes Control.1991;2:85-94.

☀ Resources

Food sources of minerals:

Calcium: Found in large amounts in a limited number of foods such as milk and dairy products. Vitamin D is necessary for its proper assimilation. So is phosphorus. The National Resource Council (NRC) recommends an intake of 800 milligrams per day. Signs of calcium deficiency are muscle cramps and numbness. In children, calcium deficiency can result in the disease rickets. A glass of milk provides about 30 percent of the RDA for calcium. One can also get calcium from cooked greens such as collards, molasses, sesame seeds, broccoli and tofu. Linus Pauling recommends a daily intake of 800 milligrams per day of calcium. The Balches recommend 1,500 mg per day of chelated calcium. Andrew Weil says 1,000-1,500 milligrams a day are a "reasonable dose."

Cesium: Widespread and fairly abundant in the earth's crust—more so than silver. There are large supplies in South Africa and Manitoba, Canada, among other places.

Magnesium: Widely distributed in foods, particularly fresh green vegetables, wheat germ, soybeans, whole grains, seafoods, figs, corn, apples, and oil-rich seeds and nuts, particularly almonds.

Manganese: This mineral is found in a form of superoxide dismutase with anti-cancer effects. This is one reason it is important to get sufficient amounts in the diet. Manganese is abundant in whole-grain cereals, egg yolks, nuts, seeds and green vegetables.

Molybdenum: Found in cereals, legumes, meats, as well as some dark-green vegetables. Content is dependent on soil content.

Selenium: Some sources are brewer's yeast, cereals, dairy, fish and shellfish, grains, organ and muscle meats.

Zinc: found in brewer's yeast, pumpkin seeds, wheat bran and whole-grain products.

Mineral supplements

Mineral supplements are inexpensive and easy to get in health food stores and pharmacies. For mail order sources, please consult resource section of the vitamin chapter. However, it is important to repeat that one cannot treat mineral supplements like water-soluble vitamins. They can potentially do much harm if taken at high levels. A few of the minerals (e.g. cesium) while promising as treatments, are rare and their biological effects poorly understood. A number of others are toxic and/or cause cancer (cadmium).

Dr. Andrew Weil cautions that calcium supplements vary greatly in content and price. Calcium citrate, he says, is a good form of the mineral, because it is easily assimilated and not expensive. Chelated calcium, oyster shells and eggshells are said to be good sources as well. But he cautions not to use dolomite or bone meal as supplements, since they may be contaminated with heavy metals. And be sure, he says, to add extra magnesium to the diet as well.

Obtaining some of the rarer chemicals is difficult. Scientists might be interested to know that a number of rare minerals are available through chemical supply companies, such as Aldrich Chemical Company, Inc., 1001 West Saint Paul Avenue, Milwaukee, WI 53233. Phone: 800-558-9160. Cesium chloride, 99.995 percent pure sells approximately $150 per 50 grams. and rubidium chloride, 99.99 percent pure, is about $75 for 10

CANCER THERAPY

grams. Aldrich is emphatic that such chemicals are offered for laboratory use only and "may NOT be used as drugs." For some chemicals, they ask the buyer to offer written assurance that the chemical will neither be purchased nor resold for an improper use.

Germanium: The indiscriminate use of Ge-132 clearly has its problems. It would be prudent to take and should only be done under the care of a knowledgeable physician who can monitor the effects (if any) on the kidneys. According to George Klabin, of Klabin Marketing, his product, "Bio-Nutritional Formulas Germanium Ge-132," is the purest in existence. This is because each batch is manufactured using a combination of six different tests on each batch, including nuclear magnetic resonance tests. Assays of his latest batch are always available from Klabin Marketing Co., 115 Central Park West, New York, NY 10023. Phone: 800-933-9440 or 212-877-3632.

Magnesium: There are many over-the-counter remedies that contain magnesium. For example, Mag-Ox (Blaire) 400 contains 241.3 milligrams of elemental magnesium.

Selenium: The recommended daily allowance (RDA) ranges between 50 and 200 micrograms per day. It is said that selenium dosages of around 250 to 300 micrograms per day (in diet and supplements) are helpful in preventing cancer. Assuming one eats about 125-150 micrograms per day (the average amount), "an additional supplement amount of 100 micrograms per day is unlikely to produce any major side effects," according to Dr. Kedar N. Prasad, in *Vitamins Against Cancer*. Multi-vitamin-mineral pills often contain about 10-20 micrograms. The toxic level, says Prasad, is about 20-30 times the human RDA. Certainly, no one is suggesting megadoses of selenium. Linus Pauling warns, "The essential minerals differ from the vitamins in that overdoses of minerals may be harmful....Limit your mineral intake to the recommended amounts." Patrick Quillin, PhD, RD, author of *Healing Nutrients*, tells people that 200–600 micrograms per day is a "safe, therapeutically preventative guideline for our heavily-polluted and cancer-laden times."

One good food source is Brazil nuts, which happen also to contain at least one other anticancer substance, ellagic acid. One large nut can provide over 50 mcg of selenium. When Cornell scientist Donald J. Lisk and his colleagues ate six Brazil nuts a day for three weeks, their blood levels of selenium rose between 100 and 350 percent.

Zinc: Found in almost all health food stores. One over-the-counter form is sublingual zinc from Sublingual Products.

Medical Centers Using Minerals

Calcium: A study is underway on the use of dietary calcium in preventing cancer in the large bowel in patients with a recent history of such tumors.

Contact: John Baron, Dartmouth-Hitchcock Medical Center
Hinmen Box 7929, One Medical Center Drive, Lebanon, NH 03756.
Phone: 603-646-5250

Selenium Testing: Testing the ability of selenium-enriched brewer's
yeast versus plain brewer's yeast in preventing the recurrence of skin
cancer. Contact: Larry C. Clark, Epidemiology Section
University of Arizona College of Medicine, 2504 East Elm Street
Tucson, AZ 85716. Phone: 602-626-4890

Researchers who have experimented with cesium and/or rubidium:
F. S. Messiha, Department of Pathology,
Texas Tech University Health Sciences Center, Lubbock, TX 79430

Carl Pinsky and R. Bose, Department of Pharmacology and Therapeutics,
Faculty of Medicine, University of Manitoba, Winnipeg, Man. R3E 0W3
Canada

For cancer treatment with the Revici method, which includes organic
selenium products:
Dr. Emanuel Revici, 26 East 36th Street
New York, New York 10016. Phone: 212-685-0111. Fax: 212 685-0112.

Nieper methods, including lithium orotates:
For information on Hans Nieper's approach to cancer one can write to the
Admiral Ruge Archives of Biophysics and Future Science, A. Keith
Brewer International Science Library, 325 North Central Avenue, Richland Center, WI 53581, Phone: 608-647-6513, Fax: 608-647-6797. They will
send a price list of lectures and articles by Nieper. Hans Nieper's outpatient clinic is located at Sedan Strasse 21, 3000 Hannover 1, Germany,
011-49-511-348-08-08. Inpatient clinic: Paracelsus Klinik at Silbersee,
Oertzeweg 24, 3012 Langenhagen, Germany. Phone: 011-49-511-733031.

Tellurium (AS-101).
Contact: B. Sredni, Bar Ilan Universitry, Ramat Gan, Israel

Special note: Beres Drops® Plus are a mineral supplement, formulated by
Dr. Josef Beres, a Hungarian agronomist. In 1990, they were approved as
a "paramedicine" by the Hungarian Institute of Pharmacy. The drops
contain iron, zinc, sodium, magnesium, manganese, potassium, copper,
molybdenum, vanadium, nickel, boron, fluorine and cobalt. (Chlorine was
removed from the formulation in late 1991, because of concerns about its
ability to cause cancer.) The drops do not exceed US RDAs. They are extremely popular in Hungary and efforts are now underway to bring them
into the US.

$\mathcal{H}$ERBS

Herbs are plants, or plant parts, valued for their medicinal, savory or aromatic qualities. Throughout most of history, herbs have been a mainstay against disease. The four great herbal traditions—Egyptian-European; Native American; Indian; and Chinese—have each contributed greatly to our collective health and well-being. It is only in the last century or so, in fact, that synthetic chemical compounds have emerged from the laboratory to challenge humanity's basic reliance on herbs.

Even so, about half of all drugs in current use are derived from plants. In cancer, such conventional agents as vincristine, vinblastine, maytansine, podophyllium and taxol are all derived from plants, some of which were native cancer remedies before being rediscovered and refined in the laboratory.

The use of herbs goes back to the dawn of human history, in fact, beyond. Numerous examples have now surfaced of animals deliberately using herbs to solve health problems ranging from parasites to infertility. In fact, the study of non-human discoveries of medicinal herbs has emerged as the field of "zoopharmacognosy." This was even the subject of a session at the 1992 American Association for the Advancement of Sciences (AAAS) annual meeting. Many wild animals (to quote *Science)* have been observed "practicing medicine without a license." Some examples:

• Chimpanzees seek out a sunflower-like plant to kill nematodes and other parasites.

• Monkeys "regulate their fertility through judicious

dietary practices."

• Muriqui monkeys in Brazil reduce their fertility by ingesting leaves containing estrogen-like substances.

"The fact that chimps are self-medicated...means that the history of the use of medicine goes back at least five to six million years," according to Harvard University anthropologist, Richard Wrangham. Actually, of course, it is the use of *medicinal herbs*, not just medicine, that goes back that far.

Herbs are also a field with a future in cancer. Conventional medicine has become impersonal, expensive and highly toxic. Millions of people around the world are rejecting this approach or find themselves unable to pay for its overrated wonders.

In the light of the crisis within Western medical science, the United Nation's World Health Organization (WHO) has called on doctors to create a "New Medicine," combining the wisdom of indigenous cultures with Western, scientific techniques. This New Medicine is ideally suited for developing countries but has increasing relevance in advanced countries as well. The scientific investigation of traditional herbs embodies this integrated approach. It is well-developed in such countries as Japan and China, but is steadily gaining adherents around the world.

The New Medicine has just begun, yet already it has demonstrated its potential in the field of cancer. The section that follows illustrates what can be achieved when scientists combine the innovative and inquiring spirit of science with a deep respect for indigenous traditions.

❦ ALOE

....

Aloe is a garden succulent commonly used as a remedy for irritations, cuts and burns. Aloe has been used medicinally since ancient times. It is mentioned in early Egyptian writings as an effective treatment for infections, skin ailments and constipation. Alexander the Great is said to have fought a war to obtain a supply of this plant for his wounded warriors.

Today, aloe has become the basis of a multi-million dollar industry, since it is a common ingredient in shampoos and lotions. Like garlic, aloe is a member of the lily family. And like garlic, it is finding a use in the treatment of cancer, generally as an adjuvant (helper) with other therapies. The best known species of aloe is "aloe vera," but there are over 200 other species as well. Most of them hail from arid regions of the globe.

The gel-like juice of the aloe is used for intestinal ailments and colon cleansing, and reputedly can help restore the bowels to normal functioning.

Aloe is so prized by many cultures that it got a reputation as a cure-all. This, in turn, created a reaction among some doctors. "Modern clinical use of the gel began in the 1930s, with reports of successful treatment of x-ray and radium burns, which led to further experimental studies using laboratory animals in the following decades," one scientist has observed. But early studies "suffered from poor experimental design and insufficiently large test samples. In addition some conflicting or inconsistent results were obtained" (2). In the last few years this attitude has changed, mainly because of extensive Russian studies.

While generally a safe substance, aloe is not completely without potential side effects. A bitter yellow substance in the bundle sheath cells is a purgative and laxative and needs to be removed in the processing. There are also reports of skin or intestinal irritation from both applying and ingesting extracts of aloe.

Aloe contains polysaccharides. In the past, such chemicals did not excite much interest among researchers. But over the last two decades, Japanese scientists in particular have shown that polysaccharides resemble natural parts of the cell walls of bacteria, and therefore can stimulate an immune response in people.

Japanese scientists have also found several other biologically active substances in the leaf juice. These include aloenin, barbaloin, magnesium lactate and succinic acid. Still other chemicals have been found in the roots (3). In 1976, scientists reported that they had broken down extracts of certain aloe-containing seeds (*Rhamnus frangula L.*) and isolated a chemical called aloe emodin. This showed "significant antileukemic activity" in mice (4).

Scientists have also studied aloe's effect on the development of various kinds of cancer in mice. They observed cures in the case of one kind of tumor and were encouraged to find that the growth rate of other kinds of animal tumors was also slowed. They used a water soluble, heat-stable polysaccharide. Again, preliminary studies indicated that it acts as a non-specific booster of the immune system, possibly by stimulating macrophages (scavenger cells) (5).

A few years ago, Russian scientists carried out an evaluation of the ability of aloe juice to stop the spread of cancer (metastases). They used three types of tumors in rodents. They concluded that while aloe juice did not affect the main tumor growth, it reduced tumor mass and the frequency of metastases at different stages of the tumor's progress (6).

In the south of Madagascar a form of aloe called

"Vahombe" has been shown to fight infection. Scientists at the Pasteur Institute of Madagascar gave mice an injection of Vahombe extract. It conferred strong protection against infections common among the elderly, the sick, the young and all those whose immune systems were weak (7).

Yet, interestingly, aloe did not kill bacteria in the test tube. The African scientists concluded that aloe protects mice by enhancing their immune system. And effectiveness was proportional to the amount of aloe injected. Protection was greatest when the mice were treated with aloe two or three days before the infection (8).

In the following year, Madagascar scientists extended these findings. An extract of Vahombe leaves was found to protect mice against many other infections: from bacteria (including the one that causes bubonic plague); parasites; and the common fungus, *Candida albicans*. Again, the protective fraction of aloe had to be administered two days before inoculation with the germs (9).

Although not directly related to cancer, these results could be significant for cancer patients. Many patients, especially those receiving toxic chemotherapy, are prone to infections. Aloe juice also increased the antitumor effect of standard chemotherapy drugs 5-FU and cyclophosphamide as components of combination chemotherapy (8).

Aloe was also found by scientists at Hoshi University in Tokyo to provide "a significant protective effect of skin injury" caused by radiation (10). Aloe can also protect the liver from poisons, such as alcohol. This finding may be of particular significance to cancer patients, too, since the liver is the principal detoxification organ of the body (11). Again, as in the Madagascar experiments, aloe excelled as a preventative, and was especially effective when given half an hour before the toxin.

ALOE

⊕ References

1. Gibbons A. Plants of the apes. Science.1991;255:921.

2. Grindlay D and Reynolds T. The aloe vera phenomenon: a review of the properties and modern uses of the leaf parenchyma gel. J Ethnopharmacol.1986;16:117-51.

3. Hirata T and Suga T. Biologically active constituents of leaves and roots of aloe arborescens var. natalensis. Z Naturforsch[c].1977;32:731-4.

4. Kupchan SM and Karim A. Tumor inhibitors. 114. Aloe emodin: antileukemic principle isolated from rhamnus frangula L. Lloydia.1976; 39:223-4.

5. Ralamboranto L, et al. [Immunomodulating properties of an extract isolated and partially purified from aloe vahombe. Study of antitumoral properties and contribution to the chemical nature and active principle]. Arch Inst Pasteur Madagascar.1982;50:227-56.

6. Gribel NV and Pashinskii VG. [Antimetastatic properties of aloe juice]. Vopr Onkol.1986;32:38-40.

7. Berkow R. The Merck manual of diagnosis and therapy (15th ed.) Rahway, NJ: Merck & Co., 1987,p. 2696.

8. Solar S, et al. [Immunostimulant properties of an extract isolated and partially purified from aloe vahombe]. Arch Inst Pasteur Madagascar. 1980;47:9-39.

9. Brossat JY, et al. [Immunostimulating properties of an extract isolated from aloe vahombe. Protection in mice by fraction F1 against infections by listeria monocytogenes, yersinia pestis, candida albicans and plasmodium berghei]. Arch Inst Pasteur Madagascar.1981;48:11-34.

10. Sato Y, et al. [Studies on chemical protectors against radiation. XXXI. Protection effects of aloe arborescens on skin injury induced by x-irradiation]. Yakugaku Zasshi.1990;110:876-84.

11. Sakai K, et al. Effect of water extracts of aloe and some herbs in decreasing blood ethanol concentration in rats. II. Chem Pharm Bull (Tokyo).1989; 37:155-9.

❧*A*STRAGALUS

....

Astragalus is an inexpensive, non-toxic herb that boosts immunity and fights cancer. It comes from the root of a pea-like plant called *Astragalus membranaceus*. (Another member of this family is the infamous 'locoweed' of the American Old West.) In China, an astragalus extract is extremely popular as a 'spleen tonic.' It is also found in various **kampo** formulas of Japanese traditional medicine. Science now confirms that astragalus is indeed a powerful immune booster.

This ability was discovered by studying its impact on the white blood (mononuclear) cells of healthy donors. Three active fractions of astragalus were eventually isolated. Chinese scientists found that such extracts boosted immune reactions in cancer patients, as well (1). In 1986, it was shown that astragalus protected animals against the well-known liver poison, carbon tetrachloride (2).

Astragalus also protects against the ravages of chemotherapy. Some of the standard anti-cancer drugs cause degeneration in the liver, which expresses itself as an elevation of key liver enzymes. But such enzyme activity was not elevated in a group of animals that received astragalus in addition to chemotherapy. Astragalus has no known toxicity of its own and, according to scientists, could be utilized along with chemotherapy to minimize side effects (3).

An alkaloid chemical called "swainsonine," which is derived from a form of Astragalus (*oxyphysus*), also inhibits distant metastases (spread) of melanoma (a deadly form of skin cancer) in mice. Scientists at Howard University's Cancer Center added this chemical to the animals' drinking water. Within 24 hours it had inhibited over 80 percent of tumor colonies in their lungs. This activity seemed due to the chemical's ability to "enhance natural killer (NK) cell function." NK cells are vital to fighting cancer. When the mice did not have healthy NK cells, the compound lost its effectiveness. This therapy was simple to administer, rapidly reached maximum effectiveness, and then was quickly cleared from the body. Howard scientists conclude that the drug could start a biological cascade which, in turn, could lead to an increase in antitumor cell activity.

Swainsonine also stimulates spleen cells to exercise an antimetastatic effect.

In 1988, the Washington, DC scientists classified swainsonine as a "new immunomodulator that has the ability...to block tumor metastasis" (4).

Swainsonine also reduced the growth rate of human melanoma cells growing in the test tube or transplanted into living animals (5). Scientists concluded in the *JNCI* that "the antimetastatic activity of swainsonine is not limited to artificial or experimentally induced metastasis nor to a single tumor type or specific organ" (6).

Some chemotherapists are already thinking of using swainsonine to increase the dosage of standard drugs. They hope to be able to allow "increased dosage and/or frequency of administration" of these agents without increasing the toxic effects in bone marrow (7).

⊕ References

1.   Chu DT, et al. Immunotherapy with Chinese medicinal herbs. I. Immune restoration of local xenogeneic graft-versus-host reaction in cancer patients by fractionated astragalus membranaceus in vitro. J Clin Lab

Immunol.1988;25:119-23.

2. Jiang J and Xiao Q. Handbook of planta medica. Beijing: People's Health Publishers, 1986.

3. Zhang ZL, et al. Hepatoprotective effects of astragalus root. J Ethnopharmacol.1990;30:145-9.

4. Humphries MJ, et al. Augmentation of murine natural killer cell activity by swainsonine, a new antimetastatic immunomodulator. Cancer Res.1988;48:1410-5.

5. Dennis JW, et al. Growth inhibition of human melanoma tumor xenografts in athymic nude mice by swainsonine. Cancer Res.1990; 50:1867-72.

6. Bertino JR. Swainsonine inhibition of spontaneous metastasis. J Natl Cancer Inst.1989;81:1024-8.

7. Newton SA, et al. Protective effects of swainsonine on murine survival and bone marrow proliferation during cytotoxic chemotherapy. J Natl Cancer Inst.1991;83:1149-56.

ꝁ𝒜YUR-𝒱EDA

Ayur-Veda is an ancient system of medicine that originated in India several thousand years ago. In India today, Ayurvedic medicine is said to be taught at 108 medical colleges and command the allegiance of over 300,000 doctors. In the US, Ayurvedic medicine has been adopted by followers of the Maharishi Mahesh Yoga, the well-known guru whose US operations are based in Fairfield, Iowa.

"Maharishi Ayur-Veda" is proposed as a combination of Indian traditions and Western science. Its most prominent advocate is a charismatic, Harvard-trained doctor named Deepak Chopra, MD, who has written several best-selling books on the topic. Chopra claims that Ayurvedic medicine is the world's oldest medical tradition, but that it has particular relevance to modern times.

Many people were amazed when the sober voice of organized medicine, *JAMA*, carried a highly favorable article on Ayur-veda by Chopra and others in May 1991 (1). The article was later attacked as a "marketing scheme" and a hoax within the pages of *JAMA* itself (2,3). The main charge was that Chopra had failed to disclose his own past and present financial interests in the therapy.

Ayurvedic medicine, the original article explained, emphasizes "biological individuality," i.e. the concept that every person and each person's disease is unique. Diseases arise from an imbalance and disruption of the body's own immune mechanisms. Ayur-Veda places its emphasis on mental and emotional factors, which it sees as critical in causing such imbalances. Ayur-Veda uses pulse diagnosis to a degree unknown in modern Western science.

Of special importance to people with cancer are the herbal compounds known as rasayanas. Such substances are said to increase the body's resistance to disease and promote longevity. These effects are not limited to cancer. But some recent studies indicate their potential use. For example, scientists at several midwestern US universities have found that two rasayana compounds, called M-4 and M-5, are particularly active against cancer in animal systems. (The M stands for Maharishi.) Participating research institutions include Ohio State University, Columbus; Indiana University, Indianapolis; University of Kansas, Kansas City; South Dakota College of Pharmacy, Brookings; and the University of Colorado, Denver.

According to Chopra's *JAMA* article, "Both (M-4 and M-5) have been found to reduce the incidence of chemically induced mammary carcinoma [breast cancer] in up to 88 percent of experimental animals and caused up to 60 percent of fully formed tumors in control animals to regress when the animals were subsequently given the compounds" (1).

In addition, M-4 was said to prevent lung cancer metastases in up to 65 percent of the experimental animals tested, according to an abstract presented at a major 1990 scientific meeting (FASEB). M-5 also induced differentiation in 75 percent of neuroblastoma cells in culture, meaning that it could help turn cancer cells back into normal cells. It also boosted immunity and had a number of other beneficial effects in animals.

Chemical analysis of both compounds shows that they contain a mixture of antioxidants. This is no surprise, since many naturally-occurring anticancer agents work by preventing the destructive activity of free oxygen radicals.

⊕ References

1.   Sharma HM, et al. Maharishi Ayur-Veda: modern insights into ancient medicine [published erratum appears in JAMA 1991;266:798]. JAMA.1991;265:2633-4.

2.   Various authors. Maharishi Ayur-Veda [letters]. JAMA.1991; 266: 1769-74.

3.   Skolnick AA. Maharishi Ayur-Veda: Guru's marketing scheme promises the world eternal 'perfect health' [news]. JAMA.1991;266:1741-2.

⚛ *C*ANNABIS

The most controversial herb of course has to be marijuana. There have been a number of reports that marijuana causes health problems, including possibly cancer. But in a *JNCI* article in 1975, scientists reported the surprising finding that several marijuana derivatives retarded the growth of lung cancer in mice. Animals treated for ten straight days with one of these drugs showed reduced tumor growth. Mice treated for 20 days had reduced primary tumor size. Several of these marijuana substances increased survival time by up to 36 percent. Another, given daily for ten days, significantly inhibited spleen enlargement, caused by a mouse leukemia virus, by 71 percent (4).

But the main use of marijuana in cancer stems from its remarkable ability at fighting nausea and other side effects of conventional chemotherapy.

There are three kinds of nausea and vomiting induced by chemotherapy: acute, delayed and anticipatory. A variety of drugs have been tried to control these effects. For years, doctors relied on two kinds of drugs—phenothiazines and butyrophenones— as the mainstays in treating the nausea or vomiting associated with chemotherapy (1). They frequently were used in combination (2).

The drug metoclopramide is given in high doses to control the effects of the toxic anticancer agent cisplatin. Drugs called glucocorticoids are also used, in combination with other agents (3).

These agents "unfortunately have only partially controlled nausea and vomiting." The same scientists admit that "Cannabinoids [marijuana derivatives] appear to be superior to these drugs," but they worry that the drug "must be given in doses that also cause central nervous system side effects."

Many patients have been so repelled by the side effects of chemotherapy, that they have dropped out of conventional drug treatment programs. Chemotherapists believe that "more effective management of chemotherapy-induced nausea and vomiting" would "enhance patient compliance" (1).

And the most effective candidates are cannabinoids, the derivatives of marijuana. Since the 1980s, scientists have been testing synthetic cannabinoids such as dronabinol and nabilone (5).

In one controlled study, nabilone was used on a group of 23 children who were receiving nausea-causing chemotherapy. Eighteen of the 23 completed the trial and they had fewer vomiting episodes and less nausea. Two-thirds expressed a preference for this drug over other medications.

The most common side effects were sleepiness and dizziness. One patient experienced hallucinations. The scientists concluded that nabilone is an effective antinausea medication for children, even young ones, undergoing chemotherapy, It seems better than the drug it was compared to—domperidone—although it had a higher rate of the familiar side effects of smoking 'weed' (6).

⊕ References

1.   Stoudemire A, et al. Recent advances in the pharmacologic and behavioral management of chemotherapy-induced emesis. Arch Intern Med.1984;144:1029-33.

2.   Tortorice PV and O'Connell MB. Management of chemotherapy-induced nausea and vomiting. Pharmacotherapy.1990;10:129-45.

3.   Eyre HJ and Ward JH. Control of cancer chemotherapy-induced nausea and vomiting. Cancer.1984;54:2642-8.

4.   Munson AE, et al. Antineoplastic activity of cannabinoids. J Natl Cancer Inst.1975;55:597-602.

5.   Lane M, et al. Dronabinol and prochlorperazine alone and in combination as antiemetic agents for cancer chemotherapy. Am J Clin Oncol.1990;13:480-4.

6.   Dalzell AM, et al. Nabilone: an alternative antiemetic for cancer chemotherapy. Arch Dis Child.1986;61:502-5.

CHAPARRAL

❡ CHAPARRAL

Chaparral tea is prepared from a perennial evergreen shrub called the greasewood or creosote bush of the American Southwest (*Larrea divaricata, mexicana* or *tridentata,* or *Covillea tridentata*). The active ingredient of the creosote bush is NDGA (nordihydroguaiaretic acid) which is found in the resinous coating of the plant's stems and leaves. NDGA was isolated from creosote in 1945 and since then has been used as an industrial antioxidant in fats and oils.

A number of laboratories have also explored the anti-cancer properties of NDGA. For example, when a chemical that routinely causes colon cancer was given to 14 rats, NDGA prevented the appearance of the disease in nine of animals (1). In an experiment in Mysore, India, various agents were studied for their ability to protect against damage to the genes. NDGA provided 83 percent protection against a carcinogen (2).

One week after a single injection of another powerful carcinogen, rats were given varying doses of NDGA. They all "developed significantly fewer mammary cancers" than controls. Scientists at Chicago's IIT Research Institute saw "no gross or organ-specific toxicity" following even high doses of NDGA. The scientists suggest that the chaparral-derived agent could become a new chemo-preventive drug (3).

In 1989, scientists at the University of Florida tested the effects of NDGA on three test tube cultures of leukemia cells. All three cell lines were inhibited (4).

When glioma (i.e., brain cancer) cells were incubated for just four hours with small amounts of NDGA, the chemical inhibited DNA synthesis. (Such inhibition can be a sign of

137

anticancer effects.) "Prolonged incubation [for 72 hours] of the rat and human glioma cells with NDGA markedly decreased cell proliferation," scientists at Rush-Presbyterian-St. Luke's Medical Center in Chicago, said. The scientists concluded that NDGA was an important controller of glioma cell division (5). In 1984, the extract also killed two different strains of cancer cells in the test tube (6).

Chaparral's resin also contains other promising chemicals, such as flavones, which have also been shown to exert anticancer effects. Four of the chaparral flavones demonstrated potent antiviral activity (7).

Fluid extracts of this Western bush have also been shown to have germicidal activity against five different kinds of bacteria (8).

Side Effects: Contact with the resins of the creosote bush can cause an allergic skin reaction called "contact dermatitis" (9). Taken internally, NDGA's ability to harm the kidneys has also been known for years. It is especially dangerous when combined with endotoxins, a byproduct of bacteria sometimes found in biological drugs (10).

There was a report from Canada of a 33-year-old woman who developed signs of liver damage after taking a product called Chaparral Leaf for several months. Symptoms first appeared three months after she began taking the tablets. The doctors who wrote the article warned that "the public and the medical profession must be wary of all 'harmless' nonprescription medications, whether purchased in pharmacies or elsewhere" (11).

Chaparral tea has a long and controversial history in American medicine, as well. The creosote bush figures in many Native American remedies. It was "quite generally used by southwestern tribes," according to Virgil J. Vogel, in his classic account, *American Indian Medicine* (Norman: University of Oklahoma Press, 1972). Papago Indian women boiled a preparation of salted chaparral leaves to wash wounds. Pima and Maricopa Indians drank a decoction of the branches for diarrhea and stomach troubles in general. Creosote was originally derived from this plant, and remained on the official lists of US medicines (the USP and NF) for over 100 years. Creosote carbonate, a chemical derivative, is still sometimes used as an expectorant and antiseptic, and is said to be better tolerated by the stomach and kidneys than creosote itself.

In a celebrated case in the 1960s, an 85-year-old man came to the University of Utah and was diagnosed as having melanoma on his right cheek. He refused surgery but instead treated himself with chaparral tea (12). "He returned eight months later, with marked regression of the cancer," according to an American Cancer Society account.

Utah scientists then tried the tea on other patients. "Four patients have responded to some extent to treatment with the tea, including two with melanomas, one with choriocarcinoma metastatic to the lungs and one with widespread lymphosarcoma....One of the other melanoma patients experienced a 95 percent regression," whereupon the remaining growth was removed by surgical excision, according to the ACS report (13).

Laboratory research then performed at NCI showed that "this was a very active agent against cancer," in the words of Dr. Charles R. Smart, associate professor of surgery at the University of Utah Medical Center (see *The Cancer Industry*, chapter 6).

In his initial report on the melanoma regressions, Dr. Smart warned that in some cases patients with advanced diseases did not respond to the tea.

⊕ References

1.   Birkenfeld S, et al. Antitumor effects of inhibitors of arachidonic acid cascade on experimentally induced intestinal tumors. Dis Colon Rectum.1987;30:43-6.

2.   Shalini VK and Srinivas L. Fuel smoke condensate induced DNA damage in human lymphocytes and protection by turmeric (Curcuma longa). Mol Cell Biochem.1990;95:21-30.

3.   McCormick DL and Spicer AM. Nordihydroguaiaretic acid suppression of rat mammary carcinogenesis induced by N-methyl-N-nitrosourea. Cancer Lett.1987;37:139-46.

4.   Miller AM, et al. Effects of lipoxygenase and glutathione pathway inhibitors on leukemic cell line growth. J Lab Clin Med.1989;113:355-61.

5.   Wilson DE, et al. Effect of nordihydroguaiaretic acid on cultured rat and human glioma cell proliferation. J Neurosurg.1989;71:551-7.

6.   Zamora J. Cytotoxic, antimicrobial and phytochemical properties of Larrea tridentata, Cav. [PhD dissertation.] Auburn University, 1984.

7.   Vanden Berghe D, et al. Advances in medicinal plant research. Stuttgart: Wissenschaftliche Verlagsgesellschaft, 1985.

8.   Train P. Medicinal use of plants by Indian tribes of Nevada. Lawrence, MA: Quarterman Publishers, Inc., 1982.

9.   Shasky DR. Contact dermatitis from Larrea tridentata (creosote bush) [letter]. J Am Acad Dermatol.1986;15:302.

10. Gardner KJ, et al. Endotoxin provocation of experimental renal cystic disease. Kidney Int.1987;32:329-34.

11. Katz M and Saibil F. Herbal hepatitis: subacute hepatic necrosis secondary to chaparral leaf. J Clin Gastroenterol.1990;12:203-6.

12. Smart CR, et al. An interesting observation on nordihydroguaiaretic acid (NSC-4291; NDGA) and a patient with malignant melanoma—a preliminary report. Cancer Chemother Rep.1969;53:147-51.

13. ACS. Unproven methods of cancer management. New York: American Cancer Society, 1971.

❦ CHINESE HERBS

Chinese herbs and other traditional medicines are now being shown to have dramatic effects against cancer. Such products can boost the immune system and increase the efficacy of chemotherapy, while decreasing side effects. Although still little known outside China, such traditional products and practices are slowly making their way into Western medical practice. One main avenue is through Japanese **kampo** prescriptions.

Chinese medicine is based on a set of philosophical ideas quite foreign to Western thinking. Central is the notion of *qi*, which Western authors generally translate as vital energy. Things that increase *qi* are considered good for the health. This Chinese tradition goes back at least 4,000 years, making it one of the oldest medical traditions in the world. But Western medicine has generally denegrated Chinese influences as superstitious and unscientific.

President Richard M. Nixon's visit to China in 1972 led to a 'rediscovery' of Asian medicine, particularly acupuncture. Today, there is also widescale interest in acupressure, moxibustion and traditional drugs, which are derived from vegetables, herbs, sea creatures and even insects. Chinese scientists are vigorously investigating their heritage, applying modern methods to the study of ancient traditions.

The greatest impetus to this integration has come from the World Health Organization (WHO). The 30th World Health Assembly adopted a resolution (WHA30.49) calling for a rebirth of ancient medical traditions. It urged governments to give "adequate importance to the utilization of their traditional systems of medicine with appropriate regulations as suited to their national health systems." In

China as well as in Japan, Russia, Mexico, Zimbabwe and many other countries, this mandate has been enthusiastically carried out. A turning point was the Seventeenth International Internal Medicine Medical Association meeting in Kyoto, Japan, in 1984. Representatives of 56 countries spoke on "Internal Medicine of the East and West—A View of Tomorrow." There were numerous presentations on Chinese and Japanese herbs, including some effective against cancer.

For instance, actinidia is a root used in traditional Chinese folk medicine. In 1988, Chinese scientists discovered a polysaccharide called ACPS-R in this root. Such polysaccharides can normalize the immune system and are considered "prominent candidates for an adjuvant tumor therapy" (1). When Actinidia was injected into mice, almost 90 percent of their tumors stopped growing. Almost 50 percent of liver cancers were also inhibited. This compound prolonged the life of cancer-bearing mice, and increased the percentage of tumor-free mice.

When ACPS-R was used in combination with the standard anticancer drug 5-FU, the antitumor effect was enhanced compared to the use of 5-FU alone. The immune system was also returned to nearly normal after treatment with ACPS-R. Scientists at the Zhejiang College of Traditional Chinese Medicine in Hangzhou concluded that "ACPS-R acts as a new antitumor polysaccharide, and the treatment effect of Actinidia root in folk medicine is probably related to ACPS-R" (2).

One hundred and fifteen patients with inoperable cancer of the esophagus (very common in parts of China) were treated either with chemotherapy alone or with chemotherapy plus another herb, *Rabdosia rubescens*.

In the first group, there were two partial responses (greater than 50 percent tumor regression) and 8 minimal responses out of 31 patients. But in the group that received the herb as well as chemotherapy, out of 84 patients there were 59 responses, or a total of over 70 percent. Of these, 10 showed complete response (100 percent tumor regression), as well as 16 partial response and 33 minimal response. The one-year survival rates of the chemotherapy-alone group was 13.6 percent but in the chemotherapy-plus-herb group it was 41.3 percent. There was no difference between the two groups in regard to toxicity. Since this trial involved toxic drugs, not surprisingly there were significant side effects, including baldness, wasting and nausea in about 30 percent of the patients. And two patients died of damage to their lungs, attributed to the chemotherapy (3).

Another newly discovered plant chemical is Baohuoside-1. It is a **bioflavonoid,** a kind of natural plant pigment. Baohuoside-1 was shown to stop the growth of, and then kill, six separate cancer cell lines. It appeared to work by interfering with DNA synthesis (4).

Chinese Fly: Mylabris is not an herb, but the dried body of the Chinese blister beetle. As unappetizing as this may sound, beetles once formed part of the traditional medicine in many cultures. Some kinds of beetle irritate the urinary tract. In Europe they are best known as ingredients in the notorious aphrodisiac, 'Spanish fly.' In China, beetle parts have been used as a folk remedy for more than 2,000 years, to the present day. The active constituent of the blister beetle has been identified as a chemical named cantharidin.

In the 1950s, a beetle derivative was used to treat warts, which are after all a form of nonmalignant growth (5). In recent years, scientists have found that mylabris possesses antitumor properties as well and increases the number of white blood cells.

In order to find a less-toxic formulation which still has anticancer effects, scientists at the Institute of Pharmacy of Beijing's Fourth Pharmaceutical Works synthesized two new compounds, disodium cantharidate and norcantharidin. These two compounds, and especially norcantharidin, have been found to be active against liver cancer. As hoped, both showed much less urinary irritation than the traditional beetle preparation. Luckily, the irritating portion of the compound turn out to be separate from its anticancer effects. All of these compounds are now being produced as experimental antitumor agents in China (6).

Patients with small cell lung cancer were also given a traditional Chinese kidney tonic called Liu Wei Di Huang (Six Flavor Tea) or Jin Gui Shen Qi (Golden Book Tea) along with chemotherapy or radiotherapy. Patients were divided into two groups: half got these herbal tonics, the others served as controls. Doctors at the Beijing Institute for Cancer Research found a significant difference in the response rate as well as survival time between the two groups.

A full 91.5 percent of the patients who received both chemotherapy and the Chinese teas responded with tumor shrinkage, compared to 46.9 percent in those receiving just chemotherapy.

The median survival for the group receiving both treatments was 16 months compared to 10 months for the control group. Ten patients in the Chinese herb group were alive more than two years after starting the treatment. In 1990, Beijing scientists reported that "four patients in the Chinese herb group" but only "one in the control group are still enjoying their disease-free life for more than seven years."

Blood problems were observed much more frequently in the patients receiving just chemotherapy than in those also getting the teas. Animal experiments with the same traditional medicine as used in the clinic have also shown normalization of their immune system. These results show that traditional Chinese kidney tonics may be useful in enhancing immunity and in helping to treat patients with solid tumors (7).

Buzhong Yiqi (Bu Zhong Qi Wan, also called the "Central Qi Pill") is another traditional medicine being investigated for its anticancer activity. It appears to work well with the standard anticancer agent, cyclophosphamide. Results showed that this tonic "significantly increased the anticancer activity and simultaneously decreased the toxicity" of this conventional Western drug (8).

⊕ References

1. Franz G. Polysaccharides in pharmacy: current applications and future concepts. Planta Med.1989;55:493-7.

2. Lin PF. [Antitumor effect of actinidia chinensis polysaccharide on murine tumor]. Chung Hua Chung Liu Tsa Chih.1988;10:441-4.

3. Wang RL, et al. [Potentiation by rabdosia rubescens on chemotherapy of advanced esophageal carcinoma]. Chung Hua Chung Liu Tsa Chih.1986;8:297-9.

4. Li SY, et al. Effects of the plant flavonoid baohuoside-1 on cancer cells in vitro. Cancer Lett.1990;53:175-81.

5. Epstein J and Kligman A. Treatment of warts with cantharadin. AMA Arch of Derm.1958;77:508-511.

6. Wang GS. Medical uses of mylabris in ancient China and recent studies. J Ethnopharmacol.1989;26:147-62.

7. Liu XY and Ang NQ. [Effect of liu wei di huang or jin gui shen qi decoction as on adjuvant treatment in small cell lung cancer]. Chung Hsi I Chieh Ho Tsa Chih.1990;10:720-2.

8. Ji YB, et al. [Effects of buzhong yiqi decoction on the anticancer activity and toxicity induced by cyclophosphamide]. Chung Kuo Chung Yao Tsa Chih.1989;14:48-51.

❦ ESSIAC

Essiac is an herbal cancer treatment developed by a Canadian nurse, Renée Caisse (1888-1978). (Essiac is Caisse spelled backwards.) Ms. Caisse claimed that the formula had been given to her in 1922 by a patient whose breast cancer had been cured by a traditional native American healer in Ontario.

Thousands of patients have since been treated with this herbal mixture, most of them at Caisse's own Bracebridge Clinic in Ontario. While this clinic was shut down in 1942, the controversy over Essiac simmered for years. Charles Brusch, MD—President Kennedy's physician—is said to have declared in 1959 that "Essiac has merit in the treatment of cancer."

Essiac cannot be freely marketed in either the US or Canada. However, a company in Ontario is allowed to provide Essiac to Canadian patients under a special arrangement with health officials there. One problem is that Caisse never made the formula public in her lifetime. A number of companies now sell competing "original" Essiac in the form of a tea, but the authenticity of some of these formulas are open to question.

Essiac was tested at both Memorial Sloan-Kettering (MSKCC) and the US National Cancer Institute (NCI) in the 1970s and was said to have no anticancer activity in animal systems. But the mixture remains worth investigating, not just because of persistent anecdotal reports, but because most of its identifiable components have individually shown anticancer properties in independent tests.

The four main herbs in Essiac are:

• Burdock (*Arctium lappa*): There have been several studies showing antitumor activity of burdock in animal systems (1, 2). (Other studies showed no such effects.) An antimutation factor has also been isolated, which is resistant to both heat and protein-digesting enzymes. Scientists at Kawasaki Medical School, Okayama, Japan, called this "the burdock factor" (3). Burdock has also been found to be active in the test tube against the human immunodeficiency virus (HIV) (4). **Benzaldehyde,** also present in burdock, has been shown to have significant anticancer effects in humans. (Intriguingly, burdock independently was included in another famous 'secret' herbal remedy, the **Hoxsey** treatment.)

• Indian rhubarb (*Rheum palmatum*): This plant has been demonstrated to have antitumor activity in the sarcoma 37 test system (5). (Again, conflicting tests did not show such activity.) Certain chemicals in Indian rhubarb, such as aloe emodin, catechin and rhein, "have shown antitumor activity in some animal test systems," according to the Office of Technology Assessment report on unconventional cancer treatments (6).

• Sorrel: NCI is said to have tested one sample of Taiwanese sorrel and found no activity against mouse leukemia. But again, aloe emodin, isolated from sorrel, does show "significant antileukemic activity" (7, 8).

• Slippery elm: NCI tested slippery elm and found no activity. But slippery elm contains beta-sitosterol and a polysaccharide, both of which have shown activity (9).

Several cases of poisoning have been reported from drinking commercial burdock root tea (10). "It is important to consider plant sources in the differential diagnosis of the poisoned patient," Arizona doctors wrote. No acute toxicity was seen with Essiac in the MSKCC tests, although there was said to be a slight weight loss in treated animals. NCI, however, claimed to see lethal toxicity at the highest concentrations of Essiac given to animals.

⊕ References

1. Foldeak S and Dombradi G. Tumor-growth inhibiting substances of plant origin. I. Isolation of the active principle of Arctium lappa. Acta Phys Chem.1964;10:91-93.

2. Dombradi C and Foldeak S. Screening report on the antitumor activity of purified Arctium lappa extracts. Tumori.1966;52:173.

3. Morita K, et al. A desmutagenic factor isolated from burdock (Arctium lappa Linne). Mutat Res.1984;129:25-31.

4. WHO. In vitro screening of traditional medicines for anti-HIV activity: memorandum from a WHO meeting. Bul. WHO (Switzerland), 1989;67:613-618.

5. Belkin M and Fitzgerald D. Tumor damaging capacity of plant materials. 1. Plants used as cathartics. J Natl Cancer Inst.1952;13:139-155.

6. US Congress, Office of Technology Assessment (OTA). Unconventional cancer treatments. Washington, DC: US Government Printing Office, 1990.

7. Kupchan SM and Karim A. Tumor inhibitors. Aloe emodin: antileukemic principle isolated from Rhamnus frangula L. Lloydia.1976;39:223-4.

8. Morita H, et al. Cytotoxic and mutagenic effects of emodin on cultured mouse carcinoma FM3A cells. Mutat Res.1988;204:329-32.

9. Pettit GR, et al. Antineoplastic agents. The yellow jacket Vespula pensylvanica. Lloydia.1977;40:247-52.

10. Rhoads P, et al. Anticholinergic poisonings associated with commercial burdock root tea. J Toxicol.1984-85;22:581-584.

❦ GARLIC

Garlic (*Allium sativum*) is a well-known European bulbous herb of the lily family, closely related to onions, scallions and leeks. Thousands of years ago, garlic originated as a wild plant in the deserts of Western Russia. Its use as food and medicine spread west and southward with wandering tribes. We know that it was already being cultivated in the Middle East 5,000 years ago, making it one of humanity's first cultivated plants.

The 'father of history,' Herodotus (484-425 BC), told of seeing an inscription on the Egyptian pyramids that recorded the amount of garlic consumed by the monuments' builders. Cloves of garlic were discovered in the tomb of Pharaoh Tutankhamen. Pliny the Elder (23-79 AD), the Roman encyclopedist, wrote that "garlic has powerful properties."

Today, garlic is grown all over the world and has justly been called the "quintessential medicinal food." It has been employed to control dysentery, fight parasites, detoxify, fight fever and stomach aches, and many of these traditional usages have been confirmed by scientific experiments.

In the past, it was thought the single beneficial element in garlic that conferred the plant's health benefits was allicin (1). This compound is formed when the garlic bulb is crushed or bruised. It is strongly antibacterial and is mainly responsible for garlic's characteristic odor. Allicin is rather unstable, according to Varro Tyler in *The New Honest Herbal* (Philadelphia: G.F. Stickley, 1987).

In addition to allicin, garlic also contains 32 other sulfur compounds, 17 amino acids, **germanium, calcium,** copper, iron, **potassium, magnesium, selenium, zinc,** as well as small amounts of **vitamin A, vitamin B$_1$** and **vitamin C** (2).

The main active components seem to be the sulfur compounds. These include not just allicin, but allixin, diallyl disulfide, and diallyl trisulfide (3) and thioallyl amino acids, as well as other compounds formed during preparation and cooking. It is a complex picture, still under investigation.

Garlic has a broad spectrum of activities: it stops the clumping of platelets, thus exerting a beneficial effect on the circulatory system, similar to aspirin. It lowers cholesterol, regulates blood sugar and high blood pressure and helps in a host of other ailments (4).

Over 1,000 articles are said to have been published on various aspects of this remarkable plant in the last twenty years (5). Although most of this work has been done on garlic's beneficial effects on the heart and circulation, in a small pilot study, AIDS patients with weakened natural killer (NK) cells were given garlic for ten weeks.

Six out of seven AIDS patients were found to have normal Natural Killer cells six weeks later.

Four out of seven also had improvements in the ratio of helper cells to suppressor cells. Most also experienced reduction of diarrhea, genital herpes, candida infections and recurrent fevers (6).

The main flavor component in garlic is diallyl sulfide (DAS), which has been shown to inhibit chemically-caused cancers of stomach and lungs of mice. Scientists do not yet know the exact mechanism by which DAS exerts this anticancer activity. They studied different levels on the enzyme systems in mice and noted a significant increase in these detoxifying enzymes in the stomach of mice treated with DAS. The more garlic, the greater the effect. These results suggest that garlic may exert its anticancer effect through a key detoxification system, glutathione-S-transferase (7).

In cancer research, garlic has been found to shorten the cell-doubling time and stimulate the growth and proliferation of some beneficial cells (8). In an extensive review of 30 studies it was shown that garlic and onion consumption was associated with reduced deaths from cancer.

A major turning point in garlic studies was the "First World Congress on the Health Significance of Garlic and Garlic Constituents," held in Washington, DC in 1990. Sponsored by Nutrition International Company, makers of Kyolic® brand aged garlic, and co-sponsored by

Pennsylvania State University and the US Department of Agriculture, this Congress brought together scientists from around the globe to present the growing body of evidence on garlic's remarkable properties.

For example, it was shown that aged garlic extract may protect against radiation damage. Rats and rabbits were first given cobalt-60 gamma radiation. Those which were also given aged garlic extract had lower death rates; less leakage of intracellular enzymes into the blood; and decreased loss of white blood cells and platelets (9).

Two scientists at Penn State found that aged garlic extract powder "significantly delayed the onset of tumors and reduced the total number of rats developing mammary cancer."

The incidence of breast cancer was 90 percent in rats fed a normal diet, but only 35 percent in mice given garlic in their diet for two weeks before and after receiving a carcinogen.

Garlic seemed capable of stopping breast tissue from turning this carcinogen into a substance capable of binding in a harmful way to genetic material (10).

The incidence of melanoma is increasing rapidly, especially in the developed world. This form of skin cancer is deadly because it metastasizes easily and is very difficult to treat. Doctors at UCLA studied the effects of aged garlic extract on melanoma cells growing in the test tube. Garlic inhibited cancer cell growth by more than 50 percent, but had no such effect on normal white blood cells.

More remarkably, treating melanoma cells with garlic altered the shape of these cancer cells to an appearance "resembling precursor cells of melanoma, melanocytes." In other words, cancer cells began to differentiate, or revert to normal, under garlic's influence. The UCLA scientists said that aged garlic extract "appears to be a more potent or an equivalent inducer of differentiation of melanoma compared to some known cytokines and agents" (11). In other words, it was as good as, if not better, than synthetic and toxic drugs.

In addition, garlic suppressed the promoting effects of a known carcinogen (TPA) on skin cancer in mice. This worked only at the initial stage of the promoting process, however. A scientists at the Kyoto Prefectural University of Medicine reported that "garlic is proved to have potent antitumor-promoting activity." A number of key ingredients are responsible for these antitumor effects, including allicin.

There is no data in the National Toxicology Program on the toxicity of garlic, although some negative health effects at high doses have been reported. The ancient Chinese actually classified garlic as a moderately-toxic herb. This was because too much raw garlic can lead to stomach upset and intestinal gas.

Some garlic companies, catering to the false impression that allicin is the main active constituent in garlic, may soon try to fortify their products with this readily-made compound. But "excessive consumption of allicin and/or allicin decomposition products may cause toxicity" (1).

⊕ References

1.   Lin R. Myths, theories and facts about garlic's health benefits. First World Congress on the Health Significance of Garlic and Garlic Constituents. Washington, DC, 1990.

2.   Abdullah TH, et al. Garlic revisited: therapeutic for the major diseases of our time? Journal of the National Medical Association.1988; 80:439-445.

3.   Leung AY. Encyclopedia of common natural ingredients used in foods, drugs and cosmetics. New York: John Wiley and Sons, 1980.

4.   Foster S. Garlic (Allium sativum) (1st. ed.) Austin, TX: American Botanical Council, 1991:7 (AB Council, Botanical Series; vol. 311).

5.   Fenwick GR and Hanley AB. The Genus Allium. CRC Crit. Rev. Food Sci. Nutr.1985;22:199 and 23:1.

6.   Abdullah TH, et al. Enhancement of natural killer cell activity in AIDS with garlic. Deutsch Zeitschrfit für Onkologie.1989;21:52-53.

7.   Nair SC, et al. Differential induction of glutathione transferase isoenzymes of mice stomach by diallyl sulfide, a naturally occurring anticarcinogen. Cancer Lett.1991;57:121-9.

8.   Fujita E, et al. Stimulation of cell growth and proliferation in NIH-3T3 cells by onion and garlic oils. Cell Biol Toxicol.1986;2:369-78.

9.   Lin R. Antioxidant, pro-oxidant, antifree radical, and radiation protective properties of garlic extracts. First World Congress on the Health Significance of Garlic and Garlic Constituents. Washington, DC, 1990.

10.   Milner J and Liu J. Prevention of 7,12-dimethylbenz(α)anthracene (DMBA) induced mammary tumors by dietary garlic powder supplementation. First World Congress on the Health Significance of Garlic and Garlic Constituents. Washington, DC, 1990.

11.   Hoon S, et al. Modulation of cancer antigens and growth of human melanoma by aged garlic extract. First World Congress on Health Significance of Garlic and Garlic Constituents. Washington, DC, 1990.

❦ GINSENG

The most famous of all Chinese medicines, ginseng, has been used in Asia for thousands of years. Its reputation as a cure-all has spread its fame but worked against it with some scientists. Only recently have Westerners begun to take this remarkable plant seriously and to confirm many of its traditional uses.

There are two major problems in evaluating ginseng's health benefits. The first is that there are several different plants that go by the same basic name:

• Oriental ginseng, or *Panax ginseng;*

- American ginseng, or *Panax quinquefolius;* and
- Siberian ginseng, or *Eleutherococcus senticosus.*

Each has somewhat different properties and uses and each has its share of the burgeoning ginseng market.

The second problem is that there are no standards for ginseng purity and strength. A ginseng capsule, tablet or extract could conceivably contain little (or even no) ginseng at all. There are ways around this dilemma, however (see Resources).

To add to the confusion, Japanese and Russian scientists who did most of the work on this "panacea," chose different names for the various compounds they discovered. The Japanese called them ginsenosides, while the Russians named them panaxosides. There are so many active ingredients in this plant, however, that when the two research teams compared notes they found that only one ginsenoside was identical to a panaxoside.

In addition to starch and sugars, ginseng contains steroids, pectin, many **B vitamins**, such as B_1, B_2, B_{12}, nicotinic and pantothenic acids, and biotin, as well as the minerals **zinc**, manganese, **calcium**, iron and copper. It also contains choline, fats, and trace amounts of a volatile oil, among other things, according to Dr. A. Leung in his informative book, *Chinese Herbal Remedies* (New York: Phaidon Universe, 1984).

After hundreds of research reports, however, scientists still do not understand exactly what ginseng does in the body. According to a celebrated Russian theory, ginseng is not so much a medicine as an "adaptogen," i.e., a substance that brings the organism into equilibrium. Thus, ginseng might increase the blood pressure of someone with low blood pressure, while decreasing it in people with hypertension. The adaptogen theory is based on many scientific observations over decades. Yet it "sounds as if it has been taken directly out of a page of a book on the theory of Chinese medicine," Dr. Leung remarks.

Ginseng has been regarded as generally beneficial to cancer patients. But some recent studies show that ginseng may fight cancer in particular.

Its most remarkable quality is in the differentiation of cancer cells. Like **garlic, DMSO** and **HMBA,** a crude extract of Panax ginseng can not only stop the growth of malignant liver cells in the test tube, but can turn them back to normal (1, 2). Both in terms of function and shape, Japanese scientists said, the once-cancerous cells now resembled "original normal liver cells." Pathologists at Kanazawa Medical University called this process "decarcinogenesis." These scientists also reported in the US journal *Cancer Research* that a single chemical found in ginseng (the ginsenoside Rh2) could also make melanoma skin cancer cells revert to normal (3).

Working with the Siberian variety of ginseng, *Eleutherococcus senticosus*, scientists found that it produced an immune-boosting effect on white blood cells in both cancer patients and healthy controls. This study pointed to Siberian ginseng's ability to stimulate resistance and boost the immune system in patients undergoing chemotherapy and radiation for breast cancer. Since even prolonged exposure to *Eleutherococcus* is not toxic, it can be recommended for most patients receiving intensive anticancer therapy. But the drug concentration should be tailored to the individual, Russian scientists said (4).

In a Korean study, rats were given a carcinogen with or without four food substances: red pepper, salt, maejoo (a spice mixture) and ginseng extract. After 40 weeks the impact on cancers of the gastrointestinal tract was dramatic:

Type of Diet	% of animals with tumors
Untreated controls	44.0
Salt	61.9
Red pepper	57.0
Maejoo (spices)	14.8
Ginseng	3.4

Ginseng was obviously the best such compound.

It is worth noting that hot red pepper, although a good source of vitamin C, performed worse than the untreated controls. And in fact this was not the first time that such peppers were suspected of being carcinogenic.

The finding on salt was even more significant. In the chapters on **potassium** and on the **Gerson diet** we deal with the implications of the sodium-potassium balance for the occurrence of cancer (5). Interestingly, these Korean scientists were not looking for a cancer treatment but to explain the high rate of stomach cancer among Asian people.

Ginseng is generally a harmless and beneficial substance. However, there is much confusion over its labelling and purity. In the late 1970s, *JAMA* published a letter about an alleged "ginseng abuse syndrome," among mentally-ill people who were said to be so enamored of this substance that they began injecting it into their veins (6).

In 1991, *JAMA* also published a letter alleging that a girl baby was born with body hair in a mother who was a habitual drinker of ginseng tea. The letter alleged that hormone-like substances in the ginseng were responsible for this "neonatal androgenization" (7). The report seemed confused, however, as to the actual nature of the ginseng consumed. There were other questions raised about its accuracy (8). However, until such questions are cleared up, it might be wise for pregnant or breast-feeding women to abstain from this otherwise safe herb.

⊕ References

1. Odashima S, et al. Induction of phenotypic reverse transformation by ginsenosides in cultured Morris hepatoma cells. Eur J Cancer.1979; 15:885-92.

2. Abe H, et al. Ultrastructural studies of Morris hepatoma cells reversely transformed by ginsenosides. Experientia.1979;35:1647-9.

3. Ota T, et al. Plant-glycoside modulation of cell surface related to control of differentiation in cultured B16 melanoma cells. Cancer Res.1987; 47:3863-7.

4. Kupin VI and Polevaia EB. [Stimulation of the immunological reactivity of cancer patients by Eleutherococcus extract]. Vopr Onkol.1986; 32:21-6.

5. Kim JP, et al. Co-carcinogenic effects of several Korean foods on gastric cancer induced by N-methyl-N'-nitro-N-nitrosoguanidine in rats. Jpn J Surg.1985;15:427-37.

6. Siegel RK. Ginseng abuse syndrome. Problems with the panacea. JAMA.1979;241:1614-5.

7. Koren G, et al. Maternal ginseng use associated with neonatal androgenization [letter] [see comments]. JAMA.1990;264:2866.

8. Awang DV. Maternal use of ginseng and neonatal androgenization [letter; comment]. JAMA.1991;266:363.

❦ GREEN TEA

Scientists have discovered a remarkable substance that prevents many kinds of cancer in experimental animals. It is non-toxic, easy to take and inexpensive. It is green tea, one of the most popular drinks in Asia. Tea has long been considered "that Excellent and by All Physicians approved China drink" (1658). Doctors began the present study to understand why the Japanese have the highest smoking rate, but the lowest lung cancer rate in the developed world. In fact, Japanese men have less than one-third the lung cancer of their American counterparts.

Green tea is unfermented, while the more common black

tea is fermented. (Oolong is a mixture of the two.) In the late 1980s, Japanese scientists reported that they had isolated a chemical from green tea that lowered cholesterol and inhibited the growth of cancer (1). This chemical is epigallocatechin gallate (EGCG) and it is one of the main constituents of the green tea infusion. It was shown to inhibit tumor promotion in the skin and gastrointestinal tract of experimental mice (2, 3).

Mice given EGCG develop far less cancer of the lung as well, scientists reported at the Fourth Chemical Congress of North America, held in New York City in late August, 1991. In mice specially bred to develop liver cancer, tumors simply would not appear when they ingested this remarkable drink.

Dr. Hirota Fujiki of the National Cancer Center Research Institute in Tokyo, reported that a tea-lover in Japan may ingest about one gram of EGCG per day in green tea. A diet containing EGCG reduced tumor development in mice given a carcinogen as well as injections of liver cancer cells. Application of EGCG to mouse skin immediately reduced the binding of known carcinogens and tumor promoters to cells.

"We think that EGCG is a practical cancer chemopreventive agent to be implemented in everyday life," Dr. Fujiki said (4).

"Green tea cannot prevent every cancer," he added. "But it's the cheapest and most practical method for cancer prevention available to the general public."

Dr. Chung S. Yang and his colleagues at Rutgers University's Laboratory for Cancer Research found that giving green tea to mice "significantly inhibited" stomach and lung cancer induced by the known carcinogen, NDEA. More than 90 percent of the control mice developed cancer.

But in the mice that drank the tea as their sole source of liquid, tumors were reduced by 60 to 63 percent (5). "There aren't that many things that have as broad a spectrum," a Rutgers scientist told the *New York Times*.

In work at the American Health Foundation, in Valhalla, NY, scientists found that green tea could limit the ravages of smoking. A chemical in smoke, NNK, is believed to be one of the principal causes of lung cancer. NNK-treated mice which also received green tea (or EGCG) had approximately half the lung tumors as mice that did not get tea products. Tea-treated mice weighed a bit less but otherwise "no apparent toxicity was seen" (6).

EGCG appears to be a 'free radical scavenger,' neutralizing highly reactive molecules that attack DNA and trigger cancer. The American Health Foundation report suggests that green tea and/or EGCG prevents the activation of carcinogens. Less is known about the contribution of other constituents, such as **chlorophyll,** which independently has anticancer effects.

In addition, all tea is considered healthful. For example, another ingredient of tea is theophylline, a chemical closely related to caffeine. Theophylline was "found to act synergistically" with chlorambucil, increasing the potency of that conventional anticancer drug (7).

Tea also contains tannic acid which has been used both topically and internally as an experimental cancer treatment (8-9).

⊕ References

1. Chisaka T, et al. The effect of crude drugs on experimental hypercholesteremia: mode of action of (-)-epigallocatechin gallate in tea leaves. Chem Pharm Bull (Tokyo).1988;36:227-33.
2. Fujita Y, et al. Inhibitory effect of (-)-epigallocatechin gallate on carcinogenesis with N-ethyl-N'-nitro-N-nitrosoguanidine in mouse duode-

num. Jpn J Cancer Res.1989;80:503-5.

3.   Fujiki H, et al. New antitumor promoters: (-)-epigallocatechin gallate and sarcophytols A and B. Basic Life Sci.1990;52:205-12.

4.   Fujiki H. (-)-epigallocatechin gallate (EGCG), a cancer preventive agent. Fourth Chemical Congress of North America. New York: American Chemical Society, 1991.

5.   Yang C, et al. Protection against stomach, lung and esophageal carcinogenesis by green tea. Fourth Chemical Congress of North America. New York: American Chemical Society, 1991.

6.   Chung P, et al. Protection against tobacco-specific nitrosamine-induced lung tumorigenesis by green tea and its components. Fourth Chemical Congress of North America. New York: American Chemical Society, 1991.

7.   Mourelatos D, et al. Synergistic induction of sister-chromatid exchanges in lymphocytes from normal subjects and from patients under cytostatic therapy by inhibitors of poly(ADP-ribose)polymerase and antitumour agents. Mutat Res.1985;143:225-30.

8.   Gali HU, et al. Inhibition of tumor promoter-inducer ornithine decarboxylase activity by tannic acid and other polyphenols in mouse epidermis in vivo. Cancer Res. 1991;51:2820-5.

9.   Gali HU, et al. Antitumor-promoting activities of hydrolyzable tannins in mouse skin. Carcinogenesis. 1992;13:715-8.

❦ HOXSEY THERAPY

The Hoxsey treatment is a combination of herbs that has been in use as an unconventional cancer treatment for nearly 100 years.

Harry Hoxsey was a colorful character who looked the part of a "snake oil salesman." For decades, he was a thorn in the side of the American medical establishment. At one time he broadcast his anti-AMA message through his own Iowa radio station. *JAMA*'s celebrated editor, Morris Fishbein, MD called Hoxsey a ghoul who fed "on the bodies of the dead and the dying." After a series of legal battles, Hoxsey's chain of cancer clinics were shut down by the US medical authorities.

Decades after his death, Hoxsey's treatment still survives at the Tijuana, Mexico Bio-Medical Center, under the aegis of his nurse, Mildred Nelson, RN. Yet despite decades of controversy, no clinical trials have ever been performed by either supporters or detractors.

As with **Essiac,** which it resembles, the constituent parts of this therapy have shown anticancer activity. "More recent literature leaves no doubt that Hoxsey's formula...does indeed contain many plant substances of marked therapeutic activity," according to a paper on Hoxsey's method, prepared by historian Patricia Spain Ward, PhD for the Office of Technology Assessment (1).

Hoxsey claimed his formula was passed down to him by his dying father, who got it from his own father. He, in turn, had watched a horse cure itself of a life-threatening illness by eating certain rarely-consumed plants. The idea that an animal could point the way to a cancer treatment was long derided as arrant nonsense and the Hoxsey method is still dismissed as the height of quackery (2). But this tale, while it sounds apocryphal, is consonant with the field of "zoopharmacognosy" discussed in the introduction to this section.

In 1950, at the FDA's insistence, Hoxsey revealed what he said was his proprietary formula. To a basic solution of cascara (*Rhamnus purshiana*) and potassium iodide one or more of the following herbs was added:
• poke root (*Phytolacca americana*);
• burdock root (*Arctium lappa*);
• barberry or berberis root (*Berberis vulgaris*);
• buckthorn bark (*Rhamnus frangula*);
• stillingia root (*Stillingia sylvatica*), also known as queen's, yaw or silver root ; and
• prickly ash bark (*Zanthoxylum americanum*).

As Ward stated, individually most of these herbs do show biological activity at a level that could not have been suspected decades ago.

Poke root: This is used in conventional medicine as an antirheumatic, emetic and killer of external parasites (3). It has also become a standby tool in immunological research for its ability to stimulate a kind of mitogenic (immune) response (4-6). Poke root can also kill plant viruses (7), act as a spermicide (8), and stimulate inter-leukin production (9). Polysaccharides derived from a related substance (*Phytolacca acinosa*) have "significant enhancing activity" on the ability of macrophages (scavenger cells) to kill sarcomas and malignant fibroblasts.

When macrophages were incubated with pokeweed derivatives, they produced two powerful anticancer biological response modifiers, **tumor necrosis factor** (TNF) and interleukin-1 (IL-1). The optimal time for TNF production was found on the eighth day.

"Significant increases in TNF and IL-1 were observed," scientists from the Second Military Medical University of Shanghai, China wrote. A pokeweed-derived substance, called PEP-1, was as good as the known immune booster **BCG** (Bacillus Calmette-Guerin) in stimulating the production of TNF. And it was better than BCG in its effect on IL-1 production (10).

Burdock: This herb is used in conventional medicine as a skin treatment (3). The presence of burdock in the Hoxsey treatment is interesting, because it is also a constituent in that other famous North American herbal folk remedy, **Essiac.** In 1984, Japanese scientists found a substance in burdock that reduced the harmfulness of a wide range of mutation-causing substances. This "burdock factor," as it was called, proved resistant to heat and protein-digesting enzymes (11). In preliminary tests, burdock has also proven to have an "inhibitory activity against HIV" virus, according to the World Health Organization (12).

Barberry: Also known as berberis bark, jaundice berry,

woodsour, sowberry, pepperidge bush and sour spine, this plant yields several chemicals, including berberine, berbamine, oxyacanthine, tannin, wax, fat and resin. Berberine has been the subject of intense research as an antibacterial, antimalarial and fever-reducing drug. Derivatives have also been reported to have anticancer effects (18).

Buckthorn: Buckthorn bark yields frangulin, emodin, and chrysophanic acid (3). Frangulin was first prepared in 1933 from the bark of the alder buckthorn. It is used as a purgative agent, as is emodin. Emodin was also "found to show significant antileukemic activity against the P388 lymphocytic leukemia in mice," according to chemists at the University of Virginia in Charlottesville (13).

Stillingia: Not much research has been done on this herb, but it is known to be an emetic and carthartic (3).

Prickly ash bark: A member of this tree's family has yielded a chemical with anti-inflammatory action (14). Crystals isolated from another form have yielded a painkiller (15).

How safe are these herbs? "Phytolacca," the root of the pokeweed plant is said to be dangerous. At least two cases of poisoning have been reported, one in Denver and the other in Arizona, from the consumption of commercial burdock tea (16, 17).

Hoxsey also sold a salve for the treatment of external cancers. This is what was known as an "escharotic," a kind of burning paste made up of zinc chloride, antimony trisulfide and blood root. A related orthodox version of this treatment, Mohs's microsurgery, is now standard for certain forms of skin cancers. According to the OTA report, "Mohs reported high rates of success with this method— e.g., a 99 percent cure rate for all primary basal cell carcinomas he treated" (19).

Ambitious claims have been made for this type of external agent in the treatment of skin cancer. Since over half a million Americans alone undergo surgical or radiation treatment for skin cancer each year, a relatively inexpensive paste would be a breakthrough. However, although variations on this therapy are available, there are not many reports in the current peer-reviewed literature on the use of such alternative treatments.

⊕ References

1.   US Congress Office of Technology Assessment (OTA). Unconventional cancer treatments. Washington, DC: US Government Printing Office, 1990.

2.   ACS. Hoxsey method/Bio-medical center. Ca.1990;40:51-5.

3.   Budavari S, et al (Eds.). The Merck index: an encyclopedia of chemicals, drugs, and biologicals. Rahway, NJ: Merck & Co., Inc., 1989, p. 1606.

4.   Yokoyama K, et al. Purification and biological activities of pokeweed (Phytolacca americana) mitogens. Biochim Biophys Acta.1976;427:443-52.

5.   Bodger MP, et al. Mitogenic proteins of pokeweed. I. Purification, characterization and mitogenic activity of two proteins from pokeweed (Phytolacca octandra). Immunology.1979;37:785-92.

6.   Bodger MP, et al. Mitogenic proteins of pokeweed. II. The differentiation of human peripheral blood B lymphocytes stimulated with purified pokeweed mitogens (Po-2 and Po-6) from pokeweed, Phytolacca octandra. Immunology.1979;37:793-9.

7.   Owens RA, et al. A possible mechanism for the inhibition of plant viruses by a peptide from Phytolacca americana. Virology.1973;56:390-3.

8.   Stolzenberg SJ and Parkhurst RM. Spermicidal actions of extracts and compounds from Phytolacca dodecandra. Contraception.1974; 10:135-43.

9.   Basham TY, et al. A series of murine interleukin molecules which stimulate both murine and human lymphocytes. Production by Phytolacca americana (pokeweed) lectin 2 (Pa-2)-stimulated thymus and thymus-derived cells. Cell Immunol.1981;63:118-33.

10. Zhang JP, et al. [Effects of Phytolacca acinosa polysaccharides I on cytotoxicity of macrophages and its production of tumor necrosis factor and interleukin 1]. Chung Kuo Yao Li Hsueh Pao.1990;11:375-7.

11. Morita K, et al. A desmutagenic factor isolated from burdock (Arctium lappa Linne). Mutat Res.1984;129:25-31.

12. WHO. In vitro screening of traditional medicines for anti-HIV activ-

ity: Memorandum from a WHO meeting. Bul. WHO (Switzerland), 1989;67:613-618.

13. Kupchan SM and Karim A. Tumor inhibitors. 114. Aloe emodin: antileukemic principle isolated from Rhamnus frangula L. Lloydia.1976; 39:223-4.

14. Oriowo MA. Anti-inflammatory activity of piperonyl-4-acrylic isobutyl amide, an extractive from Zanthoxylum zanthoxyloides. Planta Med.1982; 44:54-6.

15. Hong GX and Zeng XY. [Studies on the mechanism of analgesic action of crystal-8 isolated from Zanthoxylum nitidum (Roxb.) DC]. Yao Hsueh Hsueh Pao.1983;18:227-30.

16. Bryson P, et al. Burdock root tea poisoning. Case report involving a commercial preparation. JAMA.1978;239:20.

17. Rhoads P, et al. Anticholinergic poisonings associated with commercial burdock root tea. J Toxicol.1984/85;22:581-584.

18. Hoshi A, et al. Antitumor activity of berberine derivatives. Japan J Cancer Res. (Gann).1976;67:321-25.

19. Mohs FE. Chemosurgical treatment of cancer of the skin. A microscopically controlled method of excision. JAMA.1948;138:564-9.

❦ KAMPO

••

Kampo (or kan po) refers to the Japanese version of traditional Chinese herbal medicine. Chinese herbal medicine has deep roots in ancient history. Asian scientists have now begun to purge non-scientific elements from this extremely valuable tradition.

Herbs in kampo medicine are never taken alone, but usually involve complicated prescriptions of ten plants, or more. Such herbs are said to work synergistically.

Many constituents of kampo prescriptions have been found to have significant biological effects. Scientific studies in this area are vigorous and promising. Most cancer research has focused on three kampo preparations: *juzen-taiho-to; shi-un-kou;* and *sho-saiko-to.* But there are over 140 kampo preparations, a goldmine for researchers.

Juzen-taiho-to: This kampo recipe is traditionally given to patients suffering from anemia or chronic exhaustion. Juzen-taiho-to is composed of **Astragalus,** Cinnamon, Foxglove, Nettle, Peony root, Angelica, **Ginseng,** Licorice, and other herbs.

Fractions of this mixture are known to be able to stimulate cells to divide (1). It was tried in 23 cancer patients who had previously had their stomachs or colons removed. Surgeons at the Kanagawa Cancer Center Hospital in Japan saw a "remarkable elevation" in Natural Killer cell activity three to six months after drug administration (2).

Scientists were able to significantly reduce the the toxicity of platinum-containing drugs by giving this herb mixture to mice with bladder cancer. Without it, the mice suffered "lethal toxicity," from kidney and liver damage and suppression of their bone marrow. With the prescription, the mice could take much more of the platinum drug without being killed by its toxicity. Together, there was "significantly greater inhibition of the tumor growth" and prolongation of survival. Japanese doctors concluded that Juzen-taiho-to lessens the toxic side effects of this form of chemotherapy and enhances its effects in animals. It could therefore be classified as a biological response modifier (3).

Juzen-taiho-to as well as several other kampo medicines (*Hochu-ekki-to* and *Sho-saiko-to*) were found to stimulate the production of **tumor necrosis factor** (TNF) in the body. Pretreatment with such drugs prevents the usual side effects of recombinant human TNF, without decreasing its antitumor activity. Kampo medicines can also decrease the harmfulness of free radicals and stabilize cell membranes. These kampo medicines were modified by scientists at the Department of Internal Medicine of the University of Tokyo (4).

Juzen-taiho-to may now present "new advantages with little toxicity in combination with chemotherapy or radiation therapy." Promising results have been obtained in preventing leukemia in cancer patients who have taken antitumor agents, according to scientists at the Kitasato Institute (Oriental Medicine Research Center). Combined with the conventional antibiotic drug, mitomycin C, this kampo medicine produced significantly longer survival in mice with cancer than did mitomycin C alone.

Juzen-taiho-to also decreased the side effects of this conventional drug, including destruction of white blood cells and weight loss. How this happens is still unclear, however. The kampo recipe fed to mice enhanced their antibody production and activated macrophages (5, 6).

Shi-un-kou: This is another Kampo prescription, made up of three main herbs: *Lithospermum erythrorhizon*, *Macrotomia euchroma* and *Angelica acutiloba*. This prescription was studied in the test tube for its ability to inhibit the Epstein-Barr virus which had been activated by a tumor promoting chemical, TPA. The crude drugs did inhibit the virus, especially when *Macrotomia* and *Angelica* were given together. In animals, "Shi-un-kou markedly inhibited TPA-induced skin tumor formation in mice," according to scientists at the Institute of Osaka Oriental Medicine Co., Ltd (7).

Keis-bukuryo-gan (as well as *Simotuto*) were found to be effective in treating various kinds of prostate problems. In prostatitis, the clinical effects of Kampo treatment was considered "excellent" in 21.3 percent of cases, and the overall efficacy rating was 67.2 percent. Kampo medicine proved much better than Western medicine, which has few effective therapies for nonbacterial prostate ailments. In "prostatitis-like syndrome," kampo alone worked as well as kampo plus Western antiinflammatory agents. In cases of chronic non-bacterial prostatitis, kampo plus Western

CANCER THERAPY

medicine worked better than either route alone. There were few side effects (8).

Sho-saiko-to: This prescription enhances immune responses through at least two different routes. It eliminates the inhibition of white blood cells by the hormone-like substance prostaglandin E_2 and it presents antigens (foreign proteins) to the white blood cells more efficiently (9). Sho-saiko-to also boosts the natural production of interferon, an internally-produced chemical called a cytokine that fights viruses and cancer. As an externally administered drug, toxicity limits interferon's use.

Xiao-chai-hu-tang also brings about interferon production in mice. White blood cells removed from the spleens of mice would produce interferon when they were put in the same test tube with this herbal extract. When spleen cells from these herb-treated mice were injected into mice that hadn't received this compound, the untreated mice's cells also produced more interferon. And even putting the herb in the animals' feed increased their production of interferon. While interferon production wore off when the drug was given by injection, there was no such decrease when it was given by mouth.

"These results showed that shosaiko-to is an [interferon] inducer," said scientists at the Traditional Chinese Medicine Research Laboratories of the Kanebo Co. in Osaka, and is "capable of repeated peroral administration" (i.e., by mouth) (3). Doctors at Kanazawa University also found that sho-saiko-to resulted in "effective inhibition of EBV [Epstein-Barr Virus]-antigen induction" (10).

Sho-saiko-to has also been used to treat chronic hepatitis. Studies at Nagoya City University suggest that it makes the liver more sensitive to a steroid-like glucocorticoid, by some unknown mechanism (11).

Sho-saiko-to enhanced the immune system's response to hepatitis B virus. Scientists studied its effect on antibody and on interferon-gamma production in the white blood cells of hepatitis patients. Both were "significantly increased." The activity was dependent on the dose given. These findings may account for the efficacy of sho-saiko-to in treating type B chronic hepatitis, scientists at Nagoya University School of Medicine said (12).

Side effects: With many herbs, especially such little-known ones, side effects are always possible. In general, the scientific studies remark on the harmlessness of these preparations. But large doses of the herb 'skullcap' (in sho-saiko-to) can cause dizziness, erratic pulse and mental confusion. A prudent person would proceed with caution, preferably under the supervision of a qualified health care professional.

⊕ References

1.   Kiyohara H, et al. Characterization of mitogenic pectic polysaccharides from Kampo (Japanese herbal) medicine "juzen-taiho-to." Planta Med.1991;57:254-9.

2.   Okamoto T, et al. [Clinical effects of Juzen-taiho-to on immunologic and fatty metabolic states in postoperative patients with gastrointestinal cancer]. Gan To Kagaku Ryoho.1989;16:1533-7.

3.   Ebisuno S, et al. [Basal studies on combination of Chinese medicine in cancer chemotherapy: protective effects on the toxic side effects of CDDP and antitumor effects with CDDP on murine bladder tumor (MBT-2)]. Nippon Gan Chiryo Gakkai Shi.1989;24:1305-12.

4.   Satomi N, et al. Japanese modified traditional Chinese medicines as preventive drugs of the side effects induced by tumor necrosis factor and lipopolysaccharide. Mol Biother.1989;1:155-62.

5.   Yamada H. [Chemical characterization and biological activity of the immunologically active substances in Juzen-taiho-to (Japanese kampo prescription)]. Gan To Kagaku Ryoho.1989;16:1500-5.

6.   Yamada H, et al. Fractionation and characterization of mitogenic and anticomplementary active fractions from Kampo (Japanese Herbal) medicine "juzen-taiho-to". Planta Med.1990;56:386-91.

7.   Konoshima T, et al. [Antitumor promoting activities and inhibitory effects on Epstein-Barr virus activation of Shi-un-kou and its constituents]. Yakugaku Zasshi.1989;109:843-6.

8. Ikeuchi T. [Clinical studies on chronic prostatitis and prostatitis-like syndrome (4). The Kampo treatment for intractable prostatitis]. Hinyokika Kiyo.1990;36:801-6.

9. Nagatsu Y, et al. Modification of macrophage functions by Shosaikoto (Kampo medicine) leads to enhancement of immune response. Chem Pharm Bull (Tokyo).1989;37:1540-2.

10. Furukawa M, et al. Inhibitory effects of Kampo medicine on Epstein-Barr virus antigen induction by tumor promoter. Auris Nasus Larynx.1990;17:49-54.

11. Inoue M, et al. Response of liver to glucocorticoid is altered by administration of Shosaikoto (Kampo medicine). Chem Pharm Bull (Tokyo). 1990;38:418-21.

12. Kakumu S, et al. Effects of TJ-9 Sho-saiko-to (kampo medicine) on interferon gamma and antibody production specific for hepatitis B virus antigen in patients with type B chronic hepatitis. Int J Immunopharmacol.1991;13:141-6.

℞ PAU D'ARCO

Pau d'arco is a tea made from the inner bark of a tree found in South American rain forests. The tree that yields pau d'arco is a member of the bignonia plant family, which includes Surinam greenheart, Taigu wood and Lapacho heartwood. Scientifically it is known as *Lapacho colorado* or *Lapacho morado* but is popularly called taheebo, ipes, lapacho and trumpet bush. In Brazil, where the bark is used as medicine, it is known as ipe roxo.

The active ingredient in pau d'arco appears to be lapachol, which was discovered in 1857 and synthesized in 1927. Although it resembles **vitamin K,** lapachol does not have any effect on coagulation. Another chemical in the bark, lapachic acid, was discussed in a book on Argentina at the 1876 Philadelphia World's Fair. According to another Brazilian report, one of the Russian tsars and Mohatma Gandhi both drank pau d'arco. In 1864, Bayer introduced a pau d'arco tincture to treat dizziness, indigestion, malaria, tuberculosis and ulcers. Indians in Argentina, Brazil, Bolivia, Paraguay and Peru have also reputedly used this bark tea to treat asthma, bronchitis, diabetes, infections and even some kinds of cancer, according to a story in a popular magazine (F. Murray, "Pau d'arco: the herbal healer," *Better Nutrition for Today's Living*, July, 1990).

There have also been stories in American and Brazilian newspapers about pau d'arco being used to successfully to treat leukemia and other cancers. A water extract of the bark of *L. colorado* inhibited the growth of animal tumors by 44 percent after doses of one-fifth of a gram per kilogram in rats, according to the *Lawrence Review of Natural Products* (May, 1986). Lapachol also inhibited two experimental tumors, Yoshida sarcoma and Walker 256 carcinoma (1, 2), by 82 percent and 50 percent, respectively.

The NCI's Natural Products Branch, which studies anticancer plants from around the world, has investigated extracts from *L. Colorado* and *L. morado*. They initially reported minor antitumor activity from the plants, but have not continued research.

On the basis of positive animal results with lapachol, it was examined in at least two clinical studies. NCI sponsored a phase I study of oral doses. In that study, 19 patients with advanced tumors and two with chronic myelocytic leukemia in relapse were given 250 to 2,750 mg per day by mouth. According to the OTA report, one patient with metastatic breast cancer had a regression in one of several bone lesions (3).

In addition to its widescale use in cancer, pau d'arco is also included in some holistic protocols for yeast infection, as used by John Parks Trowbridge, MD, of Texas and Robert Atkins, MD of New York City. It is also being used in the treatment of AIDS: four to six drops of pau d'arco tincture, three times a day as prescribed by Ian Brighthope, MD, an Australian physician who treats many

AIDS patients in Australia.

Pau d'arco is one of the most popular folk remedies for cancer. Many cancer patients take the tea, which appears to be without side effects, as an adjuvant (helper) treatment for cancer. In general, however, its use is not well supported by scientific data at the present time.

⊕ References

1. Rao KV. Quinone natural products: streptonigrin (NSC-45383) and lapachol (NSC-11905) structure-activity relationships. Cancer Chemother Rep [2].1974;4:11-7.

2. Budavari S, et al. (Eds.). The Merck index: an encyclopedia of chemicals, drugs, and biologicals. Rahway, NJ: Merck & Co., Inc., 1989, p. 1606.

3. Block JB, et al. Early clinical studies with lapachol (NSC-11905). Cancer Chemother Reports Part 2, 1974;4:27-28.

⚕ SPICES

Various spices used in cooking, especially in Indian cuisine, have been found to have surprising anticancer effects.

Most prominent of these is turmeric (*Curcuma longa*), a spice derived from the root of a perennial tropical plant, similar to ginger. Because of its brilliant orange-yellow color and low price, it is sometimes known as the poor man's saffron. Turmeric gives color to curries, mustards, mayonnaises, pickles and sauces. Although relatively new to the West, turmeric has been used in southeast Asia for thousands of years. It is now also cultivated in many tropical countries, including Indonesia, Haiti and Jamaica.

To produce the spice, the roots are dug in the fall, cleaned, boiled, then dried in the sun and powdered. It is considered the most important and sacred spice of Hindus, used in various religious and social rituals.

In ancient Indian medicine, turmeric was used as a cleansing herb for the whole body. It has also been used medically as a digestive aid, a treatment for infections, arthritis, jaundice and other liver problems (1). Turmeric is also widely employed in Chinese medicine, where it is known as "yellow ginger" (*huang jiang*). Traditional Chinese doctors use it to treat liver and gallbladder problems. It has many other medical uses: to promote bile secretions, increase appetite, lower blood pressure, alleviate pain and reduce inflammation. A Chinese scientific study even showed that it was "100 percent effective in preventing pregnancy in female rats," according to Dr. A. Leung, in *Chinese Herbal Remedies* (New York: Phaidon Universe, 1984). The traditional Chinese dose is three to six grams (0.1 to 0.3 oz.) taken in the form of a decoction, pill or powder.

Turmeric contains carbohydrates, protein, fats, minerals (especially potassium) and vitamins (especially **vitamin C**). But the greatest interest has been in its yellow pigment curcumin, first isolated in 1842. Routinely used in paper production, scientists have recently discovered that curcumin is an effective topical agent and anti-inflammatory drug (2). It is considered highly protective against stomach ulcers, including those caused by alcohol (3). And, more to the point, it inhibits the growth and promotion of tumors.

In 1985, Indian scientists found that curcumin reduced the development of animal tumors. It was toxic to cancer cells but also to lymphocytes in general. This effect was found within 30 minutes at room temperature (4).

It also has value in skin cancer. A poultice of turmeric is a standard traditional Chinese recipe for skin pain or itching from sores or ringworms.

An alcohol extract of turmeric as well as a curcumin ointment has now been shown to produce what scientists called "remarkable symptomatic relief" in patients with external cancerous lesions (5).

A reduction of offensive odors were noted in 90 percent of the cases and a reduction in itching in almost all the patients. Lesions dried up in 70 percent of the cases, and one-tenth of patients actually had a reduction in the size and pain of the skin growths. In many of the patients these effects lasted for several months. An adverse side effect was seen in only one of the 62 patients treated (5).

A study at the College of Pharmacy of Rutgers University, New Brunswick, NJ, showed that a topical application of curcumin, at the highest dose, inhibited the number of carcinogen-induced tumors in mice by up to 98 percent (6).

Curcumin is also a very effective antioxidant, protecting cells from damage to their genetic material. In a study of antioxidants, it was shown to be as effective as the highly-effective commercial antioxidant, BHA. The scientists also showed that there had to be at least one other antioxidant in turmeric besides curcumin. A water solution of turmeric extended 80 percent protection to DNA against oxidative injury (7). It also has been shown to provide 90 percent protection against harmful carcinogens such as those in fuel smoke (8) and to be a "potent inhibitor" of inflammation in mouse skin (9).

At the levels of use common in India, China and many other countries, turmeric appears to be a "natural, non-toxic food constituent" (10), which has been well-tolerated for thousands of years. It does not cause mutations in standard tests (11). At very high levels, however, it may pose problems. For example, pigs given large amounts of the spice suffered weight loss and other harmful changes after several months of constant feeding (12). At levels about one hundred times normal, the spice or its active constituent seemed capable of becoming toxic (13).

Other spices: That **garlic** given to mice with cancer extends their life spans is not surprising. But in one experiment, three other spices did even better (15).

Spice	Extension of life (% more than controls)
Black pepper	64.7
Asafoetida	52.9
Pippali	47.0
Garlic	41.1

This finding may strike some people as odd, because another study has suggested that black pepper is mutagenic, and therefore probably carcinogenic (14). Further research is clearly needed to clarify the impact of this common dietary item on health.

Giving spices in injectable form did not produce any significant reduction in tumor growth except for sesame, which caused nearly 40 percent decrease. Garlic and asafoetida extracts were also found to inhibit cancer on the skin of the mice, with significant reduction in papilloma (wart-like) growths.

"These results," said Dr. R. Kuttan, who led the Indian team, "indicate the potential use of spices as anticancer agents as well as antitumour promoters" (15).

Out of various Indian spices screened as protective agents against carcinogens, the following caused at least a 78 percent increase in anticancer enzyme systems: cumin seeds, poppy seeds, asafoetida, turmeric, kandathipili, neem flowers, manathakkali leaves, drumstick leaves, basil leaves and ponnakanni. Almost all of these also protected against chromosome damage caused by carcinogens.

"The results suggest that these nine plant products are likely to suppress carcinogenesis and can act as protective agents against cancer," according to a 1990 study at the Cancer Institute of Madras, India (16).

Cinnamon: This fragrant bark and its derivatives have long had many industrial and medical uses. In 1989, Japanese researchers found a new polysaccharide in dried cinnamon bark, which they called cinnamon AX. It showed what the scientists called "remarkable" immune system boosting activity (17).

⊕ References

1.   Srivastava KC. Extracts from two frequently consumed spices—cumin (Cuminum cyminum) and turmeric (Curcuma longa)—inhibit platelet aggregation and alter eicosanoid biosynthesis in human blood platelets. Prostaglandins Leukot Essent Fatty Acids.1989;37:57-64.

2.   Satoskar RR, et al. Evaluation of anti-inflammatory property of curcumin (diferuloyl methane) in patients with postoperative inflammation. Int J Clin Pharmacol Ther Toxicol.1986;24:651-4.

3.   Rafatullah S, et al. Evaluation of turmeric (Curcuma longa) for gastric and duodenal antiulcer activity in rats. J Ethnopharmacol.1990;29:25-34.

4.   Kuttan R, et al. Potential anticancer activity of turmeric (Curcuma longa). Cancer Lett.1985;29:197-202.

5.   Kuttan R, et al. Turmeric and curcumin as topical agents in cancer therapy. Tumori.1987;73:29-31.

6.   Huang MT, et al. Inhibitory effect of curcumin, chlorogenic acid, caffeic acid, and ferulic acid on tumor promotion in mouse skin by 12-O-tetradecanoylphorbol-13-acetate. Cancer Res.1988;48:5941-6.

7.   Shalini VK and Srinivas L. Lipid peroxide induced DNA damage: protection by turmeric (Curcuma longa). Mol Cell Biochem.1987;77:3-10.

8.   Shalini VK and Srinivas L. Fuel smoke condensate induced DNA damage in human lymphocytes and protection by turmeric (Curcuma longa). Mol Cell Biochem.1990;95:21-30.

9.   Conney AH, et al. Inhibitory effect of curcumin and some related dietary compounds on tumor promotion and arachidonic acid metabolism in mouse skin. Adv Enzyme Regul.1991;31:385-96.

10. Tonnesen HH, et al. Studies on curcumin and curcuminoids. IX:

Investigation of the photobiological activity of curcumin using bacterial indicator systems. J Pharm Sci.1987;76:371-3.

11.   Vijayalaxmi. Genetic effects of turmeric and curcumin in mice and rats. Mutat Res.1980;79:125-32.

12.   Bille N, et al. Subchronic oral toxicity of turmeric oleoresin in pigs. Food Chem Toxicol.1985;23:967-73.

13.   Donatus IA, et al. Cytotoxic and cytoprotective activities of curcumin. Effects on paracetamol-induced cytotoxicity, lipid peroxidation and glutathione depletion in rat hepatocytes. Biochem Pharmacol. 1990;39:1869-75.

14.   Ames BN. Dietary carcinogens and anticarcinogens. Oxygen radicals and degenerative diseases. Science.1983;221:1256-64.

15.   Kuttan R, et al. Tumour reducing and anticarcinogenic activity of selected spices. Cancer Lett.1990;51:85-9.

16.   Aruna K and Sivaramakrishnan VM. Plant products as protective agents against cancer. Indian J Exp Biol.1990;28:1008-11.

17.   Kanari M, et al. A reticuloendothelial system-activating arabinoxylan from the bark of Cinnamomum cassia. Chem Pharm Bull (Tokyo).1989; 37:3191-4.

Resources

Herbs and spices have been used medicinally for thousands of years. Many conventional medicines were originally derived from herbs, including aspirin (white willow bark), digitalis (foxglove) and vincristine (periwinkle). Today, every shopping mall has its health food store with racks of powdered herbs. But some doctors prefer either fresh herbs, when available; tinctures in alcohol or vinegar; or freeze-dried herbs.

The best source we have discovered of freeze-dried extracts is the Eclectic Institute, an affiliate of the National College of Naturopathic Medicine. It also makes herbal tinctures. Eclectic Institute's has a catalogue available. Their address is 11231 S.E. Market Street, Portland, OR 97216. Phone: 800-332-4372.

Aloe products are readily available in health food stores and through catalogues. Two well-known brands, recommended by the Balches, are Aerobic's and George's Aloe Vera Juice. The latter needs no refrigeration and tastes almost like plain water. "Aloe-Ace" a concentrated, organic whole leaf aloe vera juice is marketed by Klabin Marketing, 115 Central Park West, New York, NY 10023. Phone: 800-933-9440, in NY 212-877-3632.

Astragalus tablets are available in health food stores or from catalogues. Freeze-dried extracts are available from the Eclectic Institute (see above). Their alcohol-based liquid extract costs $4.50 per ounce, with bulk discounts up to 20 percent. Kyolic makes a Super Formula 103 capsule. It contains astragalus plus aged garlic extract powder (220 milligrams), vitamin C, and calcium. Kyolic is organically-grown in northern Japan and then aged for 20 months. Many people take two capsules, three times a day.

Available from:Wakunaga of America Ltd., 23501 Madero, Mission Viejo, CA 92691. Phone: 714-855-2776

Ayurvedic herbs: Ayurvedic herbs are available from the Ayur-Veda Herb Co., Nature's Herbs (a division of Twinlabs), Box 336, Orem, UT 84059. One may write for a free catalog. For further information on Ayur-Veda, one can contact the American Association of Ayurvedic Medicine, Box 282, Fairfield, IA 52556. Phone: 515-472-5866. For orders: 800 255-8332. A *Journal of the Central Council for Ayur-veda and Siddha Medicine* is published in New Delhi, India.

Ayurvedic practitioners in the United States include:
Scott Gerson, MD, Ayurvedic Medicine of New York, 13 West 9th St, New York, NY 10011. Phone: 212-505-8971.

Karta Purkh Khalsa, Khalsa Health Center, 1305 Northeast 45th St., Suite 205, Seattle, WA Phone: 206-547-2007, Fax: 206-547-4240. In-person consultation, $45; telephone consultation, $25.

Cannabis: Not only is this illegal for recreational use, but in recent years the Reagan and Bush administrations have made it virtually impossible to obtain, even by cancer patients undergoing chemotherapy. Check with NCI at 1-800-4-CANCER for latest rulings.

Chaparral: Many people complain that chaparral tastes and smells bad. They prefer a more palatable health food product called "Jason Winter's Tea," which contains red clover and Chinese herbs, in addition to chaparral. Jason Winters products are available from Tri-Sun North America, 109½ Broadway, Box 1606, Fargo, ND 58107 Phone: 800-447-0235 or 701-234-9654. Fax: 701-235-9762. A package of 16 tea bags sells for $5.95 retail. They offer Tribalene, a tablet containing chaparral, at $15.95 per 100. They also sell other products that may be of interest to readers of this book.

Dr. Andrew Weil recommends the use of chaparral tea as a douche (a teaspoon of tincture of chaparral to a quart of warm water) for the precancerous condition, cervical dysplasia. In addition one can take beta-carotene and folic acid supplements by mouth. He gives the following 'recipe' to prepare the douche: simmer a small handful of leaves or four capsules in a quart of water, covered, for fifteen minutes. Strain out the particles and allow it to cool. If the Pap test is normal after this, Weil suggests a 25,000 IU dose of beta-carotene and a 2 milligram dose of folic acid daily. He advises women who have had cervical dysplasia to stay on this maintenance dose indefinitely. If the Pap smear is still abnormal, he advises women to continue the regimen for one more month and then have another smear. If that is still abnormal, he suggests conventional treatment.

Chinese medicine: Many traditional medications are available in specialty herb shops in the Chinatowns of larger cities. One comprehensive mail order source is Nuherbs, but will they sell only to medical professionals

HERB RESOURCES

(including pharmacists). This should not present an insurmountable problem to determined patients, however. Nuherbs Co., 3820 Penniman Ave., Oakland, CA 94619. Phone: 800-233-4307. In California: 415-534-HERB. Fax: 415-534-4384. They sell Chinese medicines. For example, Liu Wei di Huang Wan (Six Flavor Tea) and Jin Kui Shen Qi Wan each cost $2.25 for 200 pills. Bu Zhong Yi Qi Wan (Central Qi Pill) costs $1.35 for a 100 pill bottle.

A source of Min Tong® Chinese herbal extract is Tashi Enterprises, 3252 Ramona St., Pinole, CA 94564. Phone: 800-888-9998 (24 hours). Fax: 510-758-0223.

Mrs. Tsong's Herbal Tonic Soups®, containing 19 different Chinese herbs in different combinations, is available from the Very Good Soup Company, 379A Clementina St., San Francisco, CA 94103. Phone: 415-441-5505. Fax: 415-243-0194.

Practitioners of Traditional Chinese Medicine:
Betances Health Unit, 281 East Broadway, New York, NY 10002. Phone: 212-227-8843. Holistically-oriented clinic in New York's Chinatown that uses acupuncture, herbs, etc. They accept Medicare and Medicaid.

Dr. Daniel Hsu, c/o Oriental Healing Arts Institute, 1945 Palo Verde Ave., Suite 208, Long Beach, CA 90815. Phone: 310-431-3544 Publishes the book by Dr. Hong-yen Hsu, *Treating Cancer with Chinese Herbs* ($12.95) and other materials. Ask for catalog.

Miki Shima, OMD, Lic. Ac.
(Doctor of Oriental Medicine, Licensed Acupuncturist)
21 Tamal Vista Boulevard, Suite 110, Corte Madera, CA 94925
Phone: 415-924-2910. Fax: 415-924-5072. Contact: Diana or Brenda.

Dr. Binyan Sun, 463 James Road, Palo Alto, CA 94306. Phone: 415-858-0320. Chinese speakers only: 415-858-2520.
Dr. Sun is author of *Cancer Treatment and Prevention with Traditional Chinese Medicine* (available from Offete Enterprises, 1306 South "B" Street, San Mateo, CA 94402., 164 pp. $20.00). At this writing, he is planning to leave for China. All patients will then be seen by Dr. Miriam Lee, OMD, and Esther Su, a California-licensed acupuncturist.

Dr. Qing Cai Zang, M.D (China) and Lic.Ac. 87-89 Fifth Avenue, #604, New York, NY 10003. Phone: 212-675-9343.

Essiac: Available from Claude Corson, c/o Totem Products, PO Box 638, White Pigeon, MI 49099. Phone: 616-483-7644. It costs $35 a pint for a 14-day supply. (Add $5 per order for shipping and handling.) Essiac is sold as a food supplement only. Some of the Essiac ingredients are available separately. Burdock root is available as a botanical liquid extract or fresh freeze-dried from Eclectic Institute (see above). According to standard herbals, "turkey rhubarb" is another name for the kind of rhubarb (*Rheum palmatum*) found in most food markets fresh in the spring and frozen the year round. The stalk is edible, but one must not eat the leaf blades, since they contain enough oxalic acid to cause poisoning.

Garlic is of course readily available. For those who find garlic's breath odor unpleasant, there are a number of odor-free or "sociable" garlics on the market. Since the chemicals DCPA, DDT, ethion, diazinon and malathion have been detected in regular commercial garlic, it is preferable to buy organic. See Astragalus (above) for Kyolic brand. Some other sources:

Arizona Natural Products, Michael Hanna, 8281 E. Evans Rd., #104, Scottsdale, AZ 85260. Phone: 602-991-4414. Claims not to use pesticides. Sells onions and garlic and ships within 48 hours. Has catalogue. Has the first US patent on odorless garlic. ANP offers a money-back guarantee and free literature with orders.

Pleasant Groves Farms. Ed or Wynette Sills. PO Box 636, Pleasant Grove, CA 95668. Phone: 916-655-3391. Sells huge "elephant garlic" by mail order to the public. Their produce is certified 70 percent organic by the California Certified Organic Farmers.

Walnut Acres. Onions and other root crops available by mail. Walnut Acres Road, Penns Creek, PA, 17862. Phone: 800-433-3998 or 717-837-0601. Produce is 100 percent organic, and orders shipped within three days. One of the oldest organic farms in the country (1946), Walnut Acres is one of the top rated sources of chemical-free food of all kind.

Ginseng: The selection and preparation of ginseng is an art. The easiest way to take ginseng is in the little foil-based packets of "instant Korean ginseng tea." These contain two grams of ginseng extract and glucose, and cost about $15 per hundred in Asian markets. There are many brands. "Gae Poong" is one of them, distributed by Jin Han International, Inc., Brooklyn, NY 11211 and Pacific Foods, Inc., Los Angeles, CA 90011.

In New York's Chinatown, four ounces of lower-grade Chinese ginseng cost $12.50. American ginseng is about double that. (Some Korean ginseng costs $30 per ounce and up.) One way to be assured of the quality of ginseng extract is to make it oneself. Three or four ounces of ginseng can be chopped up (e.g., in a food processor) and put in a bottle of high-quality, high-proof vodka. Honey can be added to taste. Set this bottle in a dark, cool cabinet for at least six weeks. The end product is potent indeed and is meant for sipping, not guzzling. Siberian ginseng (*Eleutherococcus sentiocosus* leaves) from Hokkaido Island, Japan, are made into a tasty tea by YSK International Corp., Kyoto, Japan, and marketed in the US by Sun Chlorella, Torrance CA.

Green tea is widely available in health food stores, since reports of its benefits appeared in newspapers in 1991. One excellent and inexpensive variety is the "Golden Sail Brand," from Guangdong, China, available from Wah Yin Hong Enterprises, 232 Canal Street, New York, NY 10013, Phone: 212-941-8954. The American Health Foundation, 1 Dana Road, Valhalla, NY 10595, Phone: 914-592-2600, Fax: 914-592-6317, will send out scientific information on the health benefis of tea. International symposia on this topic are planned for India in 1993 and New York in 1994.

Hoxsey: Bio-Medical Center clinic is in Tijuana, PO Box 727, General Ferreira #615, Col. Juarez, Tijuana, B.C., Mexico. Phone: 706-684-9011, -9081, -9082 or -9376. The treatment program costs $3,500. That includes a week at the clinic, return visits, and a lifetime supply of the tonic and the external "salve." Thirty percent of this amount must be paid on the first visit. This fee represents treatment for as long as necessary (life time).

A sympathetic film about Hoxsey, *When Healing Becomes a Crime*, had its premiere at the Margaret Mead Film Festival at New York's Museum of Natural History, aired on Home Box Office's Cinemax movie channel and was favorably reviewed in the *New York Times*. Available from Realidad Productions, PO Box 1644, Santa Fe, NM 87504 Phone: (505) 989-8575 Fax: (505) 983-8957. Film costs $39.95 plus $3.00 shipping and handling per tape.

A product similar to Hoxsey's external salve is currently marketed by Lenex Laboratory, PO Box 358, Watersmeet, MI 49969 Phone: 906-358-4802, Richard Ross, President. The product is called Herb Veil 8. It is a form of zinc chlorate. A quarter ounce bottle costs $49.95. Money back guarantee.

Kampo: Nuherbs (see Chinese Medicine resources, above) is one source of kampo herbs. Interested readers are advised to consult Akira Tsumura's book, *Kampo: How the Japanese Updated Traditional Herbal Medicine* (ISBN 0-87040-792-9), published by Japan Publications, Inc. and distributed in the US by Kodansha America, Inc., Phone: 212-727-6460. The book is also available through the Kinokuniya Bookstores in New York (212-765-1461), Los Angeles (213-687-4447) and San Francisco (415-567-7625). Mr. Tsumura's Japanese company, Tsumura, Inc. is described as a "leading supplier of herbal medicinals."

Pau d'Arco: Available in health food stores or through a catalogue from Lindberg Nutrition, Torrance, CA. Phone: 800-338-797. Fax: 310-371-8177. Pau d'Arco is also known as ipe roxo or taheebo. In health food stores, 24 tea bags generally sell for around $3.00.

Spices: Turmeric and other spices are available in most markets and certainly in Indian specialty shops. Turmeric costs about $1.00 per ounce.

$\mathcal{D}$IETS

What follows are several diets that should be of great interest to people with cancer. They differ from one another and sometimes contradict each other in particulars. But the underlying theme of all of them is that our modern way of eating has gone wrong and contributes to cancer. We generally eat too much, especially of the wrong things such as saturated fats, protein and calories. And, in general, the food supply is overprocessed and robbed of nutrients. Most dietary approaches to cancer recommend:

• eating fresh, whole, raw organically grown foods as much as possible;

• drinking and cooking with purified, not tap, water; and

• eliminating exposure to carcinogens and other toxic chemicals in the home, on the job, in the air, food and water.

$\mathcal{C}$ALORIE $\mathcal{B}$ALANCE

For many years, there has been a great debate over what is the best diet for people with cancer. One school of thought maintains that cancer patients are basically malnourished and that nothing should be done to diminish their nutritional intake. In fact, their diets should be supplemented in various ways. A minority view has held that such patients already get too much of some nutrients and should be put on diets restricted in these components.

At one time, a famous scientist called any linkage of diet

and cancer "the hallmark of quackery." Then came the 1978 McGovern Report on nutrition, which led to huge changes in the public's perception of the link between food and disease.

Many scientists lagged behind. In 1984, participants at an ACS conference were still "divided on what advice the public should be given regarding diet, nutrition, and cancer." Two-thirds said that "no advice was warranted or that general advice stressing the desirability of eating in moderation was adequate" (1). In 1992, the National Cancer Institute launched its "5 A Day Program." This is to encourage Americans to eat five servings or more of fruits and vegetables as part of a low-fat, high-fiber diet. According to an NCI press release (7/1/92), "an estimated thirty-five percent" of all cancer deaths "may be related to diet."

The 'cancer establishment' has made the leap to dietary prevention. The subject of treating cancer with diet remains taboo. Yet for many years, innovative scientists have been investigating the role of dietary intake, especially protein and calories, on the outcome of already-existing cancers.

"Calorie restriction is one of the oldest, best-documented, and most effective ways known to reduce cancer risk in rodents," Dr. Michael W. Pariza of the University of Wisconsin, Madison has said. But, he added, "it has had little impact on modern cancer research" because scientists believe that hefty lab rodents, who eat their fill of protein and calories, are "normal," whereas those put on a calorie restricted diet are abnormally slim.

In the late 1930s, scientists showed that fully-fed mice became obese, and 88 percent of the females developed breast cancer. But similar mice that were exercised, and whose weight was carefully maintained at their initial, young adult level, had only a 16 percent rate of cancer (2). Between 1940 and 1950, these findings were extended in a famous series of experiments by Dr. Albert Tannenbaum of the Michael Reese Hospital in Chicago.

Tannenbaum (3) showed that by underfeeding a stock diet to mice he could dramaticaly reduce cancer incidence. This finding is complicated by the fact that cancer itself may reduce the desire to eat and that standard treatments "contribute further to disturbances of nutrition" (4).

According to Pariza, restricting calories increases production of the hormone ACTH and decreases production of another class of hormones, the gonadotrophins. These changes may come about from restrictions of the time during which feeding is allowed, in addition to restrictions put on the intake of the food itself.

There are also differences in the way animals use various energy sources. In particular, fat calories are used more efficiently than those from carbohydrates. Some scientists regard saturated fat per se as harmful. But Pariza believes that fat is carcinogenic because mice get more calories from the fat. This effect can be abolished by a "moderate calorie restriction of only 15 to 20 percent" (5).

The application of this knowledge to human cancer treatment is still uncertain, however. Should cancer patients go on a calorie rectricted diet? It is known, for instance, that weight loss has an negative impact on cancer patient survival. This led in the 1970s to feeding patients through an intravenous drip. However, there is no proof that giving more calories intravenously (as part of total parenteral nutrition, or TPN) actually improves the outcome in chemotherapy patients.

In clinical tests, "no significant improvement in either response or survival" was seen with TPN for adult patients with lymphoma, sarcoma, colon cancer, adenocarcinoma and small cell carcinoma of the lung, or testicular carcinoma. In fact, in two instances, TPN was associated with decreased survival. This raised the spectre that increasing calories without concurrently providing an effective antitumor program "might stimulate cancer growth" (6).

According to Rowan Chlebowski, MD, PhD, studies demonstrate that leaner patients do better. The UCLA scientist suggests some new strategies for nutritional intervention. For example, low testosterone levels have been seen in men with advanced cancer. This in turn is connected to weight loss and poor outcome. This has led to trials of replacement therapy with a male hormone. Similarly, the abnormal glucose metabolism often seen in the patients with the 'wasting' syndrome (cachexia) has led to clinical tests with agents such as **hydrazine sulfate** and **Megace®** (6).

In 1991, the relationship between energy intake, selected nutrients and cancer of the colon and the rectum was reported from Majorca, a Spanish island in the Western Mediterranean. From 1984 to 1988, food frequency questionnaires had been given to 286 islanders with this type of cancer. Estimates were made of the intake of 29 nutrients as well as of total calories. Colorectal cancer was found associated with a higher dietary intake of total calories and cholesterol. Increased risk was also found with increased intake of protein, especially animal protein, and carbohydrates. A protective effect was associated with the intake of fiber from legumes such as peas, beans and lentils and of folic acid (a **B vitamin**) (7).

Can low protein intake be dangerous? Two groups of mice with breast cancer were fed normal or low protein diets. The conventional anticancer drug 5-FU was then given daily for three weeks. As expected, tumors shrank in both groups. However, the protein-deprived mice did not live as long. All protein-deprived mice were dead within two weeks. In another part of the study, two immune boosters (OK-432 and **Lentinan**) were given daily for three weeks. Tumor growth was inhibited on the fourteenth day in the mice receiving the normal amount of protein. However, tumor growth was "paradoxically" accelerated after giving these immune boosters to protein-deprived mice. Natural killer (NK) cell activity was increased in the normal group, but no such change was seen in the deprived group (8). Extrapolating to humans, these findings suggest that cutting back on protein while undergoing therapy is a questionable idea.

It is difficult to summarize such varied results. The most likely conclusion is that a low-calorie, low-protein diet is beneficial for the prevention of cancer. But once cancer is established, such deprivation might be harmful, especially if the patient is simultaneously receiving chemotherapy.

⊕ References

1.   Pariza MW. A perspective on diet, nutrition, and cancer. JAMA.1984;251:1455-8.

2.   Silvertsen I and Hastings W. A preliminary report on the influence of food and function on the incidence of mammary gland tumor in A stock albino mice. Minn Med.1938;21:873-875.

3.   Tannenbaum A. The initiation and growth of tumors. Am J Cancer.1940;38:335-350.

4.   Henriksson R, et al. [The effect of diet on the treatment of malignant diseases]. Nord Med.1990;105:289-91.

5.   Pariza M. Calorie restriction, ad libitum feeding, and cancer. Proc Soc Exp Biol Med.1986;183:293-8.

6.   Chlebowski RT. Critical evaluation of the role of nutritional support with chemotherapy. Cancer.1985;55:268-72.

7.   Benito E, et al. Nutritional factors in colorectal cancer risk: a case-control study in Majorca. Int J Cancer.1991;49:161-7.

8.   Akimoto M, et al. [Effects of protein calorie intake on immuno- and chemotherapy]. Gan To Kagaku Ryoho.1982;9:1387-93.

❧ GERSON DIET

The Gerson diet is one of the best-known and and best doc-umented alternative treatment programs. It is a nutrition-based "salt and water management" program devised by the German-born physician, Dr. Max Gerson (1881-1959). Gerson was a 1907 graduate of the University of Freiburg Medical School, who practiced medicine in Germany, Aus-tria and France before coming to the United States as a refugee from fascism in 1936. He remained a licensed med-ical doctor in New York until his death (1).

As a young man Gerson himself suffered from debilitat-ing migraine headaches. While still in medical school, he cured these headaches through the use of an experimental low-salt diet that was rich in fresh fruits and vegetables. As a physician, he then tried this diet on tuberculosis and then on cancer. There appeared to be improvement in some cases (2, 3). Gerson later refined his approach with a num-ber of other therapeutic principles.

Some of these were fairly conventional at the time, but appear strange today because of the rapid changes in medicine. For example, it was Gerson who introduced the coffee enema, which is now considered emblematic of far-out quackery, into cancer therapy. But this procedure was based on proper German research of the 1920s and 1930s, had a plausible scientific rationale and in fact remained in the *Merck Manual* until 1972 (albeit not as a treatment for cancer) (4).

As time progressed, Gerson and his work were attacked and maligned. In 1949, the AMA took a swipe not just at Gerson but at the entire notion of dietary control of cancer which he represented: "There is no scientific evidence whatsoever to indicate that modification in the dietary intake of food or other nutritional essentials are of any specific value in the control of cancer," they said. Such words are richly ironic in this age of the officially-sanctioned "chemoprevention" of cancer by nutritional factors.

Yet, if the link between diet and cancer has been rehabilitated, its greatest pioneer has not been. That is partly because of the all-to-human tendency to appropriate the ideas of rivals without credit or attribution. That process was already underway at the time of Max Gerson's death in 1959.

One of his celebrated patients, Nobel laureate Albert Schweitzer, MD, wrote: "I see in him one of the most eminent medical geniuses in the history of medicine."

"Many of his basic ideas have been adopted without having his name connected with them," Schweitzer continued. "He leaves a legacy which commands attention and which will assure him his due place."

Although there has been unprecedented enthusiasm in recent years for dietary prevention, conventional science still balks at the notion of treating cancer through diet (4). The Gerson method, supervised by his daughter Charlotte Gerson in Tijuana, "is considered unacceptable by the medical establishment" and is scorned by authorities (3,5).

Gerson himself did publish in the scientific literature when he could (6-10). In fact, Gar Hildenbrand of the Gerson Institute and Michael Blake of the Harvard University Library of Medicine have assembled a bibliography of over 300 peer-reviewed articles on Gerson's treatment. Towards the latter part of his career, when most journals were closed to him, Gerson also wrote a popular book, *A Cancer Therapy: Fifty Cases*, in which he detailed his successes. Many of these cases were presented in celebrated testimony to a committee of the US Congress in 1946.

Gerson's philosophy was that our basic nutritional biology is derived from our past as wild animals, when we ate not only other wild animals but especially foraged for plants. With the development of civilization, our food supply became denatured and devitalized, lacking in essential nutritional value. Gerson was also among the first doctors to warn of the dangers of man-made pesticides and fertilizer residues in food. It is only by getting back to an elemental kind of diet, featuring fresh organic vegetables and fruits, he taught, that we will be able to overcome the chronic diseases that are the inevitable result of our over-refined way of life.

The Gerson regimen is divided into two components:
• the detoxification of wastes and toxins that interfere with healing and normal metabolism; and
• an intensive nutritional program to flood the body with healing nutrients.

This program is a low-fat, low-animal protein and high-carbohydrate diet obtained through organic fruits, vegetables and grain.

Some of the specific elements of the Gerson diet include:
• over a dozen glasses a day of freshly pressed vegetable and fruit juices (primarily carrot juice);
• a daily vegetable soup;
• a low-sodium, high-potassium diet, with potassium supplements;
• iodine supplements (Lugol's solution) for some patients;
• patient education and mutual support; and
• coffee enemas every three to four hours; and
• raw liver juice (discontinued at the Gerson hospital since 1989, because of bacterial and parasitic contamination of most commercially-available liver).

The coffee enema is the hallmark of the Gerson program. It bears some explanation. An enema is a fluid injected into the rectum for the purpose of clearing out the bowel, or administering drugs or food. It is one of the most ancient medical procecures still in current use. This procedure was known to all the major ancient civilization. One of the first uses of rubber in the world was for enema bags among pre-Columbian South American Indians. On the other side of the world, the Egyptian Pharaoh had a special "shepherd of the anus" to administer the royal flush.

Enemas were once a routine home remedy. Doctors still employ them before surgery and childbirth and barium enemas are given before colonic X rays. But within our lifetime, self-administered enemas have largely died out.

And why coffee? Coffee enemas appeared in the medical literature as early as 1917. In the 1920s German scientists found that a caffeine solution administered rectally would stimulate the production of bile in experimental animals. Gerson then used coffee enemas as part of his general detoxification regimen, first for tuberculosis, then for cancer. The caffeine, he said, travels up the veins of the rectum to the liver, where it stimulates that vital organ.

Gerson noted some remarkable effects through the use of this procedure. For instance, some patients could dispense with pain-killers or remarked on the paradoxical calming effect of this caffeinated treatment. Gerson advised: "Patients have to know that the coffee enemas are not given for the function of the intestines but for the stimulation of the liver."

Gerson's theories about coffee anticipated the work of Wattenberg and others on the anticancer agents present in coffee (17).

The work of Dr. Denis Burkitt and others on the protective effect on colon cancer of a high **fiber,** low fat diet can be seen as a confirmation of Gerson's concepts (11). As we have shown, protein and **calorie restriction** has been shown in many animal experiments to prevent the development of cancer and to dramatically extend life time (12-13). All of this was elaborated by Gerson fifty or more years ago.

So too, the intense interest in the carotenes, such as **beta-carotene** (14-16), which are abundant in carrot juice and green leafy vegetables in the standard Gerson broth.

In general, the Gerson thesis seems to be borne out by a growing body of evidence that links the typical Western diet with the increase in chronic illnesses such as cancer. A scientist in Uganda has written that "dramatic differences occur in the diets in the North and South of the country." The industrial regions have generated cancer, cardiovascular and other degenerative diseases. The author concludes that "in the course of agriculture we have changed the balance of nutrients offered by wild plants and animals." We have particularly changed our "diet in the direction of a high refined carbohydrate food structure" (18).

Gerson's emphasis on the beneficial effects of potassium in the diet, and the harmfulness of sodium, were far-sighted. This theory has been confirmed by the work of a number of independent researchers (19-22). Dr. Birger Jansson of the M.D. Anderson Cancer Center, Houston, TX noted that people in Seneca County, NY have less cancer than those in surrounding counties. He tied this, among other things, to the high concentration of potassium in the soil of that particular county (23).

This tipping of the balance towards sodium and away from potassium is a relatively modern phenomenon.

It is Jansson's contention that the ratio between sodium and potassium is a crucial element in the formation of cancer (24). He wrote:

"One of the greatest changes in the human diet, a change that has occurred only within the past few thousand years, is the immense increase in the intake of sodium caused by use of table salt."

"At the same time," he continued, "man's intake of potassium has decreased" (24).

The primitive Yanomamo Indians in South America (who live mainly on unsalted cooking bananas) have a potassium to sodium ratio about 100 to 200 times greater than so-called civilized people. But since physical evolution takes much more time than cultural evolution, our sophisticated minds inhabit rather primitive bodies. This imbalance "has caused increased rates of a number of diseases in civilized man, among them cancer."

The dietary ratio of potassium to sodium should be more than one-to-one, Jannson says, and preferably should be five or higher. Jansson notes that only five percent of our sodium comes naturally in our food. The rest comes from industrial processing (e.g. freezing and canning) and food preparation. Only five percent is added as a condiment at the table. The Houston scientist says that eating more fruit and steamed vegetables would significantly increase this critical ratio (25).

Only a few clinical studies have been done on the Gerson diet. Peter Lechner, MD, of the Second Department of Surgery of the Landeskrankenhaus in Graz, Austria has carried out a long-term study of Gerson's methods, including "the strict reduction of salt" and an "adequate supply of fluids, vitamins and trace elements through fruit juices."

His general summary is that "the patients treated with the adjuvant nutritional therapy are in a better general condition, with less risk of complications, and they also tolerate radiation and chemotherapy better than patients who do not follow the diet" (26). He concluded that cachexia (wasting) "can, in most cases, be prevented or at least significantly delayed" on this diet. Patients have less need for analgesics (pain killers) and psychotropic drugs (used in the treatment of mental illness). There was a slower progression of existing liver metastases and less marked occurrence of effusions from the tumor, all important parameters in the clinical control of cancer.

In 1990, the *Lancet* carried a short evaluation of the Gerson program by physicians at Maudsley and Hammersmith Hospitals. They examined the case histories of 149 patients of the Gerson clinic. Of these, 27 had independent documentation, and they disregarded 20 of these as "nonassessable." Of the 7 cases that were actually evaluated, 3 (43 percent) were found to be in complete remission. One striking feature of the Gerson program, they wrote, was:

"The high degree of control the patients felt they had over their health, and, perhaps as a consequence, their high ratings for mood and confidence."

They found "particularly intriguing" the "low pain scores and analgesic requirements for all the patients," despite the fact that most had extensive metastatic disease.

"We could find little objective evidence of an antitumor effect from the Gerson therapy," they wrote, but they added that "most patients were not assessable because of concomitant conventional therapy." However, they said "in a few patients definite tumor regression was documented." Noting that a "fighting spirit" is associated with a better outcome for some cancers, they suggested that "the improvement in the Gerson patients' sense of well-being may take on a greater importance....These approaches may suggest ways forward for oncologists in the management of desperate cancer patients and their families" (3).

⊕ References

1. Seifter E and Winzweig J. Contribution of Dr. Max Gerson to nutritional chemistry. American Chemical Society abstract, 1985.

2. Bishop B. Organic food in cancer therapy. Nutr Health.1988;6:105-9.

3. Reed A, et al. Juices, coffee enemas, and cancer. The Lancet.1990; 336:667-668.

4. US Congress. OTA. Unconventional cancer treatments. Washington, DC: US Government Printing Office, 1990.

5. ACS. Gerson Method. Ca.1990;40:252-6.

6. Gerson M. Dietary considerations in malignant neoplastic disease. Rev Gastroent.1945;12:419-425.

7. Gerson M. Effects of a combined dietary regimen on patients with malignant tumors. Exp Med Surg.1949;7:299-317.

8. Gerson M. No cancer in normal metabolism. Medizinische Klinik. 1954;5:175-179.

9. Gerson M. Cancer, a problem of metabolism. Medizinische Klinik. 1954;5:1028-1032.

10. Gerson M. The cure of advanced cancer by diet therapy: a summary of 30 years of clinical experimentation. Physiol Chem Phys.1978;10: 449-464.

11. Burkitt DP. Colonic-rectal cancer: fiber and other dietary factors. Am J Clin Nutr.1978;31:S58-S64.

12. Chlebowski RT. Critical evaluation of the role of nutritional support with chemotherapy. Cancer.1985;55:268-72.

13. Pariza M. Calorie restriction, ad libitum feeding, and cancer. Proc Soc Exp Biol Med.1986;183:293-8.

14. Peto R, et al. Can dietary beta-carotene materially reduce human cancer rates? Nature.1981;290:201-8.

15. Bendich A and Shapiro SS. Effect of beta-carotene and canthaxanthin on the immune responses of the rat. J Nutr.1986;116:2254-62.

16. Bendich A and Olson JA. Biological actions of carotenoids. FASEB J.1989;3:1927-32.

17. Lam LK, et al. Effects of derivatives of kahweol and cafestol on the activity of glutathione S-transferase in mice. J Med Chem.1987;30: 1399-403.

18. Crawford MA. Nutritional control of heart disease and cancer: are different diets necessary. Nutr Health.1985;4:7-15.

19. Cope F. A medical application of the Ling association-induction hypothesis: the high potassium, low sodium diet of the Gerson cancer therapy. Physiol Chem Phys.1978;10:465-468.

20. McCarty MF. Cytostatic and reverse-transforming therapies of cancer – a brief review and future prospects. Med Hypotheses.1982;8:589-612.

21. Ling G. The association-induction hypothesis. Agressologie.1983; 24: 293-302.

22. Zs.-Nagy I, et al. Correlations of malignancy with the intracellular Na+:K+ ratio in human thyroid tumors. Cancer Res.1983;43:5395-5402.

23. Jansson B. Seneca County, New York: an area with low cancer mortality rates. Cancer.1981;48:2542-6.

24. Jansson B. Geographic cancer risk and intracellular potassium/sodium ratios. Cancer Detect Prev.1986;9:171-94.

25. Jansson B. Dietary, total body and intracellular postassium-to-sodium rations and their influence on cancer. Cancer Detection and Prevention.1990;14:563-565.

26. Lechner P and Kronberger I. Experiences with the use of dietary therapy in surgical oncology. Aktuelle Ernaehrungsmedizin. 1990;2:15.

℣ℳACROBIOTICS

Macrobiotics literally means "long life." The macrobiotic diet is basically an adaptation of the traditional Japanese diet, brought to America and Europe by a man named George Ohsawa in the 1950s. Its best known proponent, however, has been Michio Kushi.

Kushi was born in Japan and studied law and political science at Tokyo University. He came to the United States in 1949 and founded the Kushi Institute, the Kushi Foundation and One Peaceful World. From a base in Massachusetts, Kushi has travelled all over the world spreading the gospel of macrobiotics. He has published little in the scientific literature (1) but has written a number of popular health books.

Macrobiotics is a controversial philosophy, with social, political and spiritual aspects, as well as medical ones. Decades before Western research discovered 'chemoprevention,' macrobiotics was preaching an Eastern version. It claimed that the increase in cancer and other chronic diseases could be linked to the typical Western diet. Moreover, Kushi suggested that "a macrobiotically balanced diet may positively influence the outcome of existing cancers." Cancer does not strike at random, he said, but is the direct result of the choices people make, especially in food. Cancer is preventable and caused by faulty life-style.

"Cancer is a symptom of modern society," especially unhealthy diet, artificial farming practices and a "preoccupation with short-term gain at the expense of long-term health and well-being" (1).

Macrobiotics also believes that "sickness is actually a sign that some aspect of our daily lives is causing us to become out of alignment with nature." Followers tend to believe, therefore, that in some sense cancer, when it strikes, is a kind of retribution for life style errors.

The standard macrobiotic diet consists by volume of 50 to 60 percent whole grains; 25 to 30 percent vegetables; 5 to 10 percent beans and **seaweed**; and five percent soups. In addition, they supplement their diet with fish and other seafood; seasonal fruit; condiments and seasonings; beverages; and occasional healthy snacks.

The whole grains include brown rice, barley, millet, oats, corn, rye, wheat and buckwheat. Soups are made from vegetables, seaweed, grains and beans. Seasonings can include miso and tamari soy sauce. Vegetables include various local and organically grown cabbages (see **indoles**), kale, broccoli, cauliflower, collards, pumpkin, watercress, bok choy, dandelion, mustard greens, daikon, scallion, onions, turnips, acorn squash, butternut squash, burdock and carrots.

Some vegetables are avoided, such as potatoes, sweet

potatoes, tomatoes, eggplant, peppers, asparagus, spinach, beets, zucchini and avocado. Mayonnaise is also forbidden.

Tiny azuki beans, chickpeas and lentils are also eaten, but other kinds of beans are only used occasionally. Such soy bean products as tofu, tempeh and natto are included. Fish is allowed in small amounts one to three times a week.

Drinks include roasted bancha twig tea, and various other roasted teas, but not black tea or coffee. Well water is allowed, but not iced. While preparing all this food can be a daunting task, Kushi cautions his followers to "live each day happily without being preoccupied with your health."

Few scientific studies have been done on the benefits of macrobiotics for cancer patients. There are so many elements to this program that designing a well-controlled study is difficult. Nonetheless, one can see at a glance that there are areas of profound agreement between recent scientific findings and macrobiotics. Just a few examples:

• Macrobiotics discourages consumption of red meat. Fatty red meat is now widely believed to promote various common forms of cancer, such as that of the bowel (2).

• A whole grain–vegetable diet promotes colon movement and regularity. This is consistent with increasing stool bulk to prevent colon and other cancers (3).

Regular intake of yellow and green vegetables, as well as foods containing **calcium, selenium** and other micronutrients, lowers the risk of colon cancer. Macrobiotics features precisely such vegetables.

On the other hand, the greatest source of calcium, a most necessary nutrient, is dairy foods, which are usually eliminated on the macrobiotic diet. Other sources, such as seafood, green leafy vegetables, broccoli, cabbage, turnip greens, are generally allowed in the diet, however.

• Macrobiotics popularized the use of **seaweed** in the West. Many such sea products have been shown to contain polysaccharides and other anticancer substances (4).

• Macrobiotics uses soy products, such as tofu, and tamari (soy sauce) as seasoning. Studies have shown that soy sauce helps prevent cancer promotion in mice (5, 6). Soybeans are being investigated as anticarcinogens by Mark Messina and colleagues at the National Cancer Institute. Soy contains phytate and protease inhibitors and are a unique source of isoflavones, antihormones that inhibit the production of cancer genes (7, 8).

• Macrobiotics has championed burdock root as a vegetable. In Japan, burdock (gobo) is believed to act as a tonic. It protects against cancer-causing mutations (9). Burdock was once the 'root' in root beer, but its use has largely died out. (It is found in herbal-based treatments **Essiac** and **Hoxsey**.)

• Macrobiotics encourages the consumption of Bancha instead of black or oolong tea, or coffee. Bancha, a variety of **green tea**, contains EGCG, which protects against various kinds of cancer (10, 11).

One reason that macrobiotics has been controversial is its rigorous exclusion of certain foods (dairy, red meats, etc.). It is feared that such exclusion could lead to serious nutritional deficiencies in adults and, especially, children. Except for vitamin B_{12} deficiencies, vegetarian diets in general do not produce other deficiencies, if they are correctly followed and if adherents get at least the recommended daily allowances (RDAs) of basic nutrients. Nevertheless, when macrobiotics is followed in a rigid way, it can be the cause of dietary deficiencies, especially in children and pregnant women (12).

Scientists in the Netherlands were concerned about the lack of fat, protein and some vitamins in the strict macrobiotic diet. They attempted to get macrobiotic followers to add certain substances to their diet. In an "intervention study" in 27 cases of infants with "clear nutritional deficiencies" the health workers distributed information on the nutritional content of foods, gave personal advice when it was requested and provided referrals to teachers in macrobiotics for further advice. They even published a newsletter.

The nutritionists recommended that macrobiotics followers include sources of fat, fatty fish and dairy in the diet (13). Unfortunately, none of this led to an improvement in nutritional intake, growth or blood values in the children. But the macrobiotic community worldwide became more aware of the need for some changes in the basic diet.

In addition, the Vitamin D status of 53 macrobiotic infants was studied. By late summer, the Dutch scientists said, the physical symptoms of rickets were present in 28 percent of macrobiotic children. By spring, 55 percent had such symptoms. The lack of calcium in the macrobiotic diet was said to be the cause of this now-rare disease. "Avoidance of milk products in combination with a high fiber intake may damage bone development in young children," said scientists at Wageningen Agricultural University (14).

One danger of macrobiotics, and indeed of all unsupplemented vegetarian diets, is a lack of vitamin B_{12}. This essential nutrient is found mainly in meat. The vitamin B_{12} status was studied in a macrobiotic community in New England. Half the adults were found to have low concentrations of vitamin B_{12} in their blood. The longer they had been macrobiotic, the lower the levels. Fifty-five percent of children also showed signs of low B_{12}. Their children were also relatively low in weight and height (15).

In general, however, many scientists would agree that a moderate macrobiotic diet is a safe and beneficial approach to the dietary prevention of cancer and other chronic diseases.

⊕ References

1. Kushi M. A cancer approach from dietetics according to the principles of macrobiotics. Farm Tijdschr Belg (Belgium). 1979;56:353-358.

2. Weisburger JH and Horn CL. Human and laboratory studies on the causes and prevention of gastrointestinal cancer. Scand J Gastroenterol Suppl.1984;104:15-26.

3. Burkitt DP. Colonic-rectal cancer: fiber and other dietary factors. Am J Clin Nutr.1978;31:S58-S64.

4. Teas J. The consumption of seaweed as a protective factor in the etiology of breast cancer. Med Hypotheses.1981;7:601-13.

5. Benjamin H, et al. Reduction of benzo[a]pyrene-induced forestomach neoplasms in mice given nitrite and dietary soy sauce. Food Chem Toxicol.1988;26:671-8.

6. Benjamin H, et al. Inhibition of benzo[a]pyrene-induced mouse forestomach neoplasia by dietary soy sauce. Cancer Res.1991;51:2940-2.

7. Messina M and Messian V. Increased use of soyfoods and their potential role in cancer prevention. J Am Diet Assoc. 1991;91:836-40.

8. Messina M and Barnes S. The role of soy products in reducing risk of cancer. J Natl Cancer Inst.1991;83:541-6.

9. Morita H, et al. Cytotoxic and mutagenic effects of emodin on cultured mouse carcinoma FM3A cells. Mutat Res.1988;204:329-32.

10. Fujiki H, et al. New antitumor promoters: (-)-epigallocatechin gallate and sarcophytols A and B. Basic Life Sci.1990;52:205-12.

11. Fujiki H (-)-epigallocatechin gallate (EGCG), a cancer preventive agent. Fourth Chemical Congress of North America. New York: American Chemical Society, 1991.

12. Debry G. [Diet peculiarities. Vegetarianism, veganism, crudivorism, macrobiotism]. Rev Prat.1991;41:967-72.

13. Dagnelie PC, et al. [Dietary intervention and follow-up study in 1-to-2-year-old children on macrobiotic diets]. Ned Tijdschr Geneeskd. 1990;134:341-5.

14. Dagnelie PC, et al. High prevalence of rickets in infants on macrobiotic diets. Am J Clin Nutr.1990;51:202-8.

15. Miller DR, et al. Vitamin B12 status in a macrobiotic community. Am J Clin Nutr.1991;53:524-9.

☀ Resources

An excellent guide to a healthier food supply is John T. Marlin, PhD and Domenick Bartelli, *The Catalogue of Healthy Food* (New York: Bantam Books, 1990, $14.95. This is an indispensable guidebook.

Gerson: For further information on the program and clinic contact The Gerson Institute, PO Box 430, Bonita, CA 92002. Phone: 619-267-1150.

Macrobiotics: Kushi Institute of the Berkshires, Box 7, Becket, MA 01233, Phone: 413-623-5742. See Michio Kushi's, *The Macrobiotic Approach to Cancer* (Garden City Park: Avery, 1991).

Livingston: Another largely-dietary treatment program is that of the late Virginia Livingston, MD. See the "Less Documented" section as well as the author's *The Cancer Industry*, chapter 13.

Metabolic Typing is another largely-dietary approach. See "Less Documented" section .

$\mathcal{F}$ROM $\mathcal{E}$ARTH & $\mathcal{S}$EA

Natural anticancer substances are being discovered not just among the traditional herbs, but among many land and sea species that are not generally thought of as edible. In this category are included a variety of substances from the earth and the sea that are yielding important new ways of influencing the immune system. They include exotic oils, unusual fish products (such as shark cartilage), algae and seaweeds. The medical use of mushrooms alone is a major development in cancer treatment. One unusual aspect of these new natural treatments is that most of them come from a single country, Japan. Many of them are also derivatives of delicacies that are well-known in the Orient and are bound to become more familiar in the West as well.

$\mathcal{A}$LGAE

There are over half a million species of marine life. Due to their unusual environment, these plants and animals produce a wide variety of substances with "unprecedented chemical structures" (1).

A wealth of natural compounds remain to be discovered beneath the sea. In recent years, natural marine substances have yielded remarkable drugs, including new antibiotics. Some of these substances are cell-killing poisons that interfere with the normal metabolism of cells. But others are non-toxic and work by stimulating the immune system. In fact, marine plants and animals harbor powerful health-promoting chemicals. These include peptides and alkaloids that have been isolated from organisms as diverse as sponges, corals, marine algae, tunicates, nudibranches and bryozoans.

Medical research has been conducted on a wide variety of exotic substances, such as a seaweed from the Enewetak Atoll in the Marshall Islands (2); a blue algae from the Caribbean (3); and a brown algae that has yielded a new anticancer agent called turbinaric acid (4). When scientists searched the Adriatic, off Trieste, they found over a dozen previously unknown algae, at least one of which "significantly inhibits the growth of cell cultures" (5).

Algae have proved to be among the richest sources of carotenes. Japanese scientists studying a beta-carotene-rich algae named Dunaliella bardawil found that it "markedly inhibited" spontaneous breast cancers in mice. In a 1991 paper, they reported that it not only stopped breast cancer, but normalized the mice's glucose tolerance and lactic acid levels. Japanese scientists concluded that the results strongly suggest that D. bardawil inhibited breast cancer by this stabilization of body chemistry as well as the antioxidant activity of **beta-carotene** (6).

Most research has been done on a one-celled alga known as Chlorella. This has been shown to have powerful antitumor effects (7-10). An oral administration of Chlorella protected between 73 and 80 percent of mice against several kinds of cancer. However, all the mice that received Chlorella that had been deprived of its protein, died.

Japanese scientists studied Chlorella (*pyrenoidosa*) as a biological response modifier. First, experimental mice were given Chlorella every other day for ten days. Then one of three kinds of cancer—breast, leukemia or Ehrlich ascites—were injected into them. All of the untreated mice died within 20 days. But over 70 percent of the treated animals survived over 60 days. Since Chlorella does not directly kill cancer cells, the scientists concluded that its effects were caused by boosting the immune response (11).

In another experiment, a group of scientists took a hot water extract of Chlorella and injected it into the body cavities of mice that had first been inoculated with tumor cells. They found that "survival times were strikingly prolonged" (7). Furthermore, when they gave mice injections of Chlorella, their cells still exhibited "an anti-tumor effect" 24 hours later. This effect remained intact even after 'T' type white blood cells and macrophage (scavenger) cells were destroyed, but it was effectively wiped out by irradiation. Chlorella's anticancer effect was thus dependent on the portion of the immune system most sensitive to x-rays.

There has also been work on the benefits of Spirulina, a blue-green algae, and Chlorella's commercial archrival. One group has studied the effect of a Spirulina extract on tumor regression. An extract of Spirulina and Dunaliella algae called phycotene was injected into tumors of hamsters induced by a potent carcinogen. Other tumors were injected with beta-carotene; another natural food pigment called **canthaxanthin**; and a vitamin A-like drug, Accutane.

Treatment	Complete Regressions (%)	Partial Regressions (%)
Algae	30	70
Beta-carotene	20	80
Canthaxanthin	15	85
Accutane	0	70
Controls	0	0

Thus, the best results were seen in the algae-treated group, with astonishing 100 percent regressions, of which 30 percent were total (12).

ALGAE

⊕ References

1. Kitagawa I and Kobayashi M. [Antitumor natural products isolated from marine organisms]. Gan To Kagaku Ryoho.1989;16:1-8.

2. Mynderse JS, et al. Antileukemia activity in the Osillatoriaceae: isolation of Debromoaplysiatoxin from Lyngbya. Science.1977;196:538-40.

3. Gerwick WH, et al. Novel cytotoxic peptides from the tropical marine cyanobacterium Hormothamnion enteromorphoides. 1. Discovery, solation and initial chemical and biological characterization of the hormothamnions from wild and cultured material. Experientia.1989;45:115-21.

4. Asari F, et al. Turbinaric acid, a cytotoxic secosqualene carboxylic acid from the brown alga Turbinaria ornata. J Nat Prod.1989;52:1167-9.

5. Kosovel V, et al. Algae as possible sources of antitumoural agents. Preliminary evaluation of the "in vitro" cytostatic activity of crude extracts. Pharmacol Res Commun.1988;5:27-31.

6. Nagasawa H, et al. Suppression by beta-carotene-rich algae Dunaliella bardawil of the progression, but not the development, of spontaneous mammary tumours in SHN virgin mice. Anticancer Res. 1991;11:713-7.

7. Konishi F, et al. Antitumor effect induced by a hot water extract of Chlorella vulgaris (CE): resistance to Meth-A tumor growth mediated by CE-induced polymorphonuclear leukocytes. Cancer Immunol Immunother.1985;19:73-8.

8. Matsueda S, et al. [Studies on antitumor active glycoprotein from Chlorella vulgaris. I]. Yakugaku Zasshi.1982;102:447-51.

9. Matsueda S, et al. [Studies on antitumor active glycoprotein from Chlorella vulgaris. II. Glycoprotein hydrolyzed with hydrolase]. Yakugaku Zasshi.1987;107:694-7.

10. Firsova NA, et al. [Inhibition of glutamine synthetase activity by biologically active derivatives of glutamic acid]. Biokhimiia.1986;51:850-5.

11. Miyazawa Y, et al. Immunomodulation by a unicellular green algae (Chlorella pyrenoidosa) in tumor-bearing mice. J Ethnopharmacol. 1988;24:135-46.

12. Schwartz J and Shklar G. Regression of experimental hamster cancer by beta carotene and algae extracts. J Oral Maxillofac Surg.1987; 45:510-5.

☙ BRYOSTATINS

Bryostatins are chemicals called lactones that have been isolated from an ocean invertebrate called *Bugula neritina*. These three-inch-long primitive animals, also called sea mats or corallines, are little known because they have virtually no commercial use to humans. But they are quite interesting to scientists since, although they are technically animals, they are very plantlike and live in underwater branching colonies.

Bryostatins have some remarkable effects in people. They seem to be involved in boosting immunity through interleukin-2 and T-type white blood cells (1). In 1990, bryostatin 1 was found to be active against mouse leukemia (2). It also inhibited three out of four leukemia cell lines from humans and acute non-lymphocytic leukemia cells from 10 out of 12 patients. In a Johns Hopkins study, the drug seemed to work by inhibiting the growth, rather than killing, such cells (2). It also made chronic myelogenous leukemia (CML) cells mature into macrophages, making it "a possible therapeutic agent" for this disease, according to researchers at the University of Washington in Seattle (3).

Bryostatin also produced "a decline in cellular proliferative activity" in some kinds of cancer cell lines. Together with another substance, ara-C, bryostatin inhibited the HL-60 cancer cell line (4). When used with a chemical called TPA, bryostatin produced a "marked reduction in the growth," according to scientists at the University of Newcastle in Newcastle upon Tyne, UK (5).

Bryostatin was tested by the Cancer Research Campaign (CRC) of the UK. In 1992, the NCI requested FDA permission to test bryostatin in humans.

⊕ References

1.   Eckert R, et al. Splenopentin (DAc-SP5)—influence on engraftment and graft-vs.-host reaction after non-H-2 bone marrow transplantation in mice. Exp Clin Endocrinol.1990;96:307-13.

2.   Jones RJ, et al. Bryostatin 1, a unique biologic response modifier: antileukemic activity in vitro. Blood.1990;75:1319-23.

3.   Lilly M, et al. Differentiation and growth modulation of chronic myelogenous leukemia cells by bryostatin. Cancer Res.1990;50:5520-5.

4.   Grant S, et al. In vitro effects of bryostatin 1 on the metabolism and cytotoxicity of 1-beta-D-arabinofuranosylcytosine in human leukemia cells. Biochem Pharmacol.1991;42:853-67.

5.   Nutt JE, et al. Phorbol ester and bryostatin effects on growth and the expression of oestrogen responsive and TGF-beta 1 genes in breast tumour cells. Br J Cancer.1991;64:671-6.

⍣ CANTHAXANTHIN

Canthaxanthin is a naturally-derived food coloring agent, also known as Food Orange 8, Roxanthin Red 10 or Carotaben plus. Like **beta-carotene,** canthaxanthin is a pigment widely distributed in nature. It was originally isolated from an edible mushroom and from flamingo feathers in the 1950s. The US patents for its isolation and synthesis were granted in the early 1960s.

Canthaxanthin's conventional medical use is to protect against the effects of sunlight in certain diseases of the skin caused by light exposure. It is also a pigment for darkening skin abnormally lightened by the "piebald" disease, vitiligo. In one study, it was judged satisfactory for this purpose by about half the patients who took it (1). Canthaxanthin's most controversial use has been as a chemical tanning, or bronzing, agent, since it will darken the skin without one having to actually sit in the sun.

Like beta-carotene, canthaxanthin has been found to be

a good immune booster in rats fed two grams per kilogram of the colorant for over a year. Most scientists ascribe the benefit of beta-carotene to the fact that it is converted into **vitamin A.** Yet, interestingly, canthaxanthin is one of those carotenes that is not converted into vitamin A in the body. Its beneficial effects must therefore be attributed to some other, little-understood "carotenoid effect," according to scientists at Roche Pharmaceuticals (2).

Researchers at the Yale University School of Medicine showed that in young chickens, at least, canthaxanthin works by enhancing **vitamin E** levels in membranes and only secondarily by serving as an antioxidant (3).

Canthaxanthin was given to rats with salivary gland tumors. While it did not have a significant effect on tumor incidence, the weights of the tumors "tended to be lower in rats fed the dietary supplements compared with the controls." In addition, "the incidence of tumor-bearing rats with large tumors was significantly lower in rats fed canthaxanthin than in the control rats." By the end of the experiment, rats receiving canthaxanthin had blood and tissue levels of vitamin A somewhat lower than controls. This was further proof that the anticancer effects of carotenes could not be dependent on vitamin A activity (4).

At the University of Hawaii, scientists studied the effects of canthaxanthin (as well as beta-carotene) on the transformation of normal mouse cells to cancerous cells. Both beta-carotene and canthaxanthin slowed this change, when it was caused by chemicals. When the food colorants were given one week after x-ray treatment, and then kept up, both agents stopped further tumors from developing. Canthaxanthin was actually more effective than beta-carotene. Upon withdrawal of both substances, however, the cancers began to grow again. This showed that they did not kill cancer cells, as much as inhibit their growth. The Honolulu scientists suggested that the carotenoids fight cancer by stopping free radical damage to fats (5). In 1991, scientists at the Veterans Affairs Medical Center in Houston called canthaxanthin an "excellent quencher" of oxygen free radical activity (6).

Local injections of canthaxanthin caused tumors in hamsters to regress. Twenty hamsters were given 250 micrograms of each agent. At the end of the experiment, tumors were counted and measured. Beta-carotene was more effective than canthaxanthin in causing tumors to regress while Accutane had no effect in this system (7).

Does canthaxanthin prevent the damage to the immune system caused by ultraviolet light? University of Arizona College of Medicine scientists put mice on a carefully-controlled diet that contained canthaxanthin, a kind of vitamin A (retinyl palmitate), or both.

The Tucson scientists then exposed them to a bank of six unfiltered ultraviolet B lamps. After more than six months of this treatment, spleen cells from these mice were injected into fresh mice that had not been exposed to this dangerous component of sunlight. Half of these fresh mice were then challenged with implants of cancer cells. Only half of the mice that received spleen cells from animals that had gotten both canthaxanthin and vitamin A developed cancer.

By contrast, mice that received spleen cells from mice that had not been so treated, got cancer more frequently. Spleen cells from animals that had received either substance alone did not provide as much beneficial effect, however (8).

When rats were given canthaxanthin in their diet three weeks before receiving a chemical that causes breast cancer, there was a "65 percent reduction in the number of mammary cancers." Some rats were given nearly four grams per kilogram of the colorant, a high dose.

"Canthaxanthin, at least in these models of mammary cancer, is active in preventing cancer initiation," the University of Alabama nutritionists said.

Although there were "very high" levels of the coloring agent in the animals' livers, Birmingham scientists judged this agent "without toxicity" and urged further evaluation for chemoprevention (9).

Until the mid-1980s, it was generally thought that the worst effects of large doses of canthaxanthin were red stools and orange palms and soles (1). But in 1985, on a routine examination, a 50-year-old Australian was found to have "small golden particles in the macular regions of both eyes." The man had taken canthaxanthin orally to chemically bronze his skin (10). These golden particles in the retina turned out to be canthaxanthin deposits, which had been absorbed by retina cells, ophthalmologist at the Medical University in Lubeck, Germany concluded (11).

There followed a flurry of concern, as reports of golden eye spots filtered in. Such reports raised the fear that this seemingly harmless substance might cause serious eye damage. And since canthaxanthin was used for medical conditions, as well as for tanning, there was widespread concern about the public health dimensions.

To examine such questions, scientists at Laval University Medical Center in Québec, examined the eyes of 19 patients who had been taking canthaxanthin. Eleven had maculopathy, i.e., a problem in the sensitive oval part of the eye called the macula retinae. The other eight did not. Patients were re-evaluated two to three years after they had ceased taking canthaxanthin.

At both testing sessions, patients with maculopathy had less sensitive retinas. The patients who did not have the maculopathy had basically normal vision. "These results suggest that canthaxanthin retinopathy can adversely

CANTHAXANTHIN

affect the neurosensory retina," the Québec scientists wrote (12).

In 1989, however, the same scientists concluded that "canthaxanthin retinopathy is reversible" (13). Scientists at the University Eye Clinic in Leiden, Holland examined 32 patients treated with canthaxanthin and beta-carotene. Eight had "gold dust" in their eyes. But "no deterioration of visual function was found in any of these patients," the Dutch scientists reported (14).

At Moorfields Eye Hospital in London, UK, doctors studied patients who had taken canthaxanthin and beta-carotene to reduce their sensitivity to sunlight. Patients took the compounds only during the summer, but were monitored for the whole year. The characteristic crystals in the retina "reduced during the winter." Again, British scientists noted that such changes "are reversible" (15).

In some countries, a drug called Phenoro® is marketed. Each capsule contains 10 milligrams of beta-carotene and 15 milligrams of canthaxanthin. Some patients have received a cumulative total of up to 178 grams of canthaxanthin in this way, over 12 years. Five years after they discontinued this treatment, some of the patients were re-examined. "There was an extensive reduction of the number of deposits," Swedish ophthalmologist reported, "confirming other reports which have demonstrated that the formation of the crystalline deposits is reversible" (16).

The most serious report of alleged toxicity appeared in a 1990 *JAMA* report. This claimed that a previously healthy young woman contracted the blood disease aplastic anemia and died after taking canthaxanthin for tanning purposes. The *JAMA* article complained that canthaxanthin "is readily available through commercial tanning salons and mail advertisements." It ominously suggested that there was an "unknown" risk of "bone marrow suppression," based on this case. Use of this drug for cosmetic purposes does

211

not justify this risk, the AMA warned (17).

Canthaxanthin appears to be a powerful anticancer agent, however, especially when combined with other carotenes and vitamin A. It is found in nature and is a legal food additive in most countries. Dutch scientists found seven patients who had gold-colored specks in their eyes, yet none of them had taken canthaxanthin-containing drugs. Leiden scientists speculated that canthaxanthin used as a food additive could have caused these spots. Some people might therefore have a "high individual tendency" to develop such crystal deposits (18).

⊕ References

1.   Gupta AK, et al. Canthaxanthin. Int J Dermatol.1985;24:528-32.

2.   Bendich A and Shapiro SS. Effect of beta-carotene and canthaxanthin on the immune responses of the rat. J Nutr.1986;116:2254-62.

3.   Mayne ST and Parker RS. Antioxidant activity of dietary canthaxanthin. Nutr Cancer.1989;12:225-36.

4.   Alam BS, et al. Effects of excess vitamin A and canthaxanthin on salivary gland tumors. Nutr Cancer.1988;11:233-41.

5.   Pung A, et al. Beta-carotene and canthaxanthin inhibit chemically- and physically-induced neoplastic transformation in 10T1/2 cells. Carcinogenesis.1988;9:1533-9.

6.   Black HS and Mathews RM. Protective role of butylated hydroxytoluene and certain carotenoids in photocarcinogenesis. Photochem Photobiol.1991;53:707-16.

7.   Schwartz J and Shklar G. Regression of experimental oral carcinomas by local injection of beta-carotene and canthaxanthin. Nutr Cancer.1988;11:35-40.

8.   Gensler HL. Reduction of immunosuppression in UV-irradiated mice by dietary retinyl palmitate plus canthaxanthin. Carcinogenesis. 1989;10:203-7.

9.   Grubbs CJ, et al. Effect of canthaxanthin on chemically induced mammary carcinogenesis. Oncology.1991;48:239-45.

10.   McGuinness R and Beaumont P. Gold dust retinopathy after the ingestion of canthaxanthine to produce skin-bronzing. Med J Aust.1985; 143:622-3.

11.   Bopp S, et al. [Canthaxanthin retinopathy and macular pucker]. J Fr

Ophtalmol.1989;12:891-6.

12. Harnois C, et al. Static perimetry in canthaxanthin maculopathy. Arch Ophthalmol.1988;106:58-60.

13. Harnois C, et al. Canthaxanthin retinopathy. Anatomic and functional reversibility. Arch Ophthalmol.1989;107:538-40.

14. Nijman NM, et al. [Canthaxanthin retinopathy]. Klin Monatsbl Augenheilkd.1989;194:48-51.

15. Arden GB, et al. Monitoring of patients taking canthaxanthin and carotene: an electroretinographic and ophthalmological survey. Hum Toxicol.1989;8:439-50.

16. Leyon H, et al. Reversibility of canthaxanthin deposits within the retina. Acta Ophthalmol (Copenh).1990;68:607-11.

17. Bluhm R, et al. Aplastic anemia associated with canthaxanthin ingested for 'tanning' purposes. JAMA.1990;264:1141-2.

18. Oosterhuis JA, et al. [Canthaxanthin retinopathy without intake of canthaxanthin]. Klin Monatsbl Augenheilkd.1989;194:110-6.

℀ *C*HLOROPHYLL

As most high school students know, chlorophyll is the substance that makes the plants green and is responsible for photosynthesis. Yet few know that common chlorophyll may also have powerful anticancer effects.

Extracts of various vegetables have been found to combat mutagenesis in the standard Ames test. It turned out that the potency of each vegetable extract was directly related to its chlorophyll content. Chlorophyllin (the sodium-copper salt of chlorophyll) showed similar levels of activity, scientists at M.D. Anderson Hospital in Houston, TX said (1).

A 1985 article in *Mutation Research* examined the effects of several food compounds in preventing mutations caused by two chemicals found in cigarette smoke (cigarette-smoke condensate and benzo[a]pyrene). Ellagic acid and riboflavin inhibited mutations. Vitamin C, beta-carotene and vitamin E did not. But the big surprise was that the most potent antimutation agent of all turned out to be chlorophyllin (2).

In the following year, chlorophyllin was again tested for antimutation ability by scientists at the National Institute of Occupational Safety and Health (NIOSH). They put it up against a variety of complex (and possibly carcinogenic) substances, such as extracts of fried beef, fried shredded pork, red grape juice, red wine, cigarette smoke, tobacco snuff, chewing tobacco, airborne particles, coal dust and diesel emission particles. Chlorophyllin stopped mutations in eight out of ten of these tests. In fact, its rate of inhibiting mutagens was an astonishing 90 to 100 percent.

"The mechanism of the antimutagenicity of chlorophyllin in these experiments is not known," the Morgantown, WV scientists said. "However, chlorophyllin is an antioxidant." And this ability to soak up harmful free radicals makes chlorophyll, especially in its slightly modified form, an agent potentially useful against cancer (3).

Three years later, these results were extended to other mutagens, including a solvent containing extracts of coal dust and diesel emission particles. Chlorophyllin inhibited over 90 percent of the mutagen activity of these substances. It was a more effective antimutagen than retinol, beta-carotene, vitamin C or vitamin E (4).

Some rats were given free access to food and water containing chlorophyllin. After five weeks University of Illinois scientists gave them a chemical that causes colon cancer. Rats that had been given chlorophyllin had significantly fewer cancer-like changes in their colon cells than rats that did not. "This implies that chlorophyllin, a known antimutagen, may have anticarcinogenic properties as well," the scientists concluded (5).

Other scientists showed that chlorophyllin, **beta-carotene** and a form of **linolenic acid** inhibited the activity of the "powerful mutagen" and anticancer drug, thio-tepa. Each of these natural protective compounds inhibited the harmful effects of this drug by 70 to 85 percent (6). Chlorophyllin also protected fruit flies from the effects of radiation, according to scientists at Brown University (7).

In 1991, scientists at the Center for Life Sciences and Toxicology, in Research Triangle Park, NC put chlorophyllin up against aflatoxin, one of the most potent carcinogens known, as well as other known mutagens. "Results showed that chlorophyllin...completely or almost completely inhibited the mutagenicity" of most of these substances. Once again, these results substantiated the remarkable effectiveness of chlorophyllin as an anticancer substance, the North Carolina scientists said (8).

⊕ References

1.   Lai C-N, et al. Antimutagenic activities of common vegetables and their chlorophyll content. Mutation Res.1980;77:245-250.

2.   Terwel L, et al. Antimutagenic activity of some naturally occurring compounds towards cigarette-smoke condensate and benzo[a]pyrene in the Salmonella/microsome assay. Mutat Res.1985;152:1-4.

3.   Ong TM, et al. Chlorophyllin: a potent antimutagen against environmental and dietary complex mixtures. Mutat Res.1986;173:111-5.

4.   Ong T, et al. Comparative antimutagenicity of 5 compounds against 5 mutagenic complex mixtures in Salmonella typhimurium strain TA98. Mutat Res.1989;222:19-25.

5.   Robins E and Nelson R. Inhibition of 1,2-dimethylhydrazine-induced nuclear damage in rat colonic epithelium by chlorophyllin. Anticancer Res.1989;9:981-986.

6.   Renner HW. In vivo effects of single or combined dietary antimutagens on mutagen-induced chromosomal aberrations. Mutat Res.1990; 244:185-8.

7.   Zimmering S, et al. Evidence for a radioprotective effect of chlorophyllin in Drosophila. Mutat Res.1990;245:47-9.

8.   Warner JR, et al. Antimutagenicity studies of chlorophyllin using the Salmonella arabinose-resistant assay system. Mutat Res.1991;262:25-30.

℣ℭOENZYME Q

Coenzyme Q (also known as CoQ10 or ubiquinone) is a "quasi-nutrient" that plays an important role in energy metabolism. It may be necessary for some people at certain stages of their life, including pregnancy, sickness and stress—and chemotherapy.

Although it can be manufactured internally from two amino acids and various vitamins, and is present in most foods, supplements are probably justified in some of the above situations, just to make sure that adequate amounts are available. Some doctors prescribe between 30 and 80 milligrams per day to increase aerobic endurance and improve disease resistance.

The most important use of CoQ10 in cancer is to counteract the highly toxic action on the heart of conventional anticancer drugs. Some studies indicate that the heart toxicity of the toxic antibiotic adriamycin is actually due to a depletion of CoQ10. The drug injured the mitochondria (microscopic energy centers) of heart muscle cells. A daily intake of 50 milligram of CoQ10, starting with the first dose of adriamycin, resulted in a decrease in heart damage. CoQ10 was found to be nontoxic and did not interfere with the antitumor activity of adriamycin (1).

Two other conventional anticancer agents, mitomycin C and 5-flourouracil (5-FU), cause disturbances in the energy metabolism of liver cells. When these agents were used in combination with CoQ10, however, the malfunction of energy metabolism in such liver cells was "significantly prevented," Japanese scientists reported in *Cancer Research* (2).

⊕ References

1.   Cortes EP, et al. Adriamycin cardiotoxicity: early detection by systolic time interval and possible prevention by coenzyme Q10. Cancer Treat Rep.1978;62:887-91.

2.   Okada K, et al. Cell injury by antineoplastic agents and influence of coenzyme Q10 on cellular potassium activity and potential difference across the membrane in rat liver cells. Cancer Res.1980;40:1663-7.

❦ EVENING PRIMROSE

Evening primrose oil (EPO) is extracted from the common evening primrose, an annual plant found in wastelands and dry meadows in the eastern half of the US. Its yellow, lemon-scented flowers open at dusk, hence the lovely name. Evening primrose has also been known as fever plant, king's cure-all, and scurvish, all indications of its various folk usages. It has also been used as a cough remedy and an anodyne for mental depression. The entire plant is edible.

Evening primrose oil stands out as an abundant source of gamma-linolenic acid (GLA). This is a form the essential fatty acid, linoleic acid, takes when it is broken down in the body. GLA is a non-toxic, readily available polyunsaturated oil with a remarkable range of therapeutic properties. The essential fatty acids "exhibit no side-effects when taken as a dietary supplement, even in large doses," scientists at the Medical University of Southern Africa report (1).

In 1980, Dr. David F. Horrobin and scientists at the Efamol Research Institute in Kentville, Nova Scotia suggested that cancer cells cannot make a substance that converts linoleic into gamma-linolenic acid. This lack "may be the critical step in the malignant change in many forms of cancer." By providing gamma linolenic acid, he said, physicians could normalize malignant cells and reverse cancer's growth. Since this approach is completely non-toxic, Horrobin suggested using it in cancer cases for which no other viable treatment was available (2). He also suggested that the hormone prostaglandin was involved in this change, a mechanism that has been questioned by other scientists (3).

In a critical test of Horrobin's theory, South African scientists showed that GLA supplements produced a "highly significant reduction" in the growth rate of human liver cancer cells in the test tube, up to 87 percent, and "requires urgent further investigation at all levels including trials in human cancer patients" (4).

Writing in the *JNCI*, Horrobin and colleagues reported that polyunsaturated fatty acids killed human breast, lung and prostate cancer cells at concentrations which had no adverse effects on normal human cells. When human cancer cells and normal cells were grown together in a test tube without such polyunsaturated fatty acids, however, malignant cells overgrew normal ones. But when GLA or other fatty acids were added to the test tube, normal cells outgrew the malignant ones. "These observations suggest," Horrobin wrote, that treatment of cancer with fatty acids "may have considerable potential while being associated with a high level of safety" (5).

Doctors at the Children's Research Hospital of Kyoto Prefectual University of Medicine, Japan, studied the effects of GLA on two types of human nerve cancer cells. Growth was inhibited and this was associated with "striking membrane fatty acid" changes. These results indicate, they said, that the anticancer effect of GLA is probably due to the "cellular dysfunction" of tumor cells after GLA was incorporated into their structures (6).

Scientists at Kumamoto University Hospital studied the effects of GLA on liver cancer cells of the rat. The growth of these cells was also "significantly suppressed" by GLA. The presence of albumin (the protein present in egg white) suppressed the cell killing ability of GLA, however (7).

Kyoto scientists concluded that GLA by itself shows antitumor activity in various cell cultures. They therefore tried combining it with various standard anticancer drugs in nerve cancer. Two standard anticancer drugs, vincristine and vinblastine, were twice as effective "when GLA was added simultaneously to the growth medium." On the other hand, platinum-containing drugs, such as cisplatin and carboplatin, were inhibited by GLA supplementation. The cell-killing activity of other anticancer agents was unaffected (8). Combining EPA with standard chemotherapy enhanced the killing ability of the toxic drugs (12).

Other results have been mixed. In 1982, South African scientists reported that GLA killed human esophagus cancer cells in the test tube (9). However, in the following year, they reported that 89 "nude mice" (a special breed that lacks normal immunity) implanted with different human tumours were injected with GLA. This route of delivery had no significant effect on the growth of any of these tumors (10). The scientists at the University of Natal themselves questioned the validity of the particular animal model used, however (11).

GLA also suppressed the growth of four kinds of nerve cancer cells (3). It also killed human breast, lung, and prostate cancer cells selectively. Normal cells were not killed, but their rate of division slowed. "The cancer cells were selectively eliminated," said Efomel scientists (12).

While scientists generally try to stop free radical activity, GLA may work by causing deadly free radicals to form in cancerous—but not in normal—cells (13). GLA was more effective than linoleic acid in this regard (14,15).

Urologists at the Aberdeen Royal Infirmary examined the composition of the essential fatty acids in the blood of 98 bladder cancer patients who came in for routine examinations. The patients were divided into two groups: those with active tumors and those with no evidence of active disease. Compared to the general population, the levels of fatty acids were "significantly lower" in bladder cancer patients.

The Scottish doctors did not see any significant difference between those patients with active and inactive disease. They concluded that blood levels "of the essential fatty acids are abnormal in patients with bladder cancer; they do not help, however, to distinguish those patients with active disease from those with inactive disease." They concluded that a fatty acid deficiency may predispose people to develop bladder cancer rather than itself be a result of the cancer (16).

Researchers at Rhodes University in South Africa studied the effects of purified linoleic acid and GLA on melanoma cells. They also looked at safflower oil (which contains linoleic acid) and evening primrose oil (which contains GLA) on melanomas grown in mice. Both were found to have equal potency in inhibiting the growth of such cells.

One noteworthy (and possibly cautionary) finding was that in the mice, evening primrose oil appeared to promote melanoma growth. The Grahamstown scientists raised the possibility that "melanomas in mice have a requirement of GLA for growth" while in the test tube excess GLA could inhibit their growth (17).

Over the years, GLAs have been reported to reduce cholesterol levels (18), relieve premenstrual syndrome (19), aid in schizophrenia (20), diabetes (21), obesity (22), as well as other conditions. Most of these reports come from

Dr. Horrobin's institute.

Failure with Liver Cancer: In a double-blind study, South African doctors used evening primrose oil (as a source of GLA) as a dietary supplement for people with liver cancer. "No statistically significant effect was observed on survival time or liver size," they reported. Some crucial enzyme levels did improve, however, and no side-effects were observed. The scientists ascribed this failure to the large size of tumors and the relatively low doses of GLA used in the test (1).

⊕ References

1. van der Merwe C, et al. The effect of gamma-linolenic acid, an in vitro cytostatic substance contained in evening primrose oil, on primary liver cancer. A double-blind placebo controlled trial. Prostaglandins Leukot Essent Fatty Acids.1990;40:199-202.

2. Horrobin DF. The reversibility of cancer: the relevance of cyclic AMP, calcium, essential fatty acids and prostaglandin E1. Med Hypotheses.1980;6:469-86.

3. Fujiwara F, et al. Antitumor effect of gamma-linolenic acid on cultured human neuroblastoma cells. Prostaglandins Leukot Med.1986;23:311-20.

4. Dippenaar N, et al. The reversibility of cancer: evidence that malignancy in human hepatoma cells is gamma-linolenic acid deficiency-dependent. S Afr Med J.1982;62:683-5.

5. Begin ME, et al. Selective killing of human cancer cells by polyunsaturated fatty acids. Prostaglandins Leukot Med.1985;19:177-86.

6. Fujiwara F, et al. Fatty acid modification of cultured neuroblastoma cells by gamma linolenic acid relevant to its antitumor effect. Prostaglandins Leukot Med.1987;30:37-49.

7. Hayashi Y, et al. Anticancer activity of free gamma-linolenic acid on AH-109A rat hepatoma cells and the effect of serum albumin on anticancer activity of gamma-linolenic acid in vitro. J Pharmacobiodyn.1990;13:705-11.

8. Ikushima S, et al. Gamma linoleic acid alters the cytotoxic activity of anticancer drugs on cultured human neuroblastoma cells. Anticancer Res.1990;10:1055-9.

9. Leary WP, et al. Some effects of gamma-linolenic acid on cultured human oesophageal carcinoma cells. S Afr Med J.1982;62:681-3.

10. Botha JH, et al. Parenteral gamma-linolenic acid administration in nude mice bearing a range of human tumour xenografts. S Afr Med J.1983;64:11-2.

11. Booyens J and Koenig L. The effect of dietary supplementation with gamma-linolenic acid on the growth of induced tumours in rats. S Afr Med J.1984;65:660-1.

12. Begin ME, et al. Differential killing of human carcinoma cells supplemented with n-3 and n-6 polyunsaturated fatty acids. J Natl Cancer Inst.1986;77:1053-62.

13. Begin ME, et al. Polyunsaturated fatty acid-induced cytotoxicity against tumor cells and its relationship to lipid peroxidation. J Natl Cancer Inst.1988;80:188-94.

14. Das UN, et al. Polyunsaturated fatty acids augment free radical generation in tumor cells in vitro. Biochem Biophys Res Commun.1987; 145:15-24.

15. Das UN, et al. Uptake and distribution of cis-unsaturated fatty acids and their effect on free radical generation in normal and tumor cells in vitro. Free Radic Biol Med.1987;3:9-14.

16. McClinton S, et al. Abnormalities of essential fatty acid distribution in the plasma phospholipids of patients with bladder cancer. Br J Cancer.1991;63:314-6.

17. Gardiner NS and Duncan JR. Possible involvement of delta-6-desaturase in control of melanoma growth by gamma-linolenic acid. Prostaglandins Leukot Essent Fatty Acids.1991;42:149-53.

18. Horrobin DF and Manku MS. How do polyunsaturated fatty acids lower plasma cholesterol levels? Lipids.1983;18:558-62.

19. Brush MG, et al. Abnormal essential fatty acid levels in plasma of women with premenstrual syndrome. Am J Obstet Gynecol.1984; 150:363-6.

20. Horrobin DF. Schizophrenia as a prostaglandin deficiency disease. Lancet.1977;1:936-7.

21. Cunnane SC, et al. Abnormal essential fatty acid composition of tissue lipids in genetically diabetic mice is partially corrected by dietary linoleic and gamma-linolenic acids. Br J Nutr.1985;53:449-58.

22. Cunnane SC, et al. N-3 Essential fatty acids decrease weight gain in genetically obese mice. Br J Nutr.1986;56:87-95.

❧ *F*IBER

Fiber is a complex mixture of indigestible carbohydrates. Early in the twentieth century, nutritionists gleefully eliminated fiber from grains and other foods to make them easier to manipulate. These foods were then promoted as 'purified' products. Today, at long last, fiber is recognized by the medical profession as a "natural and hitherto much-neglected component of the normal diet" (1).

For decades, there have been suggestions that increased fiber, or "bulk" in the diet could help prevent colon and rectal cancer, diverticulitis and other diseases of the intestines. Denis Burkitt, a medical doctor in Africa, suggested in the 1960s that the standard Western diet predisposed towards such illnesses. Africans, he noted, rarely got such diseases. They also ate far more fiber and had much bulkier stools. The prevalence of colon and rectal cancer in the West, Burkitt concluded, was related to its low-fiber, high-fat diet. And of the two factors, he considered the lack of fiber the more important (2).

Colon cancer used to be a rare disease. But by the 1970s in Western countries it accounted for about two to four percent of all deaths. In 1982-83, the age-adjusted death rate from colon cancer (for men) was 50 percent higher in the highest country, Luxembourg, than it was in the United States and about 50 times higher than in El Salvador. Various theories have been propounded to account for these dramatic differences. For instance, differences in the intakes of fat, protein, refined cereal products and sugar have been put forward as plausible causes. But in what are called "sophisticated populations," higher concentrations of fecal bile acids and sterol hormones, and the longer time it takes for food to move through the digestive tract (the so-called transit time), favor the production of carcinogens. The Luxembourgeois have an extremely tasty cuisine, but it is sadly lacking in fiber, certainly when compared to the rice and bean diet common in Central America.

Why has it taken so long for the link between diet and intestinal disease to be acknowledged? Nutritional theories of cancer prevention have historically been considered quackery (see **Gerson Diet**). But Denis Burkitt was a very famous doctor ("Burkitt's lymphoma" is named in his honor) and so he could not easily be dismissed, the way a Max Gerson could be.

As early as 1978, experiments confirmed Burkitt's theory. For example, he had suggested that Western populations with long life expectancies, such as Seventh Day Adventists, Mormons and rural Finns, should be intensively studied (3). And, indeed, when biochemists at Loma Linda University, Riverside, CA studied Adventists they found that total vegetarians had high levels of potentially-dangerous estrogen hormones in their feces (4). This was encouraging, for higher fecal levels meant that an enhanced fiber diet was helping to eliminate cancer-promoting hormones.

Scientists at Fox Chase Cancer Center in Pennsylvania cautioned their colleagues not to jump to conclusions: the protective effect could come from a combination of fiber with some non-fiber elements (such as possibly vitamin C or beta-carotene) in the vegetables (5).

But there were good scientific reasons that fiber could protect against colorectal cancer, according to a scientist at the MRC Dunn Clinical Nutrition Centre in Cambridge, England (6). The feces of some people contains mutation-causing substances. Bran (a source of fiber) reduces these agents and may be an important way of preventing the onset of cancer.

One drawback of a high-fiber diet is that it produces intestinal gas in some people. But contrary to folk wisdom, unpleasant as this is, it does not represent a risk factor for colon cancer. Bile acids are particularly suspect, however. In the test tube, such internally-generated compounds can damage genetic material (DNA). This damage is "largely prevented when the bile acids are pretreated with cellulose fiber." High fiber aids in other ways:

• Cellulose converts bile acid to a biologically-inactive form (7).

• Fiber helps eliminate fatty acids (8).

• Bran reduces cancerous changes in mice receiving a drug that causes colon cancer (9).

• Psyllium husks—a popular source of fiber—strongly reduced the ability of another carcinogen to cause colon cancer. Cellulose did so, too, but only moderately. Psyllium-fed rats had the highest fecal bacteria counts and the bulkiest and most moisture-laden stools, all good things (10).

• A saccharide from rice bran (RBS) exhibits "potent anti-tumor activities" against solid sarcomas in mice, both by feeding and by injection. RBS is a white, sugar-like, pH-neutral powder. Japanese doctors believe that this activity is due to its ability to stimulate the immune system. Ingested, it was non-toxic (11).

• In most studies, fiber decreases the number of colon malignancies: the more fiber, the less fatal colon disease in rats, according to a report in *The Lancet* (12,13).

The type of fiber is important. In the late 70s, the *JNCI* reported on a study of alfalfa, pectin and wheat bran—three different sources of fiber—on colon cancer in rats. Animals fed alfalfa and then treated with a carcinogen had more colon tumors than those fed pectin or wheat bran. In this experiment, pectin (abundant in apples) and wheat bran seemed most protective (14).

In 1982, the conservative Committee on Diet, Nutrition, and Cancer of the US National Research Council concluded that a high-fat diet is associated with increased risk of breast, colon and prostate cancer. Fiber, it said, could protect against colon cancer. Frequent consumption of citrus fruits and carotene-rich and cruciferous vegetables, was also "definitely associated with a lower incidence of cancer of various types" (15).

In 1984, the American Cancer Society (ACS) decided that a large proportion of new cancer cases could be avoided if seven dietary guidelines were followed. Large-scale education programs were developed for young people, the media and the general public. These guidelines were reaffirmed in 1989 (16). Third on this list was a recommendation for people to eat more high-fiber foods such as whole grain cereals, fruits and vegetables.

"Knowledgeable patients should not die of colorectal cancer," a University of Florida surgeon has said.

By increasing the intake of dietary fiber, decreasing fat consumption, and using modern technology to detect polyps and early cancer, people can greatly decrease the death rate associated with this disease (17).

Cereal companies have seized on bran as a marketing device. But some scientists are uneasy with the quick fix implicit in the fiber theory. Dietary fiber is not the only factor that protects against colon cancer, they say. "The data suggest that the effects of fiber must be considered in the context of the total diet and interactions of dietary components," according to researchers at the Wistar Institute in Philadelphia (18). Fiber intake is not always elevated in populations at low risk of colorectal cancer. But generally colon cancer rates do increase with Westernization of the diet.

There may also be a link between breast cancer and low fiber. The National Cancer Institute of Canada conducted an analysis of studies on diet and breast cancer. These showed a strong association between the risk of breast cancer and saturated fat intake in postmenopausal women. Vitamin C was protective, as was fruit and vegetable intake in general, in part because of fiber, it is said. By changing their diets, about 20 percent of women might prevent the development of breast cancer (19). Thus, a high intake of cereal products, especially those rich in fiber, could be very healthful (20).

In a large study at Harvard, fiber was once again found protective against colon cancer. But equally significant was the positive association of animal fats with the risk of colon cancer. No association was found for oils of vegetable origin. The relative risk of colon cancer in women who ate beef, pork, or lamb as a main dish every day was about two-and-a-half times that of women who ate such foods less than once a month. Processed meats and liver were also associated with increased risk, whereas fish and chicken without skin were related to decreased risk. The Harvard Medical School scientists concluded in the *New England Journal of Medicine* that "a high intake of animal fat increases the risk of colon cancer," and they support existing recommendations to substitute fish and chicken for meats high in fat (21).

In fact, since 1980, 25 out of 32 studies have shown that fiber protects against colon cancer. Six out of seven studies of breast cancer patients also showed that fiber-rich foods were protective. For cancers of the esophagus, mouth, pharynx, stomach, rectum, endometrium and ovary, there is limited data showing a protective effect. But no one is yet sure if this protection is clearly from fiber *per se* and not from some other part of the diet. For cancer prevention, US scientists say, the emphasis should be on an entire dietary pattern rather than an isolated dietary fiber supplement (22).

Meanwhile, a case was reported in *JAMA* of a woman who developed a severe allergic reaction to a psyllium-containing breakfast cereal. Loyola University allergists warned that "physicians and consumers should be aware of potential serious reactions from eating psyllium-containing cereals even without prior history of ingestion of psyllium." However, it turned out that, as a nurse, this particular woman used to dispense a psyllium-containing laxative, which may have sensitized her to this particular form of fiber (23).

⊕ References

1. Berkow R. The Merck manual of diagnosis and therapy (15th ed.). Rahway, NJ: Merck & Co., 1987, p. 2696.

2. Burkitt DP. Colonic-rectal cancer: fiber and other dietary factors. Am J Clin Nutr.1978;S58-S64.

3. Walker AR. Colon cancer and diet, with special reference to intakes of fat and fiber. Am J Clin Nutr.1976;29:1417-26.

4. Pusateri DJ, et al. Dietary and hormonal evaluation of men at different risks for prostate cancer: plasma and fecal hormone-nutrient interrelationships. Am J Clin Nutr.1990;51:371-7.

5. Trock B, et al. Dietary fiber, vegetables, and colon cancer: critical review and meta-analyses of the epidemiologic evidence. J Natl Cancer Inst.1990;82:650-61.

6. Bingham SA. Mechanisms and experimental and epidemiological evidence relating dietary fibre (non-starch polysaccharides) and starch to protection against large bowel cancer. Proc Nutr Soc.1990;49:153-71.

7. Cheah PY and Bernstein H. Colon cancer and dietary fiber: cellulose inhibits the DNA-damaging ability of bile acids. Nutr Cancer.1990;13:51-7.

8. Cummings JH, et al. Changes in fecal composition and colonic function due to cereal fiber. Am J Clin Nutr.1976;29:1468-73.

9. Chen WF and Goldsmith HS. Colonic protection from dimethylhydrazine by a high fiber diet. Surg Gynecol Obstet.1978;147:503-6.

10. Roberts-Andersen J, et al. Reduction of DMH-induced colon tumors in rats fed psyllium husk or cellulose. Nutr Cancer.1987;10:129-36.

11. Ito E, et al. Studies on an antitumor polysaccharide RBS derived from rice bran. I. Preparation, physico-chemical properties, and biological activities of RBS. Yakugaku Zasshi (Japan).1985;105:188-193.

12. Fleiszer D, et al. Protective effect of dietary fibre against chemically induced bowel tumours in rats. Lancet.1978;2:552-3.

13. Cruse JP, et al. Failure of bran to protect against experimental colon cancer in rats. Lancet.1978;2:1278-80.

14. Watanabe K, et al. Effect of dietary alfalfa, pectin, and wheat bran on azoxymethane- or methylnitrosourea-induced colon carcinogenesis in F344 rats. J Natl Cancer Inst.1979;63:141-5.

15. Palmer S. Diet, nutrition, and cancer. Prog Food Nutr Sci.1985;9: 283-341.

16. Bal DG and Foerster SB. Changing the American diet. Impact on cancer prevention policy recommendations and program implications for the American Cancer Society [editorial]. Cancer.1991;67:2671-80.

17. Ferguson EJ and McKibben BT. Preventing colorectal cancer. South Med J.1990;83:1295-9.

18. Kritchevsky D. Fiber and cancer. Med Oncol Tumor Pharmacother. 1990;7:137-41.

19. Howe GR, et al. Dietary factors and risk of breast cancer: combined analysis of 12 case-control studies. J Natl Cancer Inst.1990;82:561-9.

20. Van t'Veer P, et al. Dietary fiber, beta-carotene and breast cancer: results from a case-control study. Int J Cancer.1990;45:825-8.

21. Willett WC, et al. Relation of meat, fat, and fiber intake to the risk of colon cancer in a prospective study among women. N Engl J Med.1990; 323:1664-72.

22. Shankar S and Lanza E. Dietary fiber and cancer prevention. Hematol Oncol Clin North Am.1991;5:25-41.

23. Lantner RR, et al. Anaphylaxis following ingestion of a psyllium-containing cereal. JAMA.1990;264:2534-6.

❦ FISH OIL

Fish oil may help prevent not only arthritis and heart disease but cancer. That is because fish oil is rich in valuable compounds called omega-3 fatty acids. This is an exciting area of nutritional research, and it is impossible to do more than summarize a small sampling of the work being done around the world.

Adding fish oil to the diet may slow the progress of pancreatic and other kinds of malignancy. Cornell University biochemist T. Colin Campbell gave young rats a single injection of a chemical that causes precancerous growths in their pancreas. After three weeks he started them on a diet that included fish oil (from the herring-like menhaden) and protein (from cod). He kept them on this regimen for the next four months. Fish protein had no effect. But the diet that included fish oil "produced a significant decrease in the development of both the size and number of preneoplastic lesions" (1).

The low-fat diet of the Japanese and the Eskimo, combined with their high intake of fish oil, seems to inhibit breast and colon cancer. At the Ludwig Institute for Cancer Research in Toronto scientists found that the more fish people ate, the less breast cancer they developed. They attributed the protective effect of fish to the omega-3 fatty acids (2).

Mice were also fed various combinations of corn oil and MaxEPA®, a fish oil product high in omega-3 fatty acids. More animals developed tumors in the groups receiving a high corn oil or a low MaxEPA diet. But mice receiving a 1:1 ratio of omega-3 (fish oil) to omega-6 (corn oil) developed the least number of tumors (3).

At the John Muir Cancer and Aging Research Institute in Walnut Creek, CA, scientists found that a diet containing MaxEPA, 11 percent by weight, reduced the rate of growth of a transplantable human breast tumor compared to mice fed equal amounts of either corn oil or lard. Whatever tumors took grew more slowly in the group receiving the fish oil than in those receiving corn oil or lard (4).

'Nude' mice (a special breed that lacks normal immunity) received injections of about 10 million human colon cancer cells. They then were given various equal calorie diets: either the standard diet; one enhanced with saturated fat in the form of 20 percent coconut oil; or one with 20 percent MaxEPA (fish oil). The MaxEPA diet "produced significant tumor growth reduction compared to the other diets," scientists at the Dudley Road Hospital in Birmingham, UK reported (5).

Another Birmingham center studied the effect of fish oil on colon cancer. The British scientists substituted fish oil for carbohydrates in the diets of these mice. They found that diets containing fish oil "significantly reduced host body weight loss." There was "almost complete protection...when the fish oil comprised 50 percent of the calories." There was also a significant reduction in tumor growth rate, they reported in *Cancer Research*, with an increase in total body fat and muscle mass. Surprisingly, fish oil was as powerful an anticancer agent as the conventional drugs cyclophosphamide and 5-FU. But while the antitumor effect of the drugs "was achieved with considerable host toxicity," treatment with fish oil produced no toxicity and almost completely abolished wasting.

"These results suggest that fish oil is a nontoxic, highly effective anticachectic agent," they concluded, "with the added advantage of antitumor activity" (6).

Mice with lymphoma and thymoma (thymus gland growth) were given either soy bean, linseed or fish oil, as four percent of their diet. While none of these supplements caused significant differences in tumor incidence or in mortality, the tumor size was decreased by diets supplying omega-3 fatty acids from fish oil or linseed oil. For example, lymphoma tumor weight was "markedly depressed" by linseed oil. Thymoma tumor weight was lowest in mice receiving fish oil.

At the same time, linseed oil caused an increase in

"good" HDL-cholesterol compared to either fish oil or soy bean oil. The mice with thymoma responded to both the linseed and fish oil diets with "greatly elevated HDL-cholesterol levels" (7).

Mice were given a chemical that causes colon cancer and then were administered four different kinds of diets. Colon cancer developed as follows:

Type of fat in diet	% developing colon cancer
Tallow (beef fat)	55
Low-fat diets	48
Safflower oil	33
Fish oil	18

Not surprisingly, cholesterol levels were "significantly higher" in mice fed tallow than in those fed fish oil (8). Such protection may have been due to the the way hormones called prostaglandins are synthesized in the body (9).

In addition, Harvard University scientists found that fish oil might reduce the severity of an autoimmune disease called glomerulonephritis (characterized by inflammation of the kidneys). Symptoms of this disease decreased in several strains of mice after feeding them fish oil. Similar protection was seen in a blood vessel disease called immune-complex induced vasculopathy. Such supplements "are potential therapeutic agents for the treatment of autoimmune diseases," the scientists wrote. They called for "careful clinical trials" (10).

⊕ References

1.   O'Connor TP, et al. Effect of dietary intake of fish oil and fish protein on the development of L-azaserine-induced preneoplastic lesions in the rat pancreas. J Natl Cancer Inst.1985;75:959-62.

2.   Kaizer L, et al. Fish consumption and breast cancer risk: an ecological study. Nutrition and Cancer.1989;12:61-68.

3.   Deschner EE, et al. The effect of dietary omega-3 fatty acids (fish oil) on azoxymethanol-induced focal areas of dysplasia and colon tumor incidence. Cancer.1990;66:2350-6.

4.   Gabor H, et al. Effect of dietary fat and monoclonal antibody therapy on the growth of human mammary adenocarcinoma MX-1 grafted in athymic mice. Cancer Lett.1990;52:173-8.

5.   Sakaguchi M, et al. Reduced tumour growth of the human colonic cancer cell lines COLO-320 and HT-29 in vivo by dietary n-3 lipids. Br J Cancer.1990;62:742-7.

6.   Tisdale M and Dhesi JK. Inhibition of weight loss by omega-3 fatty acids in an experimental cachexia model. Cancer Res.1990;50:5022-6.

7.   Yam D, et al. Insulin-tumour interrelationships in EL4-lymphoma or thymoma-bearing mice. II. Effects of dietary omega-3 and omega-6 polyunsaturated fatty acids. Br J Cancer.1990;62:897-902.

8.   Lindner MA. A fish oil diet inhibits colon cancer in mice. Nutr Cancer.1991;15:1-11.

9.   Reddy BS, et al. Effect of diets high in omega-3 and omega-6 fatty acids on initiation and postinitiation stages of colon carcinogenesis. Cancer Res.1991;51:487-91.

10.   Robinson DR. Alleviation of autoimmune disease by dietary lipids containing omega-3 fatty acids. Rheum Dis Clin North Am.1991;17: 213-22.

❦*I*NDOLES

....

Cabbages against cancer? A few years ago, that would have sounded like the height of quackery. Today, it is the official doctrine of cancer institutions around the world. The presence of cabbage, and related vegetables, in the diet have been definitively shown to enhance a particular system of enzymes that detoxify cancer-causing substances.

The roots of this 'breakthrough' are to be found in traditional folklore. Two thousand years ago, Pliny, the Roman naturalist, wrote in his *Natural History* (Book xx):

"It would be a long task to make a list of all the praises of the cabbage." Among its many uses was as a treatment for "cancerous sores, which can be healed by no other treatment."

Cabbage can increase the rate at which the body disposes of toxic drugs and carcinogens and has an effect on tumors caused by chemicals, as well. In the test tube cabbage stops mutations in bacteria. It also has a protective effect against radiation (1).

Indole glycosinate is the scientific name for a protective chemical found in cabbage, broccoli, cauliflower, and brussels sprouts. It has been shown experimentally to prevent stomach and colon cancer. In animal studies, indole derivatives have prevented precancers of the stomach as well as of the breast. They have also increased the activity of important enzymes involved in detoxification.

Whenever possible, one should eat these "cruciferous" vegetables raw. About half the indole derivatives are lost in cooking, according to *Science News* (11/25/89).

Eating raw or lightly cooked cabbage converts the hormone estrogen into its inactive form. And since estrogen can fuel the development of breast tumors, cruciferous vegetables might lower the risk of breast cancer. This may be one reason Asian women, who eat more cabbage, have so much less breast cancer than Western women.

"This may be the link between diet and protection against breast cancer,"

---

according to Christopher Longcope, of the University of Massachusetts Medical School in Wooster (*Science News*, 6/16/90.).

Brussels sprouts may also be used to help prevent, and even treat, breast cancer. Only 13 percent of rats fed a diet containing 20 percent brussels sprouts (during the initiation phase of cancer formation) developed breast tumors, compared to 77 percent of those fed a diet based on protein and starch. When the mice receiving protein and starch were then switched to brussels sprouts "there appeared to be a regression of small mammary tumors after six weeks," Cornell University scientists reported (2).

Indoles also activate a beneficial enzyme system that decreases a harmful female sex hormone. An excess of this hormone has been has been linked to an increased risk of breast cancer. Rockefeller University scientists showed that indoles were "most potent" in breaking down harmful hormones. People were then given indoles daily for a week. The results were again highly positive and indicated that indoles "strongly influence estradiol [sex hormone] metabolism in humans" and may provide a new way to control types of cancer that are dependent on female sex hormones, such as hormone-dependent breast cancer (3).

Since there is a strong association between estrogen metabolism and the incidence of breast cancer, the Rockefeller scientists also fed indoles, obtained from cruciferous vegetables such as cabbage and broccoli, to 12 healthy human volunteers for 7 days. Using three very sensitive tests, they found a decrease in harmful hormones by 50 percent during this short time of exposure. These results indicate that this compound "may provide a novel 'dietary' means for reducing cancer risk," they wrote in 1991 (4).

German scientists have modified indoles to make them into anticancer drugs. Because these substances are anti-estrogens they might find particular application in the treatment of hormone-dependent tumors, such as those of the prostate. Two such substances called "phenylindoles" were tested for their prostatic tumor-inhibiting activity. Both "exerted a strong inhibitory effect" on the weight of prostates. This effect was comparable to a standard drug, the synthetic hormone DES (diethylstilbestrol). Their tumor-inhibiting activity on prostate cancer in animals "equals that of castration" (a conventional treatment for this kind of cancer) or of DES. They "may also have low side-effects, and can therefore be of interest for the therapy of the prostatic carcinoma," University of Regensburg scientists wrote (5).

In March, 1992, a front-page story in the *New York Times* announced the discovery of a "potent anticancer compound" in broccoli. The chemical is called sulphoraphane and, according to scientists at Johns Hopkins medical school, may be the most powerful anticancer compound ever detected.

"We're very excited about this," said Prof. Paul Talalay, "and we don't excite easily."

Sulphoraphane greatly increased anticancer enzyme systems in cells, particularly one called quinone reductase. The compound is also found in other cruciferous vegetables, such as brussels sprouts, cauliflower and kale, and in such non-cruciferous vegetables as carrots and green onions. It is not destroyed by microwaving or steaming. The Johns Hopkins research was published in the March 15, 1992 issue of the *Proceedings of the National Academy of Sciences* (6,7).

⊕ References

1. Albert PM. Physiological effects of cabbage with reference to its potential as a dietary cancer-inhibitor and its use in ancient medicine. J Ethnopharmacol.1983;9:261-72.

2. Stoewsand GS, et al. Protective effect of dietary brussels sprouts against mammary carcinogenesis in Sprague-Dawley rats. Cancer Lett.1988;39:199-207.

3. Michnovicz JJ and Bradlow HL. Induction of estradiol metabolism by dietary indole-3-carbinol in humans. J Natl Cancer Inst.1990;82:947-9.

4.   Michnovicz JJ and Bradlow HL. Altered estrogen metabolism and excretion in humans following consumption of indole-3-carbinol. Nutr Cancer.1991;16:59-66.

5.   Schneider MR, et al. Antitumor activity of antiestrogenic phenylindoles on experimental prostate tumors. Eur J Cancer Clin Oncol.1987; 23:1005-15.

6.   Zhang Y, et al. A major inducer of anticarcinogenic protective enzymes from broccoli: isolation and elucidation of structure. Proc Natl Acad Sci USA.1992;89:2399-403.

7.   Prochaska HJ, et al. Rapid detection of inducers of enzymes that protect against carcinogens. Proc Natl Acad Sci USA.1992;89:2394-8.

℣ LACTOBACILLI

Lactobacilli are yeast that are often found in yogurt and other cultured milk products. Two of the most common are L. acidophilus and L. bulgaricus. These have healthful effects on the body, particularly in maintaining a healthy gut, and may also have beneficial effects in cancer.

Studies at Tufts University have shown that feeding supplements of L. acidophilus "significantly lowered" the activity of harmful fecal products in meat-eating animals (1). In addition, L. acidophilus caused a significant drop in dangerous bacterial enzymes, according to a report in the *American Journal of Clinical Nutrition*. Twenty-one people were tested for three bacterial enzymes in feces that can make certain chemicals carcinogenic. Subjects were given either plain milk or milk with live L. acidophilus cultures. There was a two-to-fourfold reduction in the activities of the three enzymes when L. acidophilus was given. "These changes were noted in all subjects and were highly significant," the Tufts scientists said. When lactobacilli feedings stopped, fecal enzyme levels returned to their usual levels in about a month (2).

The University of Nebraska at Lincoln is a center of lactobacillus studies. Three strains of L. acidophilus were isolated from the feces of mature boars. One strain caused the greatest reduction in cholesterol and inhibited various bacteria. Acidophilus yogurt reduced serum cholesterol and harmful low density lipoproteins (called LDL) (3, 4).

The rate of tumor growth was slowed by almost 75 percent in groups of mice that were fed yogurt containing live bacterial cultures, Dr. Khem Shahani, MD, of the University of Nebraska, told the Second Symposium on Lactic Acid Bacteria–Genetics, Metabolism and Applications, in Wageningen, Netherlands, September 22–25, 1987. However, yogurt feedings did not decrease death rates. Dr. Shahani has been quoted as saying that there is no doubt in his mind that "yogurt positively influences immune function."

Animal studies have also shown that feeding mice live cultures results in significant improvement in immune function. Normal indicators of immunity, such as white blood cell activity, have all been found to increase with yogurt feedings, according to the Proceedings of the Fermented Milks–Current Research, International Symposium, held in Paris, France, December, 1989.

In addition, colon cancer has been linked to conversion in the intestines of what are called primary bile acids into secondary bile acids. This conversion takes place by bacterial action. The presence of L. acidophilus was found to reduce this conversion process. The researchers suggested that the presence of L. acidophilus in the intestines may potentially reduce the onset of colon cancer.

Scientists at Tufts–New England Medical Center in Boston studied why the high-beef, high-fat, low fiber diet typical of Western societies is associated with a high risk of colon cancer. Theorizing that the intestinal microflora may play a role by metabolizing "procarcinogens" in the gut, they studied enzymes produced by fecal bacteria of people who eat a high-beef diet. These enzyme activities, they reported, can be reduced by the addition of L. acidophilus to the diet. In experimental animals, adding L. acidophilus reduced the number of colon tumors, even when the animals were given a potent carcinogen (5).

In Bulgaria, scientists have long been studying the effects of Lactobacillus bulgaricus used in making world-famous Bulgarian yogurt. Ivan Bogdanov, MD, has been researching the anticancer activity of a substance he calls Anabol in the treatment of cancer. This is derived from the LB-51 strain of L. acidophilus (6). A 1982 booklet contained the case histories of 100 advanced cancer patients who reportedly did very well on this substance. Anabol is taken orally, ten grams a day.

In a 1977 scientific paper, Bogdanov refers to the anti-tumor activity of a substance called "blastolysin," prepared from fragments of the cell wall of L. bulgaricus. Blastolysin was found to exert an anticancer effect on several experimental systems, including sarcoma, leukemia, melano-sarcoma and spontaneous tumors in mice. It is of "low toxicity," does not harm the bone marrow and appears to act quite different from standard drugs (7).

A Japanese scientist has found that another kind of Lactobacillus commonly found in milk and cheese (L. casei) "strongly inhibits" the growth of tumors in mice, in combination with standard anti-cancer drugs such as cyclophosphamide, mitomycin C, 5-fluorouracil (5-FU) and bleomycin. The combination of this Lactobacillus from cheese with cyclophosphamide "significantly prolonged the life span" of leukemic mice, but had no effect by itself (8).

It also stimulated the release of "cytostatic factors" from macrophages (scavenger cells). A number of other immune stimulants had the same effect. This sort of nutritional factor may play an important role in the release of cancer-stopping factors by activated macrophages (9).

There are "wide-ranging differences" in the anticancer activities of different strains of lactobacilli, however. Out of 23 samples, a strain called LC 9018 was found to have the strongest activities. A key indicator of anticancer activity was still elevated a day after the injection of this particular strain. Macrophages at the site of injection were held responsible for the anticancer effect. This strain could also help make bone marrow cells mature to macrophages and other kinds of white blood cells after one week.

"These matured macrophages showed strong antitumor activity."

Treatment with the LC 9018 strain serves to nurture the white blood cell system and has a potent effect on tumor cells (10).

Another culture isolated from a fermented milk product called dahi was found to be significantly toxic to cancer cells. The cell-killing substance was a protein. By refining this relatively crude product, scientists were able to get various fractions that destroyed up to 94 percent of the cancer cells in the test tube. Then, by pooling the various refined fractions, Indian scientists got even higher cell kill, showing that these various individual fractions had a "synergistic effect" with one another. The fractions, which were stable even in the presence of heat or acid, inhibited DNA synthesis in the tumor cells (11).

⊕ References

1.   Goldin B and Gorbach SL. Alterations in fecal microflora enzymes related to diet, age, lactobacillus supplements, and dimethylhydrazine. Cancer.1977;40:2421-6.

2.   Goldin BR and Gorbach SL. The effect of milk and lactobacillus feeding on human intestinal bacterial enzyme activity. Am J Clin Nutr.1984; 39:756-61.

3.   Pollmann DS, et al. Influence of Lactobacillus acidophilus inoculum on gnotobiotic and conventional pigs. J Anim Sci.1980;51:629-37.

4.   Danielson AD, et al. Anticholesteremic property of Lactobacillus acidophilus yogurt fed to mature boars. J Anim Sci.1989;67:966-74.

5.   Gorbach S. The intestinal microflora and its colon cancer connection. Infection (W Germany).1982;10:379-384.

6.   Bogdanov IG, et al. Antitumour glycopepetides from Lactobacillus bulgaricus cell wall. Febs Lett.1975;57:259-61.

7.   Bogdanov IG, et al. [Antitumor effect of glycopeptides from the cell wall of Lactobacillus bulgaricus]. Biull Eksp Biol Med.1977;84:709-12.

8.   Matsuzaki T, et al. [Augmentation of antitumor activity of Lactobacillus casei YIT 8018 (LC 9018) in combination with various antitumor drugs]. Gan To Kagaku Ryoho.1984;11:445-51.

9.   Hashimoto S, et al. In vitro and in vivo release of cytostatic factors from Lactobacillus casei-elicited peritoneal macrophages after stimulation with tumor cells and immunostimulants. Cancer Immunol Immunother.1987;24:1-7.

10.   Shimizu T, et al. Role of colony-stimulating activity in antitumor activity of Lactobacillus casei in mice. J Leukoc Biol.1987;42:204-12.

11.   Manjunath N and Ranganathan B. A cytotoxic substance produced by a wild culture of Lactobacillus casei D-34 against tumour cells. Indian J Exp Biol.1989;27:141-5.

⚘ LINSEED OIL

The substances that give fats their various flavors, melting points and textures are called "fatty acids." There are two kinds, saturated and unsaturated. The saturated—such as lard, suet, coconut oil and margarine—remain solid at room temperature. Unsaturated oils are liquids at room temperature. These are derived from vegetable sources and are generally more healthful.

There are three essential fatty acids (EFAs): linolenic, arachidonic and linoleic acids. (Collectively, these are sometimes known as vitamin F.) Since the body can make the first two if it has a sufficient supply of the latter, linoleic acid can be considered the quintessential fat for the human body.

Of all the sources of linoleic and other essential fatty acids, flaxseed oil appears to be the best. Flaxseed oil is not just rich in EFAs, but in B vitamins, protein and zinc. The "lin" in linoleic and linolenic tells us that flaxseed oil is isolated from *Linum usitatissimum,* or linseed, another name for flax. "Usitatissimum" means "most useful." Indeed, this plant has been extremely useful since ancient times as the source of linen, as well as for its deep amber oil. Even the meal left over after the oil has been expressed is fed to livestock. And, of course, the oil in most "oil paintings" is linseed.

Linseed oil has also been used in traditional Indian medicine as a stool softener, enema and skin treatment.

Orthodox medicine agrees that linoleic acid is essential and should provide at least two percent of the calories in the normal diet (three percent for babies). But it generally holds that any fatty acid deficiency is "unlikely to occur on natural diets" (1). There is even some concern that too much linoleic acid could be dangerous. Diets high in linoleic acid are said to increase cancer risk because they generate oxidizing free radicals (*Science News,* 5/21/88 and 2/15/92).

Not everyone agrees that linoleic acid is dangerous or that we even get enough of this essential component. In Central Europe, some people prize linseed's health-giving properties. Cold-pressed, virgin, unrefined raw linseed oil is more popular there. This product has now become available in US health food stores. Unrefined, it must be refrigerated after opening and only lasts about three months before turning rancid. Consumers have been advised to seek linseed oil with all the solid fats and fatty acids included.

Now, it is a well-known fact that cancer rarely develops in the small intestines. There are various explanations for this odd phenomenon. UCLA radiologists isolated a component of the intestinal lining of mice that seemed to be responsible for stopping such growths in experimental animals. Tests indicated that this substance was linoleic acid, present in the gut in "a surprisingly high concentration." Linoleic acid "was probably the major component responsible for the antitumor activity."

In further tests, using the water-soluble form of the acid called sodium linoleate, they found that it preferentially killed leukemia cells. A single injection of 1 milligram of sodium linoleate increased survival from 18 days to 48 days in mice. It also "prevented tumor growth completely in over 40 percent of the treated mice." These results indicate that linoleic acid probably keeps the small intestine from developing cancer. It also suggests, they said, "a potential role for sodium linoleate in cancer therapy" (2).

South African veterinarians used linoleic acid, together with a related compound, GLA, and vitamin E to treat two dogs with lymphoma. The dose was 40 milligrams of GLA, 350 milligrams of linoleic acid and 10 milligrams of natural vitamin E. After just one week, there was "slight to marked reduction in size of enlarged peripheral lymph nodes, spleen, skin nodules and tonsils." Both animals improved, but then deteriorated "due to complications, apparently unrelated to therapy" (3).

At Nagoya City University in Japan, scientists fed mice a related substance, "alpha linolenate." Spontaneous breast cancers were "significantly inhibited" in the animals that received alpha linolenate, but little difference was seen in the rates of lung metastasis (4).

While women are cautioned to avoid fat because it promotes breast cancer, scientists at the University of Wales cautioned that the quality of fat could be more important than quantity. Cardiff researchers gave mice dietary supplements of essential fatty acids in the form of evening primrose oil and fish oil. Olive oil as well as normal laboratory chow lacking the essential fatty acids served as the controls.

"Animals treated with essential fatty acids developed tumors which were significantly smaller" than in olive oil and regular lab chow control groups. Average tumor weights were as follows:

Type of oil received	Median weight of tumor
Fish oil	70 mg
Evening primrose oil	133 mg
Olive oil	212 mg
No EFAs (control group)	270 mg

The UK scientists concluded:

"Nutritional intervention to increase the proportion of essential fatty acids in the diet may have a role in the management of breast carcinoma" (5).

Like something out of a Woody Allen movie, scientists at University of Wisconsin–Madison have found a powerful anticancer substance in that well-known health food, "fried ground beef." This same substance was later found in milk products, including Cheese Whiz (*Science News*, 2/11/89). The agent in question is a potent free radical scavenger, with strong anticancer effects. They call it CLA (or conjugated linoleic acid). CLA is technically a long-chain, carbon-based molecule which:

• stops bacteria from mutating;

• prevents the formation of cancer in mice; and

• reduces by half the development of warts (6).

"In three independent experiments, mice treated with CLA developed only about half as many" cancers per animal as mice in the control groups, said Dr. Y. L. Ha. CLA was a more potent antioxidant than vitamin E (7). CLA, says Dr. Pariza, is "more powerful than any other fatty acids or dietary fat...in modulating tumor development." For example, CLA inhibits not just the development of malignant breast tumors, but of benign tumors as well (*Science News*, 2/15/92). Research is continuing into this promising substance (8-10).

Flaxseed oil may also be more healthful in some cases than fish oil. In a 1990 study at the University of Illinois, mice were given oil from corn, fish or flax before receiving injections of breast cancer cells. Flax oil but not fish oil reduced the growth of breast cancers and metastases, compared to the growth in those which received the corn oil. "Tumor growth was only inhibited by linseed oil," the Urbana-Champaign scientists said (11).

⊕ References

1.   Berkow R. The Merck manual of diagnosis and therapy (15th ed.). Rahway, NJ: Merck & Co., 1987, p. 2696.

2.   Norman A, et al. Antitumor activity of sodium linoleate. Nutr Cancer.1988;11:107-15.

3.   Williams JH. The use of gamma linolenic acid, linoleic acid and natural vitamin E for the treatment of multicentric lymphoma in two dogs. J S Afr Vet Assoc.1988;59:141-4.

4.   Kamano K, et al. Effects of a high-linoleate and a high-alpha-linolenate diet on spontaneous mammary tumourigenesis in mice. Anticancer Res.1989;9:1903-8.

5.   Pritchard GA, et al. Lipids in breast carcinogenesis [see comments]. Br J Surg.1989;76:1069-73.

6.   Ha YL, et al. Anticarcinogens from fried ground beef: heat-altered derivatives of linoleic acid. Carcinogenesis.1987;8:1881-7.

7.   Ha YL, et al. Inhibition of benzo(a)pyrene-induced mouse forestomach neoplasia by conjugated dienoic derivatives of linoleic acid. Cancer Res.1990;50:1097-101.

8.   Pariza MW and Ha YL. Conjugated dienoic derivatives of linoleic acid: a new class of anticarcinogens. Med Oncol Tumor Pharmacother. 1990;7:169-71.

9.   Pariza MW and Ha YL. Newly recognized anticarcinogenic fatty acids. Basic Life Sci.1990;52:167-70.

10.   Pariza MW, et al. Formation and action of anticarcinogenic fatty acids. Adv Exp Med Biol.1991;289:269-72.

11.   Fritsche KL and Johnston PV. Effect of dietary alpha-linolenic acid on growth, metastasis, fatty acid profile and prostaglandin production of two murine mammary adenocarcinomas. J Nutr.1990;120:1601-9.

⚘☙MUSHROOMS

Mushrooms first appeared on this earth about 100 million years ago, growing on trees in the mountainous regions of Asia. The ancient Chinese used a mushroom broth to treat many ailments. And, in fact, mushrooms decrease the blood pressure and cholesterol level (11).

During the Ming Dynasty of China (1368–1644 AD), the herbalist, Wu Ming, called the shiitake (black forest) mushroom the "elixir of life."

A wide variety of mushrooms, and mushroom-derived products, are still in use in China, Japan and other countries for their health-giving effects. In China over 270 species of mushrooms are believed to have medicinal properties and 50 of those are thought to have antitumor effects. There is an emerging body of scientific evidence to back up traditional claims for the virtues of such exotic food items. One of these is the maitake mushroom.

Maitake means "dancing mushroom," from the fact that people in northeastern Japan are said to dance for joy when they find one of these football-sized beauties. Legend also has it that wild monkeys, which seek out maitake mushrooms, never get high blood pressure or cancer. At a public meeting in New York on January 29, 1992, a Japanese company introduced a unique anticancer agent to America. Their product is a powder made from the rare maitake mushroom (*Grifola frondosa*) of northeastern Japan.

For years, Japanese scientists have been studying the medical properties of fungi in general and maitake in particular, according to Paul Yamasaki, a spokesperson for the company.

Extensive scientific work has been done mainly in Japan on the health benefits of these mushrooms. Maitake mushrooms in particular have been the object of intense scrutiny since the mid-1980s (1-17). Various derivatives, usually naturally occurring glucans or polysaccharides, have also been extracted and studied:

• Maitake is very effective in stopping the growth of tumors in a variety of animal systems. In a 1989 report, scientists found that feeding mice maitake powder one month after tumors had been implanted inhibited tumor growth by a remarkable 86.3 percent. Four of the ten mice were totally cured. These mice were given 20 percent of their diet in the form of mushroom powder—obviously an impractical amount. But other tests showed that much smaller doses either ingested or injected were also effective.

• Mice with Sarcoma 180 responded to small oral doses, as well. A tiny amount of the extract (1.5 milligrams) in the mice's diet inhibited cancer growth by 69 percent. Ten days of injecting one milligram of the extract also caused over

86 percent inhibition.

• Maitake did not kill cancer cells in the test tube, but worked by stimulating the immune system. It enhanced natural killer (NK) cells, increased the release of natural interleukin-1 and stimulated cytotoxic T-cells.

• Maitake also reduced high blood pressure in hypertensive rats (18).

These results were presented to NCI in 1991. Internal NCI documents show that, in their tests, maitake inhibited the growth of the HIV virus at about the same rate as the toxic drug, AZT. For reasons of its own, NCI chose to first "sulfate" maitake extract, however, rendering it toxic.

This is the fourth Japanese mushroom product to come to market since the early 1980s.

The first was PSK, one of the most widely-used drugs in the world, which has, however, never been made available in the US due to the difficulty of complying with FDA regulations.

The second was Lentinan, a shiitake extract, marketed by the giant food company, Ajinomoto. It is approved in Japan for treatment of stomach cancer.

The third is reishi (*Ganoderma lucidum*), currently available in US health food stores. It is said to have been used as a "fountain of youth" elixir for centuries. A novel protein with immunomodulating activity *in vivo* has been isolated from the mycelial extract of reishi.

Because it is called ling zhi in Chinese, the scientists called this protein ling zhi-8 (LZ-8) (28). And Prof. H. Maruyama called the antitumor activity of a water extract of reishi as well as two other mushrooms "remarkably effective for inhibition of tumor growth" (29).

But why not just *eat* maitake and other exotic mushrooms, instead of buying an expensive pill? Maybe some day fresh imported maitake will be available in Western markets. At present they are rare even in Japan and only grow in carefully-controlled environments. Paul Yamasaki succeeded in growing one football-sized maitake in his backyard, but only after six attempts, and a cost in supplies of over $100.

There have been anecdotal reports of cancer patients getting well after taking maitake powder. Clinical trials may soon get underway in Britain and Sweden, where, Yamasaki says, there is more freedom of choice than either in the US or in Japan. AIDS activists are also beginning to conduct human trials in New York City.

A variety of promising constituents of maitake and other mushrooms are being vigorously investigated in the laboratory.

For example, beta-glucan, a constituent of mushrooms, showed antitumor activity, as well as such effects on the immune system as activation of the alternative complement pathway, glucose consumption by macrophages, macrophage-mediated lysosomal enzyme activity, and interleukin-1 (IL-1) activity (17).

Scientists have isolated a lectin called GFL from the fruiting bodies of maitake. (A lectin is a protein of plant origin that resembles but is not an antibody.) This newly-discovered mushroom lectin was toxic against a kind of cancer cell widely used in experiments (19).

GF-1 is a polysaccharide from cultured fruiting bodies of maitake. It has "marked inhibitory activity" against the growth of sarcoma. A "significant antitumor activity" was also observed when GF-1 was injected on a staggered schedule or just once a week. GF-1 inhibited over 90 percent of the growth. However, oral administration was not effective. GF-1 also exhibited antitumor activity against some mouse fibrosarcomas and carcinomas (1).

Scientists studied another such glucan, LELFD, obtained from a cultured maitake broth. It too "exhibited significant antitumor effects." Two forms of leukemia were unaffected by LELFD. But like many immune system boosters, LELFD enhanced the activity of natural killer cells and macrophages in the mice. LELFD also enhanced the antibody response and activated a powerful immune system called complement (16).

Shiitake (*Lentinus edodes*) is another variety of mushroom that has yielded useful compounds, including the immune booster **lentinan.** Shiitake is highly nutritious: ounce for ounce it contains twice the protein and fiber of the typical supermarket mushroom; three times the minerals, especially **calcium**, phosphorus and iron; and high levels of the **B vitamins** and **vitamin D$_2$**. Shiitakes also contain natural chemicals called polysaccharides, other nutrients, as well as some odd virus-like particles, that inhibit the growth of various other diseases. Extracts of shiitake possess powerful anticancer and anti-infective properties (11,12,20-27).

Glucans: In 1981, Japanese scientists found antitumor activity in two glucans, natural chemicals isolated from the fruiting body of an edible mushroom called "kikurage" (Auricularia auricula-judae). A water-soluble, branched glucan called "glucan I" exhibited what the scientists called "potent, inhibitory activity" against implanted tumors in mice." Meanwhile, Glucan II showed potent antitumor activity only when it was chemically modified (30).

Grifolan: Yet another beta-glucan called "grifolan" had anticancer effects. Normally, when grifolan was injected into animals, it took days to exert any antitumor activity. But during these two days many immunological changes were seen, such as increased production of interleukin-1 (IL-1) and increased cell-killing ability. But scientists have found a way to reduce that waiting period (15).

Meanwhile, another group examined the antitumor mechanism of the grifolan dubbed NMF-5N. It did not show direct cell-killing effects on tumor cells in the test tube. However, injections of the compound increased the number of those immune cells (including T-cells), which then stopped the growth of tumor cells. In an animal study, scientists found that grifolan exerted its antitumor activity through host-mediated mechanisms and that both macrophages and T-cells play important roles in that mechanism (13).

L-glutamic acid, also called GHB, is a form of an amino acid. It is oxidized inside mushrooms into another chemical (a quinone) that inhibits cellular functions. Scientists have shown that GHB kills melanoma cells in culture. Chemotherapy drugs can be united with portions of the mushroom chemicals to make novel new compounds (33).

In 1979, Japanese scientists isolated a lectin from the mushroom, *Flammulina veltipes*. This lectin could induce the white blood cells in the mouse's spleen to undergo division (34). A few years later, they isolated several antitumor polysaccharides from the mushroom, One was a beta-glucan, similar to a lectin (35). Another was a polysaccharide called EA6 (36), deriving from the fruiting bodies of the mushroom (37). Yet another was called flammutoxin (38).

Antitumor activity of at least a dozen other Japanese mushrooms have been investigated (29-32).

Cryosurgery, a treatment that destroys tumors by freezing them, was "markedly augmented" by also injecting EA6, an extract of the enokidake mushroom. When freezing was combined with feeding the mushroom extract, prolonged survival of the mice was seen (36). It was not clear how the EA6 exerts its influence, since the immune system of the mice did not seem to be activated by the drug (39).

When EA6 was combined with a vaccine treatment, scientists found an intensification of the antitumor effect of both. Administration of EA6 prior to the injection of the vaccine, even with repeated injections, did not increase the life span of the animals. But when EA6 was given after the vaccine there was a "marked prolongation of the life span" by 223 percent (37).

Illudins are other "potent natural products derived from *Omphalotus illudins* and related fungi" (40). They were discovered by Japanese scientists in the 1960s (41). In 1990, scientists at the University of California reported that one of these, *Illudin S*, selectively and rapidly killed several different types of cancer cells. *Illudin S* has been shown to have a very different chemical structure from conventional chemotherapeutic drugs. It can kill some types of cancers with an exposure of as little as two hours. These tumor cells include myeloid leukemia as well as epidermoid, ovarian, lung, and breast carcinoma cells (40, 42, 43). Illudin's effectiveness seemed related to a unique mechanism that allows it to accumulate rapidly in relatively sensitive cells.

Mushrooms are eaten by millions with no untoward effects. But some people do experience allergic-type skin reaction to mushrooms, especially raw ones. In eight years, one team of doctors saw 30 patients with "toxicoderma" (skin disease) caused by eating mushrooms (44). Prolonged and intense exposure to shiitake spores can also be dangerous. Workers exposed to high levels of such spores have been known to develop an occupational disease known as mushroom workers' lung (45).

⊕ References

1.   Suzuki I, et al. Antitumor activity of a polysaccharide fraction extracted from cultured fruiting bodies of Grifola frondosa. J Pharmacobiodyn.1984;7:492-500.

2.   Ohno N, et al. Neutral and acidic antitumor polysaccharides extracted from cultured fruit bodies of Grifola frondosa. Chem Pharm Bull

(Tokyo).1985;33:1181-6.

3. Ohno N, et al. Structural characterization and antitumor activity of the extracts from matted mycelium of cultured Grifola frondosa. Chem Pharm Bull (Tokyo).1985;33:3395-401.

4. Suzuki I, et al. Effect of a polysaccharide fraction from Grifola frondosa on immune response in mice. J Pharmacobiodyn.1985;8:217-26.

5. Ohno N, et al. Effect of glucans on the antitumor activity of grifolan. Chem Pharm Bull (Tokyo).1986;34:2149-54.

6. Ohno N, et al. Characterization of the antitumor glucan obtained from liquid-cultured Grifola frondosa. Chem Pharm Bull (Tokyo). 1986;34:1709-15.

7. Ohno N, et al. Effect of activation or blockade of the phagocytic system on the antitumor activity of grifolan. Chem Pharm Bull (Tokyo). 1986;34:4377-81.

8. Ohno N, et al. Fractionation of acidic antitumor beta-glucan of Grifola frondosa by anion-exchange chromatography using urea solutions of low and high ionic strengths. Chem Pharm Bull (Tokyo).1986;34:3328-32.

9. Ohno N, et al. Two different confirmations of antitumor glucans obtained from Grifola frondosa. Chem Pharm Bull (Tokyo).1986;34:2555-60.

10. Adachi K, et al. Potentiation of host-mediated antitumor activity in mice by beta-glucan obtained from Grifola frondosa (maitake). Chem Pharm Bull (Tokyo).1987;35:262-70.

11. Kabir Y, et al. Effect of shiitake (Lentinus edodes) and maitake (Grifola frondosa) mushrooms on blood pressure and plasma lipids of spontaneously hypertensive rats. J Nutr Sci Vitaminol (Tokyo).1987;33:341-6.

12. Nanba H and Kuroda H. Antitumor mechanisms of orally administered shiitake fruit bodies. Chem Pharm Bull (Tokyo).1987;35:2459-64.

13. Takeyama T, et al. Host-mediated antitumor effect of grifolan NMF-5N, a polysaccharide obtained from Grifola frondosa. J Pharmacobiodyn.1987;10:644-51.

14. Hishida I, et al. Antitumor activity exhibited by orally administered extract from fruit body of Grifola frondosa (maitake). Chem Pharm Bull (Tokyo).1988;36:1819-27.

15. Nono I, et al. Modification of immunostimulating activities of grifolan by the treatment with (1–3)-beta-D-glucanase. J Pharmacobiodyn.1989; 12:671-80.

16. Suzuki I, et al. Antitumor and immunomodulating activities of a beta-glucan obtained from liquid-cultured Grifola frondosa. Chem Pharm Bull (Tokyo).1989;37:410-3.

17. Adachi Y, et al. Change of biological activities of (1–3)-beta-D-glucan from Grifola frondosa upon molecular weight reduction by heat treatment. Chem Pharm Bull (Tokyo).1990;38:477-81.

18. Adachi K, et al. Blood-pressure lowering activity present in the fruit

body of Grifola frondosa (Maitake). 1. Chem Pharm Bull.(Tokyo)1988;36.

19. Kawagishi H, et al. Isolation and characterization of a lectin from Grifola frondosa fruiting bodies. Biochem Biophys Acta.1990;1034:247-52.

20. Taguchi H and Iwai K. Characteristics of quinolinate phosphoribosyltransferase from the "Shiitake" mushroom (Lentinus edodes). J Nutr Sci Vitaminol (Tokyo).1974;20:283-91.

21. Taguchi H and Iwai K. Purification and properties of quinolinate phosphoribosyltransferase from the "Shiitake" mushroom (Lentinus edodes). J Nutr Sci Vitaminol (Tokyo).1974;20:269-81.

22. Takehara M, et al. Antiviral activity of virus-like particles from Lentinus edodes (Shiitake). Brief report. Arch Virol.1979;59:269-74.

23. Takehara M, et al. Antitumor effect of virus-like particles from Lentinus edodes (Shiitake) on Ehrlich ascites carcinoma in mice. Arch Virol.1981;68:297-301.

24. Takazawa H, et al. [An antifungal compound from "Shiitake" (Lentinus edodes)]. Yakugaku Zasshi.1982;102:489-91.

25. Takehara M, et al. Isolation and antiviral activities of the double-stranded RNA from Lentinus edodes (Shiitake). Kobe J Med Sci.1984; 30:25-34.

26. Hayakawa M and Kuzuya F. [Studies on platelet aggregation and cortinellus shiitake]. Nippon Ronen Igakkai Zasshi.1985;22:151-9.

27. Nanba H, et al. Antitumor action of shiitake (Lentinus edodes) fruit bodies orally administered to mice. Chem Pharm Bull (Tokyo). 1987;35:2453-8.

28. Kino K, et al. Isolation and characterization of a new immunomodulatory protein, ling zhi-8 (LZ-8), from Ganoderma lucidium. J Biol Chem.1989;264:472-8.

29. Maruyama H, et al. Antitumor activity of Sarcodon aspratus (Berk.) S. Ito and Ganoderma lucidum (Fr.) Karst. J Pharmacobiodyn. 1989;12:118-23.

30. Nishino H, et al. Studies on interrelation of structure and antitumor effects of polysaccharides: antitumor action of periodate-modified, branched (1–3)-beta-D-glucan of Auricularia auricula-judae, and other polysaccharides containing (1–3)-glycosidic linkages. Carbohydr. Res. 1981;92:115-29.

31. Sasaki T, et al. Antitumor polysaccharides from some polyporaceae, Ganoderma applantum (Pers.) Pat and Phellinus linteus (Berk. et Curt) Aoshima. Chem Pharm Bull (Tokyo).1971;19:4.

32. Ukai S, et al. Polysaccharides in fungi. XIII. Antitumor activity of various polysaccharides isolated from Dictyophora indusiata, Ganoderma japonicum, Cordyceps cicadae, Auricularia auricula-judae, and Auricularia species. Chem Pharm Bull (Tokyo).1983;31:741-4.

33. al Obeidi F, et al. Synthesis and actions of a melanotropin conjugate, Ac-[Nle4, Glu(gamma-4'-hydroxyanilide)5, D-Phe7]alpha-MSH4-10-NH2,

on melanocytes and melanoma cells in vitro. J Pharm Sci.1990;79:500-4.

34. Tsuda M. Purification and characterization of a lectin from the mushroom, Flammulina veltipes. J Biochem (Tokyo).1979;86:1463-8.

35. Ikekawa T, et al. Studies on antitumor polysaccharides of Flammulina velutipes (Curt. ex Fr.) Sing.II. The structure of EA3 and further purification of EA5. J Pharmacobiodyn.1982;5:576-81.

36. Ohkuma T, et al. Augmentation of antitumor activity by combined cryo-destruction of sarcoma 180 and protein-bound polysaccharide, EA6, isolated from Flammulina velutipes (Curt. ex Fr.) Sing. in ICR mice. J Pharmacobiodyn.1982;5:439-44.

37. Otagiri K, et al. Intensification of antitumor-immunity by protein-bound polysaccharide, EA6, derived from Flammulina velutipes (Curt. ex Fr.) Sing. combined with murine leukemia L1210 vaccine in animal experiments. J Pharmacobiodyn.1983;6:96-104.

38. Bernheimer AW and Oppenheim JD. Some properties of flammutoxin from the edible mushroom Flammulina velutipes. Toxicon.1987; 25:1145-52.

39. Ohkuma T, et al. Augmentation of host's immunity by combined cryodestruction of sarcoma 180 and administration of protein-bound polysaccharide, EA6, isolated from Flammulina velutipes (Curt. ex Fr.) Sing. in ICR mice. J Pharmacobiodyn.1983;6:88-95.

40. Kelner MJ, et al. Preclinical evaluation of illudins as anticancer agents: basis for selective cytotoxicity. J Natl Cancer Inst.1990;82:1562-5.

41. Matsumoto T, et al. Synthesis of illudins. I. Synthesis of the skeleton. Tetrahedron Lett.1967;42:4097-100.

42. Henderson C. Illudin S may have specific cytotoxicity (mushroom derivative drug). NCI Cancer Weekly 1990, 9-10.

43. Kelner MJ, et al. Preclinical evaluation of illudins as anticancer agents. Cancer Res.1987;47:3186-9.

44. Tarvainen K, et al. Allergy and toxicodermia from shiitake mushrooms. J Am Acad Dermatol.1991;24:64-6.

45. Nakamura T and Kobayashi A. [Toxicodermia caused by the edible mushroom shiitake (Lentinus edodes)]. Hautarzt.1985;36:591-3.

❦ $\int$EAWEED

Seaweed—more properly, sea vegetables—are edible plants that come from the ocean. Many Westerners have no taste for such aquatic plants. Even the word 'weed' in 'seaweed' reveals a bias. But marine plants can be a healthful and delicious source of nutrients as well as natural medicines.

Japanese scientists are investigating the anticancer potential of a dietary seaweed extract called "Viva Natural" (1). It has been found to contain a polysaccharide that has a positive effect on macrophage (scavenger) immune cells (2). Viva Natural is also active against lung cancer cells in mice as well as leukemia. It was found to be superior against lung cancer than the standard drug isoprinosine and this "demonstrated curative activity" in the mice.

Viva Natural also showed progress against leukemia, as did another natural substance called PTZ, an alkaloid from the narcissus plant. The activity of both was compared to standard chemotherapeutic drugs. PTZ proved superior to the toxic drug methotrexate. Mice with cancer that were given PTZ showed a 90 percent increase in survival while methotrexate-treated mice had only a 71 percent increase. Viva-Natural was also found to be the only immune system booster that was active against a common kind of leukemia. All the standard biological response modifiers were not active.

By combining either PTZ or Viva-Natural with standard drugs, Japanese scientists got better results than with either one alone. PTZ was even able to cause a complete remission of advanced leukemia (1).

Scientists also compared the effects of Viva Natural in fighting HIV infection with the standard drug AZT (azidothymidine), as well as two other substances. Mice pretreated with Viva Natural three days before inoculation with the Human Immunodeficiency Virus (HIV) showed preventative effects, while pretreatment with three other drugs showed no such effect. In the test tube, a leukemia virus could not grow and infect cells when Viva-Natural was present (3).

Dr. Jane Teas of the Harvard School of Public Health has been in the forefront of those studying the health benefits of sea vegetables. Noting that Japanese women have very low levels of breast cancer, in 1981, Teas suggested that marine vegetables (which are eaten widely in Japan) might function as a protector against breast cancer. They seem to be responsible for:

• reduction of plasma cholesterol;

• binding of biliary steroids (hormones);

• inhibition of carcinogenic bacteria in the stool;

• binding of pollutants;

• stimulation of the immune system; and

• the protective effects of beta-sitosterols.

In an experiment on sarcoma in mice, seaweed extract had definite antitumor effects.

Dr. Teas suggested that "breast cancer may be prevented and that this dietary habit among the Japanese could be an important factor in understanding the lower breast cancer rates reported in Japan" (4).

Two years later, Teas focused on a brown kelp called Laminaria. "Based on epidemiological and biological data," she said, this kelp appeared to contribute to the low breast cancer rates in Japan. Laminaria, she said serves as a source of nondigestible fiber in the diet, thereby increasing fecal bulk and decreasing bowel transit time; changes the metabolism of some hormones; contains an antibiotic that may influence bacteria in the gut; contains glucans, which alter enzymes in the bowel; and stimulates immunity. Teas suggested that Laminaria could play a role in preventing either the beginnings of breast cancer or its promotion (5,6).

As laboratory confirmation, Teas gave rats five percent Laminaria in their chow. About a month later, each rat received a carcinogen. The rats were then studied and weighed for the next half year. It was shown that the seaweed diet caused a significant delay in the time it took for the first tumor to appear. This happened at 19 weeks, compared to just 11 weeks in rats that did not receive the seaweed (7).

Another extract of brown sea algae called *Sargassum kjellmanianum* also has anticancer effects. It stopped the growth of sarcoma cells, but at first was not effective against mice with leukemia. Looking for a polysaccharide with antileukemia activity, scientists combined this algae with sulfur. The resulting compound, called sulfated SKCF, proved to be effective against leukemia. It stimulated the immune system, as do many other polysaccharides (8).

There was in addition a 13 percent reduction in the number of animals with breast cancer among those which received Laminaria. There are a number of possible explanations for this, among which is the presence of a chemical called fucoidan (7). Other scientists have found that a crude fucoidan extract is an **anticoagulant**, which might account for some of its anticancer activity (9).

Side Effects? Kombu is a widely available seaweed. It contains so much iodine that overindulgence (a daily intake of over 28 milligrams a day of iodine) can cause hyperthyroidism (from the iodine-induced disease, thyrotoxicosis). Two Japanese women, aged 42 and 59 years old, developed this condition one month and one year, respectively, after having eaten foods containing over 28 milligrams per day of iodine. All symptoms went away after the women stopped overusing kombu (10).

⊕ References

1.   Furusawa E and Furusawa S. Effect of pretazettine and viva-natural, a dietary seaweed extract, on spontaneous AKR leukemia in comparison with standard drugs. Oncology.1988;45:180-6.

2.   Sokoloff B. Anticancer potential of Viva-Natural, a dietary seaweed extract, on Lewis lung carcinoma in comparison with chemical immunomodulators and on cyclosporine-accelerated AKR leukemia. Oncology.1989;46:343-8.

3.   Furusawa E, et al. Antileukemic activity of Viva-Natural, a dietary seaweed extract, on Rauscher murine leukemia in comparison with anti-HIV agents, azidothymidine, dextran sulfate and pentosan polysulfate. Cancer Lett.1991;56:197-205.

4.   Teas J. The consumption of seaweed as a protective factor in the etiology of breast cancer. Med Hypotheses.1981;7:601-13.

5.   Yamamoto I, et al. Antitumor effect of seaweeds. I. Antitumor effect of extracts from Sargassum and Laminaria. Jpn J Exp Med.1974;44:543-6.

6.   Teas J. The dietary intake of Laminaria, a brown seaweed, and breast cancer prevention. Nutr Cancer.1983;4:217-22.

7.   Teas J, et al. Dietary seaweed (Laminaria) and mammary carcinogenesis in rats. Cancer Res.1984;44:2758-61.

8.   Yamamoto I, et al. Antitumor effect of seaweeds. IV. Enhancement of antitumor activity by sulfation of a crude fucoidan fraction from Sargassum kjellmanianum. Jpn J Exp Med.1984;54:143-51.

9.   Maruyama H, et al. A study on the anticoagulant and fibrinolytic activities of a crude fucoidan from the edible brown seaweed Laminaria religiosa, with special reference to its inhibitory effect on the growth of sarcoma-180 ascites cells subcutaneously implanted into mice. Kitasato Arch Exp Med.1987;60:105-21.

10. Ishizuki Y, et al. [Transient thyrotoxicosis induced by Japanese kombu]. Nippon Naibunpi Gakkai Zasshi.1989;65:91-8.

❧ SHARK CARTILAGE

Scientists have discovered a substance that fights cancer by interfering with the tumor's ability to create a network of new blood vessels. That substance is shark cartilage.

Tumors, like normal tissue, need blood to provide nutrients and oxygen and to get rid of toxic wastes. As tumors grow, they mobilize arteries, veins and capillaries (tiny blood vessels) in order to maintain a good supply of blood. Such growth is normally crucial for the development of embryos and for the healing processes. But cancer's capillary sprawl undermines health. Cut off a tumor's blood supply and you can cut off its growth. Any substance that could interfere with capillary growth, could be used to fight cancer, as well.

In the mid-1970s, Cambridge, MA scientists found that when a tumor cannot establish a new blood network, it cannot grow any larger than the point of a pencil. A tumor must have such a network to obtain nutrients and get rid of wastes. Tumors actually put out a substance which make capillaries (tiny blood vessels) grow.

In 1975, scientists showed that they could inhibit such capillary growth 75 percent using a form of cartilage. New blood vessel growth was prevented completely in 28 percent of the tumors. When a small amount of cartilage was implanted, it operated over a distance of up to two millimeters from the tumor. The experiments suggested that some inhibitor present in cartilage directly interfered with the growth of capillaries. They suggested this factor could prove useful in keeping tumors in check through a process they called "antiangiogenesis" (1,2).

In the following year, Dr. M. Judah Folkman and his group at Harvard Medical School found that this fraction contained several different proteins; the major one had a molecular weight of about 16,000, and it strongly inhibited the activity of protein-digesting enzymes (3).

Dr. Robert Langer, a professor at the Massachusetts Institute of Technology, followed this up by proposing the use of cartilage from the cow's shoulder blade. But Langer eventually came to believe that the shark was a better source since its skeleton contains an even more potent 'cartilage-derived inhibitor'. Powdered shark cartilage in a controlled-release pellet was shown to halt animals' tumor growth (4).

One logical way of obtaining this factor is by taking supplements of shark cartilage. Sharks have always puzzled marine biologists because they rarely get cancer, even when injected with large amounts of carcinogens. The reason has to do with the shark's all-cartilage skeleton, so unlike the calcium-based bone skeletons of most creatures. In fact, in 1977, scientists isolated two factors in the hammerhead shark that inhibited the growth of cancer (5).

In 1980, Folkman announced that vessel formation and tumor growth could be inhibited by an infusion of cartilage extract. In rabbits, the new vessel growth rate was just 3 percent that of animals receiving inert substances. The melanoma of mice receiving cartilage weighed less than 2.5 percent those of mice that only received an inert solution.

A Belgian chemotherapist, Dr. Ghanem Atassi, wrote that since new vessel growth is so clearly essential for metastases, it seems equally obvious that stopping new vessel growth might be a way to prevent the formation of secondary growths. Atassi urged the use of substances like shark cartilage as a novel form of cancer therapy, since (like other forms of cartilage) it contained natural inhibitors to the development of new tumor blood vessels.

In 1989, I. William Lane, PhD arranged for Dr. Atassi to perform tests of this theory at Belgium's Institute Jules

Bordet. Lane is a former vice president of the W. R. Grace chemical company and an international consultant on marine biology.

Atassi first injected human melanoma cells under the skin of 'nude mice,' an immune deficient animal which accepts grafts of human tissue. Two days later, half the mice were fed shark cartilage. After 21 days, the tumors in the control group had increased 2.4 times and were growing exponentially. All cancer growth in this group took place in the final seven days of the experiment, supporting the theory that tumor growth depends on the establishment of a new blood network. But in the cartilage-treated group the melanoma grafts shrank on average 35 percent.

Lane is now marketing a shark powder as a food supplement called Cartilade®. He says there are no harmful side effects and compares the product's safety to eating shark fin soup, a Chinese delicacy long reputed to have health benefits. He adds that "shark cartilage can be used along with any other type of therapy." In 1991, Lane was awarded a US patent for his method of using shark cartilage powder to inhibit angiogenesis. Lane's involvement with testing and marketing shark cartilage is outlined in his popular book, *Sharks Don't Get Cancer* (Garden City Park: Avery, 1992).

Other such substances are also on the way. Repligen Corporation, of Cambridge, MA has shown that a protein normally found in blood can also block new vessels that form in cancer. The company's drug is called Endostatin B. It is said to have potential in treating cancer, diabetes and glaucoma as well as other diseases. According to Dr. Walter Herlihy, Jr., director of research at Repligen, this work provides "a potential new therapy for solid tumors." The first use for Endostatin B will be for Kaposi's sarcoma, a skin cancer frequently associated with AIDS. Repligen's scientific director says, "The ultimate goal of our program will be to develop an Endostatin B treatment for all diseases" in which blood vessel growth plays a central role. The company expects Endostatin B to have low toxicity in people (*NCI Cancer Weekly,* 1/22/90).

Microscopic studies of the major organs as well as standard blood tests "revealed no toxic effects in any of the animals" from the use of shark cartilage. It was found that a capillary inhibitor did not retard the growth of tumor cells in the test tube, even at very high concentrations. "These results suggest that the cartilage factor does not interfere with the growth of the tumor cell population directly," Cambridge scientists said, but simply prevented tumor growth by slowing the formation of new blood vessels (4).

⊕ References

1. Brem H and Folkman J. Inhibition of tumor angiogenesis mediated by cartilage. J Exp Med.1975;141:427-39.
2. Folkman J. The vascularization of tumors. Sci Am.1976;234:58-64.
3. Langer R, et al. Isolations of a cartilage factor that inhibits tumor neovascularization. Science.1976;193:70-2.
4. Langer R, et al. Control of tumor growth in animals by infusion of an angiogenesis inhibitor. Proc Natl Acad Sci USA.1980;77:4331-5.
5. Pettit GR and Ode RH. Antineoplastic agents L: isolation and characterization of sphyrnastatins 1 and 2 from the hammerhead shark Sphyrna lewini. J Pharm Sci.1977;66:757-8.

☀ Resources

Algae: Along with its commercial archrival Spirulina, Chlorella was once widely available. But on October 5, 1991, the FDA imposed an import ban on Sun® Chlorella. At this writing, the US consumer's ability to get this non-toxic treatment remains in doubt. The FDA has also banned the importation of Mexican Spirulina, allegedly because of mercury toxicity. Since mercury-contaminated spirulina is still being smuggled into the US, one must carefully investigate the source. The Microalgae International Sales Corp (Light Force Co.) makes Spirulina from Israel and Palm

Springs, CA, both of which it claims are certified free of mercury.

Canthaxanthin is available in ten percent spray-dried beadlets from Wholesale Nutrition, PO Box 3345, Saratoga, CA 95070-1345. Phone: 800-325-2664. The price for 100 grams is $19. The reader is cautioned that canthaxanthin is responsible for possibly dangerous changes in the eye.

Chlorophyll: Abundant in green vegetables. The sodium and copper salt of chlorophyll are available in tablet form from Life Extension Foundation. This pill, called Chloroplex,® is said to contain the same copper chlorophyllins used in the NIOSH study. It also contains other antioxidants. The price is $15.00 for 100, with a 25 percent discount to members of the Life Extension Foundation. Phone: 800-544-0577. A liquid chlorophyll is available in one ounce bottles for $7.50 from Tri-Sun North America (Jason Winter's Products), 109½ Broadway, Box 1606, Fargo, ND 58107. Phone: 800-447-0235 or 701-234-9654. Fax: 701-235-9762.

Coenzyme Q (CoQ10): Generally available in health food stores.

Evening Primrose Oil: Another substance that is periodically banned by the FDA. The company that pioneered the use of this substance is Efamol Research Institute, PO Box 818, Kentville, Nova Scotia, Canada, B4N4H8, Phone: 902-678-5534. Dr. David F. Horrobin, president. At the present time it is available in some health food stores but not through the above company, which can, however, help with information. Borage and black currant oils are alternative sources of GLAs.

Fiber: This is the part of the food that is not generally digested, such as the apple's skin or the wheat kernel's husk. There are seven forms of fiber: bran, cellulose, gums, hemicellulose, lignin, mucilages and pectin. Each conveys a different effect. In addition to naturally occurring fibers, there are numerous products that provide extra amounts of one or more of the above. Some over-the-counter sources are Effer-Syllium Natural Fiber Bulking Agent (J&J, Merck Consumer); Fiberall Fiber Wafers (CIBA Consumer); and Serutan Toasted Granules (Menley & James). Patients with at least one colon polyp can contact the University of Arizona, Phoenix. Phone: 602-264-4461. Scientists there are trying to recruit 950 people to study the effects of wheat bran fiber supplements in preventing new polyps from forming.

Fish oil: Fish that are high in omega-3 fatty acids generally live in the deep water. These include bluefish, herring, eels, halibut, lake trout, mackerel, salmon, sardines and tuna. One problem is that fish pick up and concentrate pollutants, including DDT, chlordane, aldrin and dieldrin. Mercury is particularly common in lake fish. The risk of bacterial and viral infection from fish is ten times greater than from beef and seven time that from chicken. While our instinct is to seek out the freshest fish some people believe it is now actually safer to purchase fish of known quality through the mail rather than risk the local catch. Some sources of mail order fish are Aquaculture Marketing Service, 356 W. Redview Dr., Monroe, UT 84754 Phone: 801-527-4528 and Mountain Ark Trading Company, Fayetteville, AR 72701. Phone: 800-643-8909. (See *The Catalogue of Healthy Food*.)

Linseed Oil: Many people give more thought to their motor oil than their eating and cooking oil. While most food oils do contain some linoleic acid, few contain the important linolenic acid, as well. For example, safflower oil is a good source of linoleic acid, but it has little or no linolenic acid. Only linseed, soybean, pumpkin and walnut oils contain both. And of the four, linseed derives the highest percentage (72 percent) of its total fat in essential fatty acids. It therefore seems like the logical choice as a good source of EFAs, with soybean oil an inexpensive runner-up.

A book, *How to Fight Cancer and Win*, claims that an EFA deficiency is the root cause of cancer. The book claims that a deficiency of EFA and of sulphur-based proteins leads to a lack of hemoglobin and an inability to make prostaglandins. The book suggests daily consumption of one to two tablespoon of virgin linseed oil with one-half to one cup of low-fat cottage cheese. Patients who take this mixture for several months are said to show a regression of cancer. BioSan C-Leinosan is the recommended brand. It is available through New Dimensions Distributors, Inc., 16548 E. Laser St., Bldg. A-7, Fountain Hills, AZ 85268, 1-800-624-7114, x14. The oil costs $8.95 for 8.5 ounces (ask about discounts). This book also recommends grinding one tablespoon of flaxseed mixed with honey and/or grape juice (honey is not recommended for diabetics). Cold-pressed linseed oil can also be purchased in most health food stores.

Mushrooms: For more information on maitake, contact Maitake Products, Inc., PO Box 1354, Paramus, NJ 07653. Phone: 800-747-7418 or 201-612-0097. The price is $30 for 60 caplets. Many patients take four per day.

Dried shiitake mushrooms are sold in most Asian markets. Price varies, from about 50¢ to $3.50 per ounce. Fresh shiitake mushrooms are available in some specialty markets. Enokidake, too, is edible and sometimes available in speciality markets. Nuherbs Co., 3820 Penniman Avenue, Oakland, CA 94619. Phone: 800-233-4307 sells Chinese mushroom preparations. Nuherb sells only to health professionals.

Health Concerns, 2236 Mariner Square Drive, Alameda CA 94501. Phone: 415-521-7401. They sell to the public, import Ganoderma (Reishi) mushrooms and incorporate them into formulas known as Astra 8® and Power Mushrooms®. Astra 8 also contains astragalus, eleuthero ginseng and licorice. "Power Mushrooms" include shiitake and polyporus. Send for catalogue. A source of Min Tong® reishi extract, in granulated form for a tea, is Tashi Enterprises, 3252 Ramona St., Pinole, CA 94564. Phone: 800-888-9998 (24 hours). Fax: 510-758-0223. Another source of red reishi is Organotech, 7960 Cagnon Road, San Antonio, TX 78252. Phone: 800-677-8419. Fax: 512-677-8190.

Seaweed: Various seaweeds are available in Asian and macrobiotic markets. Nori is used to wrap the fish and rice in sushi. It makes a high mineral, low calories snack. Kombu comes in thick strands, and is added to soups and stews. Cheaper in Asian markets. Some brands claim to be harvested from the less polluted waters of the Atlantic Northeast.

Shark Cartilage: Cartilade® stole a march on the competition and is now found in most health food stores and distributed by Allergy Research Group. Cost is $44 per 100 pills. Phone: 800-545-9960. Some patients take 30 to 40 capsules a day.

Another 100 percent shark cartilage pill is available from Futurebiotics, 48 Elliot St., Brattleboro, VT 05301. Phone: 800-367-5433.

Alkoxyglycerol is a popular Danish product derived from shark liver oil. In 1991, oncologists at Odense Hospital surveyed their cervical cancer patients and found that one-third were also using shark liver oil preparations. They found no sign of tumor growth inhibition or reduced death rate resulting from treatment. The oncologists therefore concluded that the data "does not support the employment of alkoxyglycerol in the treatment of cancer." However, they did report that "the number of cases of irradiation damage were found to be fewer in the groups treated with alkoxyglycerol." They also found that alkoxyglycerol resulted in an increase in white blood cells.

*L*ESS *T*OXIC *D*RUGS

Not all treatments for cancer fall neatly into non-toxic or toxic chemotherapy pigeonholes. There are over a dozen prescription and over-the-counter drugs that are now being also tested as experimental treatments for cancer. None of these is entirely without side effects or dangers. Some can even kill, if taken incorrectly or in excess.

By and large, however, they are no more dangerous than drugs prescribed to millions around the world every day. In fact, aspirin and Tagamet, two of the world's most popular drugs, are in this category. Others are more exotic, such as the enzyme-like substance derived from the eggs of a common North American frog. Taken together, these substances represent a repository of new ideas for cancer therapy.

*A*MYGDALIN

Amygdalin is a chemical found naturally in over 1,200 plants around the world. It is a glycoside, a category from which some of the most useful medicines—including aspirin—have been derived. Commercially, the most important sources of amygdalin are the kernels and seeds of members of the *Prunus* family, apricots, peaches and bitter almonds. (*Amygdale* means almond in Greek, but contrary to expectations, sweet almonds contain no amygdalin.)

These seeds, and especially bitter almonds, have a long

history in folk medicine. In China, for instance, the term 'xing ren' (generally translated as almond) actually refers to apricot kernels, which are a staple of traditional Chinese medicine. Since at least the Han dynasty (206 BC to 220 AD), apricot kernels have been used medically in China. They are currently an official drug in the pharmacopeia of the People's Republic of China. Kernels are used for coughs, excess phlegm, asthma and constipation. The daily internal dose ranges from 0.2 to 0.3 oz.

In the 1970s, amygdalin became a subject of controversy as bitter as the bitterest almond when it was widely marketed in the United States as a treatment for cancer called laetrile. From the standard medical community came emotional tirades against this substance and its use. From believers came charges of conspiracy and demands for freedom of choice in cancer therapy.

"The writings of laetrile proponents are filled with erroneous and absurd statements," said one professor. "The propaganda for the doctrine of 'freedom of choice in cancer treatment' deludes many individuals with treatable cancer to reject proven methods of treatment" (1). Others called this "the deadliest delusion" and ascribed such "quackery" to a "lack of faith in the medical care system." Even today, it is impossible to mention the word laetrile without engendering heated and usually fruitless arguments.

The controversy originated in the 1950s, when some doctors in San Francisco contended that an amygdalin-like substance could be used to prevent and treat cancer. They called this substance 'Laetrile,' which stood for 'laevo-rotatory nitriloside.' This Laetrile was their patented way of preparing amygdalin, so that when light was refracted through it, it turned only in a leftward ('laevo-') direction. By the time laetrile made the cover of *Newsweek*, however, it had lost both its capital letter and its uniqueness. In fact, for better or worse, most laetrile was nothing but plain

AMYGDALIN

amygdalin and the original 'Laetrile' has not been used or tested for decades. So, the debate was actually over plain amygdalin.

Laboratory work before 1972 focused on testing amygdalin in the usual transplantable tumor systems. With few exceptions (2), all such studies found amygdalin to be without value in the treatment of experimental cancer (3-5).

Nevertheless, anecdotes of amygdalin's pain-killing and tumor-regressing power continued to circulate. When scientists at Memorial Sloan-Kettering Cancer Center (MSKCC) in New York were asked to test amygdalin, they decided to do so not just in the usual transplantable but in more natural spontaneous tumor systems.

These studies were conducted at MSKCC from 1972 to 1977 by Dr. Kanematsu Sugiura. Sugiura, who had a remarkable career of nearly 60 years in the field, "did show inhibition in the development of lung metastases," according to the Office of Technology Assessment report (6).

In repeated experiments with three different animal systems, he found that amygdalin stopped the distant spread (metastases) of cancer in mice; improved their health and well-being; and temporarily stopped the growth of small tumors. The elderly scientist's work was at first encouraged and accepted, but then attacked, by leaders of the cancer center (*The Cancer Industry*, chapters 8 and 9).

Other scientists, at the Catholic Medical Center and at Sloan-Kettering itself, claimed they could not reproduce Sugiura's results. The draft report on laetrile, released to the media in 1977, scarcely mentioned Sugiura's positive results. Any negative aspects were accentuated.

The author was assistant director of public affairs and science writer at MSKCC during this period and wrote the official media release on laetrile. In November, 1977, however, he called a media conference of his own and charged that MSKCC officials had engineered a cover-up of positive results with amygdalin. He was fired the next day for "acting in a manner that conflicts with his most basic job responsibilities" (*New York Times*, 11/24/77).

The final paper published in 1978 admits that in a series of six experiments Sugiura did see "an overall average of 21 percent of mice with lung metastases" when they were treated with amygdalin as compared to 90 percent in the control mice."

However, the paper also claimed that "the significance attributed to those early observations is seriously challenged by the negative findings of three independent investigators, by two out of three negative cooperative experiments in which Sugiura participated, and particularly by the blind experiment in which he and others under blind readings found no anticancer activity" (7). Needless to say, the accuracy of all these statements are sharply challenged in the author's book, *The Cancer Industry*.

In 1978, NCI, "in response to widespread public interest," undertook a retrospective analysis of amygdalin treatment. They sent letters to 385,000 physicians and 70,000 other health professionals, asking for cases thought to have shown objective benefit from amygdalin. Only 93 cases were submitted for evaluation, and 26 of these were eliminated due to what was called insufficient documentation. An equal number of conventionally-treated cases were then selected from NCI's files.

A panel of 12 oncologists, who had no knowledge of the actual treatments given, was then asked to evaluate the results of the treatments in abstracted records from 93 patients. This 'blinded' panel, as it is called, judged laetrile to have produced a response in six cases (two complete and four partial) but the committee claimed that "these results allow no definite conclusions supporting the anticancer activity of Laetrile" (8). However, Robert G. Houston, author of *Repression and Reform in the Evaluation of*

Alternative Cancer Therapies, points out that a close reading of the paper shows that only 22 cases were actually evaluated: the panel found remissions in 6 of these (27 percent) and stabilization in 9 others (41 percent).

After this, NCI sponsored a clinical trial at the Mayo Clinic. Amygdalin plus a "metabolic therapy" program consisting of diet, enzymes and vitamins were given to 178 patients. According to the Mayo report, the great majority were in good general condition when they began treatment and one-third had not received any previous chemotherapy. Mayo doctors concluded that "no substantive benefit was observed in terms of cure, improvement or stabilization of cancer, improvement of symptoms related to cancer, or extension of life span" (9).

Although the Mayo report stated that "the pharmaceutical preparations of amygdalin, the dosage, and the schedule were representative of past and present Laetrile practice," this claim was bitterly contested by leaders of the laetrile movement who claimed that a degraded product had been used and that Mayo had failed to consult them in carrying out the "metabolic therapy" protocol.

In the summary of the Mayo report, it is further stated that "the hazards of amygdalin therapy were evidenced in several patients by symptoms of cyanide toxicity or by blood cyanide levels approaching the lethal range. Patients exposed to this agent should be instructed about the danger of cyanide poisoning, and their blood cyanide levels should be carefully monitored. Amygdalin (Laetrile) is a toxic drug that is not effective as a cancer treatment."

However, in the body of the paper, the authors admit that "most of these reactions were either mild and transient or...possibly not drug-related." Blood levels of cyanide were seriously high with symptoms in only three (2 percent) of these patients. One was said to have taken "large amounts of raw almonds" with the amygdalin.

These have an enzyme that can release cyanide from the drug. The other two patients took double doses by mistake. The report concluded, "There were no drug-related fatalities" (9).

There is no argument that when eaten to excess or taken orally amygdalin can be dangerous. The ancient Chinese classified the kernels as toxic, but this has not stopped the Chinese from using this drug for several thousand years. Under enzymatic action, amygdalin breaks down into glucose, **benzaldehyde** and hydrogen cyanide. Laetrilists are hardly unaware of this fact but hope to exploit it to kill tumor cells, while sparing their normal counterparts.

If one were to consume a large number of apricot kernels or bitter almonds, one would eventually die of oxygen-starvation. (The red blood cells preferentially take up the cyanide, crowding out the oxygen.)

But how much is too much? In a study in rats, it was found that it would take the equivalent of almost two pounds of kernels to kill a person (10). However, in a raw slurry, far less could kill a person. Even laetrile advocates admit that 12 raw apricot kernels, taken at one time, could be dangerous.

Nor are sub-lethal amounts necessarily harmless. Like other medications, ingested amygdalin is indeed potentially dangerous, even fatal if taken in excess.

There are certainly reports about the dangers of cyanide and ingested amygdalin in the scientific literature (11). In several well-publicized cases, people have died after laetrile ingestion. For example, a woman who drank 3 grams of laetrile meant for injection appeared to have suffered severe liver damage and later died (12).

There have been several cases of children who were made sick or even died after ingesting laetrile meant for injection (13). A woman with cancer presented with nerve

AMYGDALIN

damage or "neuromyopathy." Although the woman had previously been administered the toxic drug adriamycin, doctors attributed her transient nerve damage to laetrile ingestion (14).

According to one report, it is particularly dangerous to take megadoses of vitamin C along with laetrile, since the vitamin decreases the detoxification of cyanide (15). A report in *Science* claimed that amygdalin administered orally to pregnant hamsters caused skeletal malformations in the offspring, but that intravenous laetrile did not result in such embryo defects (16).

While blood levels of cyanide are definitely released into the blood of rats following oral administration, "cyanide blood concentrations and toxicity are markedly less when amygdalin is given intravenously" (17). Amygdalin, *properly administered*, is relatively non-toxic. In Sugiura's experiments, he injected up to 2,000 milligrams per kilogram weight per day into mice daily for months. The mice seemed healthier for it. In what ways, if any, it is effective as a cancer treatment, however, must await a less politically-charged environment.

(See *The Cancer Industry*, chapters 7 and 8.)

⊕ References

1. Greenberg DM. The case against laetrile: the fraudulent cancer remedy. Cancer.1980;45:799-807.
2. Reitnauer P. Prolonged survival of tumor-bearing mice following feeding bitter almonds. Archiv Geschwulstforschung.1973;42:135.
3. Wodinsky I and Swiniarski JK. Antitumor activity of amygdalin MF (NSC-15780) as a single agent and with beta-glucosidase (NSC-128056) on a spectrum of transplantable rodent tumors. Cancer Chemother Rep. 1975;59:939-50.
4. Hill G, et al. Failure of amygdalin to arrest B16 melanoma and BW5147 AKR leukemia. Cancer Res.1976;36:2102-7.
5. Stock CC, et al. Antitumor tests of amygdalin in transplantable

animal tumor systems. J Surg Oncol.1978;10:81-8.

6.   US Congress, Office of Technology Assessment (OTA). Unconventional cancer treatments. Washington, DC: US Government Printing Office, 1990.

7.   Stock CC, et al. Antitumor tests of amygdalin in spontaneous animal tumor systems. J Surg Oncol.1978;10:89-123.

8.   Ellison NM, et al. Special report on Laetrile: the NCI Laetrile Review. Results of the National Cancer Institute's retrospective Laetrile analysis. N Engl J Med.1978;299:549-52.

9.   Moertel CG, et al. A clinical trial of amygdalin (Laetrile) in the treatment of human cancer. N Engl J Med.1982;306:201-6.

10.   Adewusi SR and Oke OL. On the metabolism of amygdalin. 1. The LD50 and biochemical changes in rats. Can J Physiol Pharmacol.1985; 63:1080-3.

11.   Beamer WC, et al. Acute cyanide poisoning from laetrile ingestion. Ann Emerg Med.1983;12:449-51.

12.   Leor R, et al. Laetrile intoxication and hepatic necrosis: a possible association. South Med J.1986;79:259-60.

13.   Hall AH, et al. Cyanide poisoning from laetrile ingestion: role of nitrite therapy. Pediatrics.1986;78:269-72.

14.   Kalyanaraman UP, et al. Neuromyopathy of cyanide intoxication due to "laetrile" (amygdalin). A clinicopathologic study. Cancer.1983;51: 2126-33.

15.   Basu TK. High-dose ascorbic acid decreases detoxification of cyanide derived from amygdalin (laetrile): studies in guinea pigs. Can J Physiol Pharmacol.1983;61:1426-30.

16.   Willhite CC. Congenital malformations induced by laetrile. Science. 1982;215:1513-5.

17.   McAnalley BH, et al. Cyanide concentrations in blood after amygdalin (laetrile) administration in rats. Vet Hum Toxicol.1980;22:400-2.

❧ cANTICOAGULANTS

Anticoagulants are drugs that reduce the clotting ability of the blood. Coumarin was the first such drug to be discovered, initially isolated from the Brazilian tonka bean, and then from lavender oil, woodruff, sweet clover and other plants. It has the characteristic odor of new mown hay and is used in some perfumes to add a scent of freshness.

As an isolated chemical, coumarin is toxic, and one well-known derivative is the rat poison warfarin. Oddly, this and similar substances are now being used to treat cancer.

Cancer generally kills by spreading to distant sites and setting up satellite growths called metastases. "Metastasis is the principal cause of failures to cure human cancers," a scientist wrote in *Science* (1).

Of the four ways that cancer spreads, moving through the blood vessels is the most ominous way. Such blood-borne spread "usually heralds a fatal outcome for the patient" (2). By blocking such secondary growths one can render most cancers non-fatal, since unless it interferes with a vital organ, a primary tumor generally cannot kill by itself.

There is a "special stickiness" to tumor cells that are shed from a primary tumor. In fact, they need this stickiness to adhere to the cell walls of organs far from the primary site (3). Their ability to spread is related to the ability of the blood to clot. A number of approaches are now being tried, using anticoagulants to stop cancer's spread, including some medically-approved substances of relatively low toxicity.

Such anticoagulants reduce tumor growth in experimental animals. By interfering with clot formation they inhibit the growth and spread of cancer. "The coagulation mechanism is commonly activated in human malignancy," according to scientists at the VA hospital in Vermont, who studied the effects of warfarin in human cancer (4).

One explanation of warfarin's effects is that cancer cells promote the formation of the clotting factor fibrin in the vicinity of tumors. Drugs that can influence such clotting could be important in controlling metastatic growth. **Vitamin K** is one such factor responsible for activating coagulation. This activity is in turn depressed by treatment with warfarin. So scientists began thinking about stopping vitamin K from helping the blood coagulate (5).

In the 1970s there were four clinical trials of anticoagulants. Although the results were divergent, they were all positive:

- In Dublin, there was a doubling of survival time;
- In Buffalo, there were impressive case histories;
- In Winnipeg, an eight-fold improvement was seen; and
- In Munich, doctors saw a ten percent improvement in the five year survival, thanks to anticoagulation.

"It is now evident," German scientists wrote, "that anticoagulant medication influences the course and healing of malignant tumors" (3).

Such medicines may cause some difficult-to-control bleeding. But any bleeding episodes are at least counterbalanced and probably far overshadowed by the general favorable effect, the German scientists said (3).

Anticoagulation therapy also improves the outcome of toxic chemotherapy and radiotherapy "in virtually hopeless cases." The Munich scientists concluded:

"The prolongation of survival time by anticoagulation is impressive. All clinical studies show the same tendency...These results can no longer be ignored" (3).

In a controlled study, warfarin prolonged survival of lung cancer patients who were also receiving conventional therapy. Survival for those receiving conventional therapy was 24 weeks while for those also getting warfarin it increased to 50 weeks. This was achieved in people who had extensive disease and no longer responded to conventional treatments. Warfarin may therefore be useful in the treatment of lung cancer (6,7).

In a study of 128 patients, it was shown that in a variety of cases, warfarin added to chemotherapy "doubled the two-year survival rate." Best results were obtained in post-menopausal women with breast cancer. However, warfarin depressed immunity, which argues against its use for cases undergoing surgery. Instead, scientists have suggested the use of **enzymes** such as Brinase or streptokinase, whose preliminary results are also favorable (8).

Heparin, first isolated from liver and now known to be part of various mammalian tissues, is another natural anticlotting agent. Heparin also produces "significant antimetastatic effects" in mice. When Natural Killer cells are suppressed, however, the antimetastatic effects of warfarin and heparin are destroyed (9). Therefore, anticoagulants work best in conjunction with drugs that enhance NK cell activity.

Cortisone given with heparin stops blood vessel formation, causes regression of large tumors and prevents metastases (12). In the 1970s, heparin (together with another drug) was given to a terminally-ill Scandinavian woman. Her brain metastasis regressed and her pleurisy (inflammation of the lining of the lung) also cleared up. One year later, the patient was free from symptoms (13).

In rats given the conventional antimetabolite drug 5-FU, more of that drug accumulated in tumors when warfarin was concurrently administered. This shows a synergistic effect between 5-FU and such anticoagulants, Japanese scientists said (10).

At the Lilly Research Laboratories scientists have studied the effects of warfarin in rats with heart disease (due to blood clots) and metastatic cancer. They found that a daily dose of half a milligram per kilogram was uniformly lethal after two weeks of treatment. But half that dose was non-toxic and not only blocked coagulation but blood clots and metastases, as well. The same drug mechanism underlies all these effects, the Indianapolis scientists concluded (11).

In addition to warfarin and heparin, a variety of similar substances have also been shown to stop clotting and therefore metastases:

• Prostacyclin is a naturally-occurring substance synthesized in the walls of blood vessels, which stops blood platelets from sticking together. In the test tube, prostacyclin was found to be a "powerful antimetastatic agent" (1). On the other hand, interfering with prostacyclin production increases metastases. Some scientists have therefore proposed its use as an antimetastatic agent (1).

• Qian-Hu is a traditional Chinese medicine that "completely suppressed tumor formation" for up to 20 weeks, without toxicity. It was found to contain a form of coumarin called Pd-II. Scientists concluded that such drugs may be useful in developing a method of preventing cancer (14).

• Anticoagulants have been recovered from the saliva of an animal with a 'professional' interest in the topic—the Mexican leech (*Haementeria officinalis*). Antistasin, a salivary protein from this leech has been found to be the active ingredient. It inhibits blood coagulation and metastasis, University of Pennsylvania scientists report (15).

• Trigramin is a peptide, rich in the amino acid cysteine, isolated from the venom of the *Trimeresurus gramineus* snake. It inhibits the adhesiveness of melanoma cells (16).

• The Chinese black tree fungus, mo-ehr, is an anticoagulant available in most Asian markets. It has been publicized for protective effects against both coronary disease and cancer. Such anticlotting substances, wrote surgeons in the *New England Journal of Medicine*, are harmless even when a patient is scheduled for any operation except one in which "the consequences of bleeding can be especially dangerous, such as neurosurgical procedures" (17).

⊕ References

1. Honn KV, et al. Prostacyclin: a potent antimetastatic agent. Science. 1981;212:1270-2.

2. Hoover HJ and Ketcham AS. Techniques for inhibiting tumor metastases. Cancer.1975;35:5-14.

3. Ludwig H. [Anticoagulants in advanced carcinoma]. Gynakologe (FRG).1974;7:204-212.

4. Zacharski LR, et al. Rationale and experimental design for the VA cooperative study of anticoagulation (warfarin) in the treatment of cancer. Cancer.1979;44:732-741.

5. Donati MB and Semeraro N. Cancer cell procoagulants and their pharmacological modulation. Haemostasis.1984;14:422-9.

6. Zacharski LR, et al. Effect of warfarin on survival in small cell carcinoma of the lung. Veterans Administration Study No. 75. JAMA. 1981;245:831-5.

7. Zacharski LR. Basis for selection of anticoagulant drugs for therapeutic trials in human malignancy. Haemostasis.1986;16:300-20.

8. Thornes RD. Adjuvant therapy of cancer via the cellular immune mechanism or fibrin by induced fibrinolysis and oral anticoagulants. Cancer. 1975;35:91-7.

9. Gorelik E. Augmentation of the antimetastatic effect of anticoagulant drugs by immunostimulation in mice. Cancer Res.1987;47:809-15.

10. Ogawa J, et al. [Experimental and clinical study of interactions between fluorinated pyrimidine derivatives and anticoagulants]. Gan To Kagaku Ryoho.1988;15:2265-71.

11. Smith GF, et al. Correlation of the in vivo anticoagulant, antithrombotic, and antimetastatic efficacy of warfarin in the rat. Thromb Res.1988;50:163-74.

12. Folkman J, et al. Angiogenesis inhibition and tumor regression caused by heparin or a heparin fragment in the presence of cortisone. Science. 1983;221:719-25.

13. Astedt B, et al. Treatment of advanced breast cancer with chemotherapeutics and inhibition of coagulation and fibrinolysis. Acta Med Scand.1977;201:491-3.

14. Zelikoff JT, et al. Studies on the antitumor-promoting activity of naturally occurring substances. IV. Pd-II [(+)anomalin, (+)praeruptorin B], a seselin-type coumarin, inhibits the promotion of skin tumor formation by 12-O-tetradecanoylphorbol-13-acetate in 7,12-dimethylbenz[a]anthracene-initiated mice. Carcinogenesis.1990;11:1557-61.

15. Tuszynski GP, et al. Isolation and characterization of antistasin. An inhibitor of metastasis and coagulation. J Biol Chem.1987;262:9718-23.

16. Knudsen KA, et al. Trigramin, an RGD-containing peptide from snake venom, inhibits cell- substratum adhesion of human melanoma cells. Exp Cell Res.1988;179:42-9.

17. George J and Shattil S. The clinical importance of acquired abnormalities of platelet function. The New England Journal of Medicine. 1991; 324:27.

✝️ℭ𝒜NTINEOPLASTONS

....

"A completely new type of antitumor agent that is non-toxic and seems to make malignant cancer cells revert to normal" is what *Oncology News* called antineoplastons in their July-August 1990 cover story. The article indicates that use of antineoplastons, a controversial peptide treatment for cancer, is at long last gaining a certain amount of respect in some scientific circles.

"The body itself has a treatment for cancer," says Stanislaw R. Burzynski, MD, PhD, who discovered anti-neoplastons in 1967, while a graduate student in Poland (1). Antineoplastons are found in normal blood and urine, but appear to be deficient in cancer patients (2-4). Burzynski uses them as a non-toxic treatment, which allegedly inhibits cancer cells and converts them to normal.

Burzynski has intensively studied these compounds, which he has variously named A2, A5, A10, and AS2-1. He has found them to be essentially non-toxic (5-7) and has also reported on preliminary clinical studies, showing that they cause tumor responses (shrinkages) in a number of difficult cases. Most of these patients had already exhausted conventional treatments (8-10).

Patients come to his Burzynski Research Institute (BRI) in Houston to receive injections or infusions with antineoplastons. They generally leave with a personal supply of the drugs, and either take them in pill form of self-administer them through an intravenous catheter.

The Burzynski treatment has been the subject of an intense medico-legal and political battle. (See *The Cancer Industry*, chapter 14). Unlike some other unconventional practitioners, Burzynski has published his results in the scientific literature, and attempted to share them with his scientific peers. Burzynski has now published scores of scientific papers and abstracts.

Independent laboratories have confimed some of his claims, as well. For example, scientists at the Medical College of Georgia found that oral antineoplaston A10 delayed the development of virally-induced breast cancers in mice. It also inhibited the growth of breast tumors in a kind of rat (13).

Doctors at Kurume University, Japan, have presented results suggesting antitumor effects of A10 on lung cancers in mice (14). Another team at Kurume found that A10 reduced the growth of human breast cancer cells in nude (athymic) mice (15).

Researchers at the Uniformed Services University of the Health Sciences in Maryland, a branch of the Department of Defense, have reported that AS2-1 promoted the maturation of leukemia cells and suppressed the cancerous qualities of some other cells (16).

Burzynski holds 20 patents on this work and has presented his results at over 20 international and U.S. conferences. In 1989, he was awarded a Special Medal by the Polish government for "achievements in the field of cancer chemotherapy." He has been granted permission to test antineoplastons by the FDA, but claims that study is being held up for lack of funding.

Scientists at Kurume University in Japan are in the third year of testing patients, and antineoplastons are also being investigated in China, Russia and Poland, as well as the US. In October 1991, site visitors from NCI examined his results in brain cancer. According to an announcement from Burzynski's institute, NCI will conduct four clinical trials with antineoplastons, starting in the summer of 1992.

Under a 1983 court order after hearings on a suit brought by the FDA, Burzynski has been allowed to treat patients with antineoplastons, but only in Texas. At this writing, he cannot ship these compounds out of state or overseas without FDA permission. To obtain antineoplastons, therefore, a patient has to go to Houston and be treated at BRI.

In February 1992, the Texas Attorney General brought suit to stop all distribution of antineoplastons and destroy existing stock. This is the latest in a long string of attempts to destroy the Burzynski clinic, including a five-year civil RICO (racketeering) suit, brought by the Aetna Insurance Co., which was thrown out of court in March, 1992.

A small percentage of patients have experienced adverse reactions during the course of treatment. These have included stomach gas, slight rashes, slight changes in blood pressure, chills and fever. Some patients report the presence of an unpleasant body odor associated with the therapy. To date no major side effects have been reported with antineoplastons.

Burzynski cannot give the treatment in-hospital. He has admitting privileges at Twelve Oaks Hospital in Houston, but is not allowed to administer antineoplastons there. Thus, if a patient requires hospitalization while in Houston, he or she will have to suspend antineoplaston therapy. This is not a comprehensive cancer management program, and while Burzynski does not oppose other treatments, one should not expect anything but antineoplastons and perhaps low doses of conventional treatments as well.

In 1992, the US National Cancer Institute announced plans to begin clinical trials in the fall of antineoplastons in four kinds of brain cancer. A statement from NCI (1/6/92) stated that "The National Cancer Institute reviewed 7 cases of primary brain tumors that were treated by Dr. Burzynski with antineoplastons A10 and AS2-1 and concluded that antitumor responses occurred."

In a negative vein: Saul Green, PhD published a full-scale attack on Burzynski and his methods as a Special Communication to *JAMA*, entitled "Antineoplastons: An Unproved Cancer Therapy" (12).

He has charged that Burzynski does not actually have a PhD. Burzynski claims to have a sworn affidavit from Professor Zdzislaw Kleinrok, President of the Medical Academy of Lublin, confirming that his PhD in biochemistry was awarded on October 16, 1968. At this writing, Burzynski has submitted a detailed rebuttal of this article to *JAMA* but there is no indication if it will be published.

Other peptides: There are other peptide treatments that show promise. Besides **bestatin,** tuftsin and trigramin, there is "mammastatin," isolated from normal human breast cells in the 1980s. This appears to be a local factor that is part of the normal balance "between growth stimulatory and growth inhibitory" factors. Mammastatin was found to inhibit the growth of five different types of breast cancer but had no effect on eleven types of cancer that were not derived from breast tissues, according to scientists at the University of Michigan Cancer Center in Ann Arbor (11).

⊕ References

1.   Burzynski S. Antineoplastons: history of the research (I). Drugs Exp Clin Res.1986;12S:1-9.

2.   Burzynski S. Biologically active peptides in human urine: I. Isolation of a group of medium-sized peptides. Physiol Chem Phys.1973;5:437.

3.   Burzynski S, et al. Biologically active peptides in human urine. III.

Inhibitors of the growth of human leukemia, osteosarcoma, and HeLa cells. Physiol Chem Phys.1976;8:13-22.

4.   Burzynski S, et al. Antineoplaston A in cancer therapy. Physiol Chem Phys.1977;9:485.

5.   Burzynski S. Toxicology studies on antineoplaston AS2-5 injections in cancer patients. Drugs Exp Clin Res.1986;12S:17-24.

6.   Burzynski S, et al. Toxicology studies on antineoplaston AS2-1 injections in cancer patients. Drugs Exp Clin Res.1986;12S:25-35.

7.   Burzynski S and Kubove E. Toxicology studies on antineoplaston A-10 injections in cancer patients with five years' follow-up. Drugs Exp Clin Res.1986;12S:47-55.

8.   Burzynski S and Kubove E. Initial clinical study with antineoplaston A2 injections in cancer patients with five years' follow-up. Drugs Exp Clin Res.1986;13S:1-12.

9.   Burzynski S and Kubove E. Initial clinical study with antineoplaston A2 injections in cancer patients with five years' follow-up. Drugs Exp Clin Res.1987;13S:1-12.

10.   Burzynski S, et al. Phase I clinical studies on antineoplaston A5 injections. Drugs Exp Clin Res.1987;13S:37-43.

11.   Ervin PJ, et al. Production of mammastatin, a tissue-specific growth inhibitor, by normal human mammary cells. Science.1989;244:1585-7.

12.   Green S. 'Antineoplastons': an unproved cancer therapy. JAMA 1992;267:2924-28.

13.   Hendry LB and Muldoon TG. Actions of an endogenous antitumorigenic agent on mammary tumor development and modeling analysis of its capacity for interacting with DNA. J Steroid Biochem.1988;30:325-28.

14.   Eriguchi N, et al. Chemopreventive effect of antineoplaston A10 on urethane-induced pulmonary neoplasm in mice. J Japan Soc Cancer Ther. 1988;23:1560-65.

15.   Hashimoto K, et al. The anticancer effect of antineoplaston A10 on human breast cancer serially transplanted to athymic mice. J Japan Soc Cancer Ther.1990;25:1-5.

16.   Samid, D, et al. Induction of phenotypic reversion and terminal differentiation in tumor cells by antineoplaston AS2-1. Abstract, 9th International Symposium on Future Trends in Chemotherapy, Geneva, Switzerland, March 1990.

ꙮc*A*RGININE

Arginine (technically, L-arginine) is an amino acid, a building block of protein. Enzymes and hormones are generally comprised of proteins, and therefore ultimately of amino acids, as well. Since many vitamins and minerals will not function without the proper amino acids being present, their importance is self-evident.

The liver is able to synthesize about 80 percent of the amino acids, but the other 20 percent must be obtained from dietary sources. These are called the essential amino acids and arginine is one of these. It is available in meat, milk and eggs, as well as nuts such as pistachios and almonds.

A lack of this amino acid causes a rare disease called argininemia, which is characterized by retardation, seizures and spasticity. Arginine also helps detoxify the liver; assists in the release of growth hormones; maintains a healthy immune system; detoxifies poisonous ammonia; increases the sperm count and muscle mass; and helps the body produce the intercellular cement, collagen.

Feeding a carcinogen to rats caused liver cancer in 50 percent of the animals after 12 to 15 months. But giving arginine along with the chemical acetamide "led to virtually complete inhibition of the carcinogenic process" (1).

In 1980, NCI scientists found that daily injections of arginine into tumor-bearing rats consistently inhibited the growth of tumors. The scientists noted:

"Within two weeks, tumor size was reduced to 80 percent of the initial size. The growth inhibition was dose-dependent. Tumor-bearing animals showed no toxic effects..." (2).

The mushroom-derived **lentinan** together with arginine made a particularly potent combination (3).

In 1985, Japanese scientists studied the effect of arginine on tumor growth and metastases. For eight days rats were fed solutions containing arginine, at the same time receiving transplants of sarcoma cells. The arginine-rich solution suppressed tumor growth in the early stages of cancer and prevented liver and kidney metastases.

Arginine maintained a positive nitrogen balance and prevented an abnormal increase in other amino acids. Its ability to suppress tumor growth "may be due to its activation of the immunologic system," e.g. macrophages (4).

One percent arginine supplements slowed the growth of nerve cancer and prolonged the average survival time, enhanced immune T-cells and increased their response to tumors. Pennsylvania scientists concluded that "supplementation of the diet with arginine...has been shown to have an antitumor effect." They added that it gave "nutritional and immunologic support to the tumor-bearing animal." Arginine may therefore have clinical importance for treating cancer patients (5).

In a study of breast cancer at Tohoku University School of Medicine, mice were fed diets with either a low, normal or high amount of arginine. NK cell activity was significantly lower in mice receiving little arginine compared to those getting normal or high amounts. An increase in NK activity was also seen after an injection of **lentinan** or another immune booster, OK-432. But no such improvement was seen in mice on a low arginine diet (3).

Interferon production by spleen cells was also significantly increased in mice that got this supplement, but significantly reduced in arginine-deprived mice. Tumor growth was also inhibited by daily administration of either lentinan or OK-432. Paradoxically, tumor growth was accelerated after administration of the same drugs into arginine-deficient mice. Japanese scientists concluded that the nutritional or hormonal environment of cancer-bearing mice plays an important role in the effect of some kinds of **biological response modifiers.**

A study of stomach cancer showed that patients treated with chemotherapy had "excellent" results with lentinan, but only if they had normal protein levels. Patients with low protein levels showed no beneficial results (3).

In late 1991, arginine figured prominently in the Texas trial of Jimmy Keller, a cancer clinic operator who claimed to have healed himself of melanoma. He was seized by US agents in Mexico, tried and sentenced to two years in federal prison for "wire fraud." One of the charges against him was that he used an unapproved arginine preparation called Tumorex.

Although arginine is basically non-toxic, it should be avoided by pregnant or lactating women, according to Dr. James and Phyllis Balch in their popular work, *Prescription for Natural Healing* (Garden City Park: Avery, 1991).

⊕ References

1.   Weisburger J. Prevention by arginine glutamate of the carcinogenicity of acetamide in rats. Toxicology and Applied Pharmacology. 1969; 14:163-75.

2.   Cha-Chung Y. Arrest of mammary tumor growth in vivo by l-arginine. Biochemical and Biophysical Research Comm.1980;95:1306-13.

3.   Akimoto M, et al. [Modulation of the antitumor effect of BRM under various nutritional or endocrine conditions]. Gan To Kagaku Ryoho. 1986;13:1270-6.

4.   Tachibana K, et al. Evaluation of the effect of arginine-enriched amino acid solution on tumor growth. Japan J Parenter Enteral Nutr.1985; 9:428-34.

5.   Reynolds J, et al. Immunologic effects of arginine supplementation in tumor-bearing and non-tumor-bearing hosts. Annals of Surgery. 1990; 211:202-209.

✿✐ASPIRIN

....

Aspirin, one of the first synthetic drugs ever manufactured, may not only prevent heart disease but guard against colon cancer, as well. While hardly health food, few people know that its original source was white willow bark, mentioned in Hippocrates. In 1763, Reverend Edward Stone of Chipping Norton, UK wrote to the Royal Society on the benefits of willow bark for fever:

"I have no other motives for publishing this valuable specific than that it may have a fair and full trial in all its variety of circumstances and situations, and that the world may reap the benefits accruing from it" (1).

Bayer introduced a purified synthetic aspirin in the 1890s. But it wasn't until 1971 that Dr. John Vane discovered that aspirin blocks the production of prostaglandins, which are compounds produced throughout the body that exhibit powerful hormone-like activity. This discovery gave humble aspirin a huge boost in prestige. Since hormonal activity is deeply involved in the growth and progression of some common forms of cancer (e.g. breast and prostate), it was logical that scientists began to look at aspirin's possible effect in cancer as well.

Aspirin is first in a class of agents called nonsteroidal anti-inflammatory drugs (NSAIDs). These include **sulindac,** which is protective against some forms of colon cancer. Much research has also been done on indomethacin (2-4).

In 1987, Russian scientists studied 106 patients with bladder cancer who had received radiotherapy. The **B vitamin** nicotinic acid (niacin) and aspirin were given at standard doses to 51 patients. Such patients showed dramatic reduction in recurrences and better five-year survival (5):

Treatment	Relapses	Five-Year Survival
Radiotherapy	76.3	27.4
with aspirin + niacin	33.3	72.5

Three population-based studies also suggested that aspirin had a protective effect on colon cancer. One was a study of over 1,300 patients with cancer of the colon or rectum. It showed that regular use of NSAIDs was associated with a 50 percent decrease in the risk of cancer at either site (6). A study from Australia showed a similar decrease in risk of colon, but not rectal, cancer (7).

Meanwhile, a California study of elderly aspirin users seemed to show a slight *increase* in colon cancer (8, 9).

In 1991, statisticians at the ACS attempted to resolve these differences through a massive study of aspirin use and colon cancer. They found that regular use of aspirin was indeed linked to a 40 to 50 percent reduction in the risk of death from either colon or rectal cancer.

The ACS study involved more than 660,000 people. Those who regularly took more than 15 aspirin tablets a month had only 60 percent the death rate from colon-rectal cancer as those who did not use aspirin. Similar results have also been seen with other NSAIDs, such as Advil® and Nuprin® (10).

ACS researchers concluded that "additional controlled trials of treatment with aspirin or other NSAIDs in people at high risk for colon cancer may be warranted" (10, 11).

Aspirin is not without side effects and risks. For example, it can also cause bleeding of the stomach.

Children should generally avoid aspirin because of the small but serious risk of Reyes Syndrome. It has also been suspected of causing birth defects. In addition, people with high blood pressure, heart disease, diabetes, thyroid disease or enlarged prostates should consult a doctor before using it.

⊕ References

1. Mills J. Aspirin, the ageless remedy? [editorial]. New Eng J Med. 1991;325:1303-4.

2. Pollard M and Luckert P. Indomethacin treatment of rats with dimethylhydrazine-induced intestinal tumors. Cancer Treat Res.1980; 64: 1323-7.

3. Kudo T, et al. Antitumor activity of indomethacin on methylazoxy-methanol-induced bowel tumors in rats. Gann.1980;71:260-4.

4. Pollard M and Luckert P. Treatment of chemically-induced intestinal cancers with indomethacin. Proc Soc Exp Biol Med.1981;167:161-4.

5. Popov AI. [Effect of the nonspecific prevention of thrombogenic complications on late results in the combined treatment of bladder cancer]. Med Radiol (Mosk).1987;32:42-5.

6. Rosenberg L, et al. A hypothesis: nonsteroidal anti-inflammatory drugs reduce the incidence of large-bowel cancer. J Natl Cancer Inst. 1991;83:355-8.

7. Kune G, et al. Colorectal cancer risk, chronic illnesses, operations, and medications: case control results from the Melbourne Colorectal Cancer Study. Cancer.1988;48:4399-4404.

8. Paganini-Hill A, et al. Aspirin use and chronic diseases: a cohort study of the elderly. BMJ.1989;229:1247-50.

9. Paganini-Hill A, et al. Aspirin use and incidence of large-bowel cancer in a California retirement community. J Natl Cancer Inst.1991; 83: 1182-3.

10. Thun M, et al. Aspirin use and reduced risk of fatal colon cancer. N Engl J Med.1991;325:1593-1596.

11. Baron JA and Greenberg ER. Could aspirin really prevent colon cancer? [editorial]. N Engl J Med.1991;325:1597.

❧ 𝒜ZELAIC 𝒜CID

Azelaic acid was originally discovered in 1943 in rancid fat (oleic acid). Since the late 1970s it has been known to interfere with mitochondria (cell energy centers) (1). Its effect on mitochondria was significantly increased by the addition of the B vitamin, **carnitine**. Carnitine reduces the time or concentration of azelaic acid needed to achieve results (2). Azelaic acid also interferes with anaerobic glycolysis, the abnormal way many cancer cells derive their energy.

In the test tube, azelaic acid shows a preference for melanoma but leaves normal skin cells unharmed (3). It has caused the regression of malignant melanoma of the skin, according to scientists at the Dermatological Institute of San Gallicano, Rome (4). It does not just kill cancer cells, but stops their growth in a selective way (3). Applied topically as a 20 percent cream, it has also been shown to benefit other skin disorders, such as acne, in which it kills the bacteria that cause this disease.

Azelaic acid was studied in 30 different human melanoma cell cultures. It curbed the growth of melanoma cells in all these systems. In addition, its interference with tumor DNA was significant in a "remarkable percentage of tumors," according to Milan scientists. While best results were seen when Italian researchers used the highest concentrations, they also achieved significant results with lower drug concentrations (5).

⊕ References

1.   Picardo M, et al. Activity of azelaic acid on cultures of lymphoma- and leukemia- derived cell lines, normal resting and stimulated lymphocytes and 3T3 fibroblasts. Biochem Pharmacol.1985;34:1653-8.

2.   Ward BJ, et al. Effect of L-carnitine on cultured murine melanoma cells exposed to azelaic acid. J Invest Dermatol.1986;86:438-41.

3.   Geier G, et al. [Effect of azelaic acid on the growth of melanoma cell cultures in comparison with fibroblast cultures]. Hautarzt.1986;37:146-8.

4.   Nazzaro PM. Azelaic acid. J Am Acad Dermatol.1987;17:1033-41.

5.   Zaffaroni N, et al. Cytotoxic activity of azelaic acid against human melanoma primary cultures and established cell lines. Anticancer Res. 1990;10:1599-602.

⚲ BENZALDEHYDE

Benzaldehyde is the essential oil of bitter almond, an aldehyde discovered in 1866. Benzaldehyde is used as an almond-like flavoring agent as well as in perfumes and dyes. It is naturally found in peach and apricot kernels as a byproduct of **amygdalin**, its presence signalled by the bitter almond taste.

Benzaldehyde has been widely studied and is generally regarded as safe in small doses. It does not cause mutations in the standard Ames test (1). But according to Dr. A.Y. Yeung in *Chinese Herbal Medicines*, 1.7 to 2.0 oz. taken internally can be fatal, due to a "slowdown of the central nervous system and respiratory failure." This is approximately 100 times the therapeutic oral dose used in the Japanese studies below.

Benzaldehyde has long been investigated as an anticancer agent. In the 1960s and 70s, it was often combined with chemotherapy (2-7). More recently, scientists have tried to exploit benzaldehyde's relatively non-toxic nature.

One clinical test, reported in NCI's *Cancer Treatment Reports*, showed dramatic effects. Using a modified form of benzaldehyde (similar to amygdalin without the cyanide), Dr. M. Kochi treated 65 patients who had inoperable cancers (8).

"The overall objective response rate was 55 percent," Japanese doctors said. "Seven patients achieved complete response, 29 achieved partial response, 24 remained stable, and 5 showed progressive disease."

Responses were seen in various cancer types and prolongation of survival was apparent in many patients. "Toxic reactions were not observed during long-term injection" with the benzaldehyde derivative, BG (8). This was confirmed at the Toyama Medical and Pharmaceutical University in 1990. Scientists there showed that BG has a unique, yet unknown, way of stopping cancer. Again, it was non-toxic (9).

Toyama scientists treated 24 patients with advanced cancer. Eleven had primary lung cancers, four had metastatic lung, five had stomach, and one each had colon, liver, pancreas and prostate tumors. Two out of the 24 patients showed a complete response to the treatment. One case of lung metastases from breast cancer disappeared, while another case showed complete disappearance of metastatic liver lesions from a primary stomach cancer.

Partial shrinkages were seen in eight and minimal responses in four others. This yielded an overall response rate of 58.3 percent. Doctors conclude that BG showed significant anticancer activity with virtually no toxicity (9).

Scientists have also synthesized an ascorbic acid form of benzaldehyde, called Zilascorb. This can inhibit the synthesis of protein, which is apparently how it exerts its anticancer effect (10). It was said to be more effective than pure benzaldehyde or other derivatives. And its effects were reversible: protein synthesis returned to normal levels within one hour after stopping treatment. Even after protracted therapy, inducing a destruction of more than 99 percent of the cancer cells, the few surviving cells appeared to be undamaged, after removal of the drug (11). This is taken as a sign of how basically safe this drug is.

In addition, benzaldehyde seems able to "detransform" malignant cells, turning them back to normal, according to a Norwegian report (12). As early as 1982, researcher Mark McCarty had suggested in *Medical Hypotheses* that benzaldehyde—as well as **beta-carotene**, interferon and **antineoplastons**—could be considered a new kind of therapy, which stops cell growth and transforms cancer back to normal, without harming the patient (13).

At Dana-Farber Cancer Institute in Boston scientists studied the effect of several benzaldehyde-type drugs in the test tube. One "exhibited significant antitumor activity" against leukemia and a large increase in life span (14).

Japanese scientists reported in *Cancer Research* that lung metastases in mice were inhibited by another benzaldehyde compound, called CDBA. The mice were treated daily with 5 milligrams per day of the drug. The effect depended on the amount given (15). Primary tumors were not affected.

But mice with cancer whose Natural Killer (NK) cells were normally depressed "showed almost as much [NK] activity as normal mice," after they were given CDBA. CDBA also increased the ability of lymphokine activated killer (LAK) cells and interleukin-2 (IL-2) to kill spleen cancer in the test tube. Toyama doctors suggested that IL-2 and CDBA could work together to kill cancer cells (16).

And although injections of the conventional antimetabolite 5-FU reduced natural killer cell (NK) activity by half,

CDBA restored it to normal. Scientists concluded that CDBA not only stopped the spread of cancer and increased NK activity but decreased the toxic side effects on the immune system of standard chemotherapy (17).

At the same time, benzaldehyde and its derivatives work well with **heat therapy**. In Japan, it has been used to increase cell sensitivity to higher temperatures, according to scientists at Fukyi Medical University (17, 18).

Since 1977, Hans Nieper, MD, an unconventional German physician, has utilized benzaldehyde for its "paralytic effect" on tumor growth. Treatment can be continued almost indefinitely, but he adds that "when the tumor is relatively large, the therapy with benzaldehyde, especially where dosage is insufficient, may result initially in the activation of tumor growth."

Nieper says that benzaldehyde must be given in a stabilized form. He cautions that "it is not possible to administer sufficient quantities of benzaldehyde by giving amygdalin," which breaks down into benzaldehyde and glucose but also hydrogen cyanide.

For melanoma, Nieper uses a related substance, acetaldehyde. Although he says that "benzaldehyde is one of the most valuable anticancer substances which is currently and practically available," he claims that acetaldehyde is "clearly superior" for melanoma.

There have been some claims that benzaldehyde is only a "weak" anticancer agent. In a treatment of 14 dogs and 11 cats with cancer, one veterinarian found that benzaldehyde at a dose of 10 milligram per kilogram caused a greater than 50 percent regression in one animal with a cancer of the mouth and another with a melanoma in the mouth. There was also a less than 50 percent regression in animals with a cancer of the sweat gland and a mast cell sarcoma. Another dog with with an oral melanoma showed tumor stabilization for eight weeks.

But the veterinarian suggested this constituted "only minimal antitumor activity at the dose studied" (19). Such relative lack of effectiveness may have been due to the low dose used. (Human subjects have received 25 to 50 times as much benzaldehyde with no major toxicity.)

In 1983, another scientist used benzaldehyde, derived from figs, against experimental tumors. It showed an inhibition of one kind of leukemia but no activity against a number of others. Against human cancer cells from 30 patients with solid tumors, cell growth was inhibited in six patients. Nevertheless, they inferred from this that benzaldehyde "lacks significant activity against most human tumors tested in these experimental systems" (20).

⊕ References

1.   Banks AR, et al. A benzylidene mannopyranoside derivative with antitumor activity in the spontaneous mammary tumor system. Neoplasma. 1982;29:589-95.

2.   Dhapalapur MG, et al. Potential anticancer angents. II. Schiff bases from benzaldehyde nitrogen mustards. J Med Chem.1968;11:1014-9.

3.   Modi JD, et al. Potential anticancer agents. 3. Schiff bases from benzaldehyde nitrogen mustards and aminophenylthiazoles. J Med Chem. 1970;13:935-41.

4.   Florvall L. Some antitumor agents derived from benzaldehyde nitrogen mustards. Acta Pharm Suec.1970;7:87-104.

5.   Modi JD, et al. Antitumor agents. Schiff bases from benzaldehyde nitrogen mustards and 2-phenyl-4-((3-amino-4-methoxy)phenyl)thiazole. J Med Chem.1971;14:450-1.

6.   Shekawat DR, et al. Potential anticancer agents. 4. Schiff bases from benzaldehyde nitrogen mustards. J Med Chem.1972;15:1196-7.

7.   Braun R and Hefter E. [On structure-activity relationships of N'methyl-N'-beta-chloroethyl-benzaldehyde hydrazones (author's transl)]. Arzneimittelforschung.1977;27:2114-7.

8.   Kochi M, et al. Antitumor activity of a benzaldehyde derivative. Cancer Treat Rep.1985;69:533-7.

9.   Tatsumura T, et al. 4, 6-0-benzylidene-D-glucopyranose (BG) in the treatment of solid malignant tumors, an extended phase I study. British J of Cancer.1990;62:436-439.

10. Pettersen EO, et al. 4,6-benzylidene-D-glucose, a benzaldehyde derivative that inhibits protein synthesis but not mitosis of NHIK 3025 cells. Cancer Research. 1985;45:2085-2091.

11. Pettersen EO, et al. Increased effect of benzaldehyde by exchanging the hydrogen in the formyl group with deuterium. Anticancer Res. 1991; 11:369-73.

12. Pettersen EO, et al. Effect on protein synthesis and cell survival of the benzaldehyde derivatives sodium benzylidene ascorbate (SBA) and the deuterated compound zilascorb(2H). Anticancer Res.1991;11:1077-81.

13. McCarty MF. Cytostatic and reverse-transforming therapies of cancer–a brief review and future prospects. Med Hypotheses.1982;8:589-612.

14. Wick MM and FitzGerald GB. Antitumor effects of biologic reducing agents related to 3,4- dihydroxybenzylamine: dihydroxybenzaldehyde, dihydroxybenzaldoxime, and dihydroxybenzonitrile. J Pharm Sci. 1987; 76:513-5.

15. Kuroki Y, et al. Augmentation of murine lymphokine-activated killer cell cytotoxicity by beta-cyclodextrin-benzaldehyde. J. Cancer Res. Clin. Oncol (Germany, Federal Republic of) .1991;2:117.

16. Masuyama K, et al. Inhibition of experimental and spontaneous pulmonary metastasis of murine RCT (+) sarcoma by beta-cyclodextrin-benzaldehyde. Jpn J Cancer Res.1987;78:705-11.

17. Kano E, et al. [Inhibition of the development of thermotolerance by combined treatment with an anticancer drug or benzylidene glucopyranose with the hyperthermia]. Gan To Kagaku Ryoho.1986;13:1377-80.

18. Kano E. [Fundamentals of thermochemotherapy of cancer]. Gan No Rinsho.1987;33:1657-63.

19. MacEwen EG. antitumor evaluation of benzaldehyde in the dog and cat. Am J Vet Res.1986;47:451-2.

20. Taetle R and Howell SB. Preclinical re-evaluation of benzaldehyde as a chemotherapeutic agent. Cancer Treatment Reports.1983;67:561-566.

❦ BUTYRIC ACID

Butyric acid is an oily liquid present (4 to 5 percent, by volume) in cow's butter. It was discovered in 1869. Although in concentrated form it has an unpleasant, rancid odor, butyric acid is now used as an artificial flavoring in liqueurs, syrups and candies. Since the late 1960s, it and

CANCER THERAPY

related compounds have been investigated as a treatment for various kinds of cancer (1, 2).

One form of the chemical, sodium butyrate, has been shown to produce profound changes in the shape, growth rate and enzyme activity of several kinds of cells in the test tube. Such effects are probably mediated by an internal cellular chemical called cyclic AMP.

"Sodium butyrate appears to have properties of a good chemotherapeutic agent for neuroblastoma tumors,"

---

said Prof. K. N. Prasad, a University of Colorado expert on nutritional therapy. This is because treatment causes the death or the "differentiation" of tumor cells. However, the compound seems to be harmless and to produce reversible changes in normal cells (3).

Butyric acid can make mouse leukemia cells differentiate in the test tube cancer (4, 5). Russian scientists tried this on cells from humans with different kinds of leukemia. The compound had the same effect in all (6).

Butyrate was the most potent form of butyric acid tested. An intravenous dose of 500 milligrams per kilograms for ten days was given to a child with acute myelogenous leukemia (AML). The child was in relapse and already resistant to all conventional therapy. This unconventional treatment resulted in:

• elimination of myeloblasts (immature cells of the bone marrow) from the circulating blood supply;

• an increase in mature myeloid cells; and

• a reduction in bone marrow myeloblasts from 70-80 percent to 20 percent.

No impairment of liver, kidney or blood coagulation were seen during the treatment. Writing in *Cancer*, the Russian scientists concluded that natural agents that make cancer cells differentiate may provide additional drugs for the clinical management of selected cases of leukemia (6).

In Seattle, sodium butyrate has gone high tech. Scientists there encapsulated it in liposome 'bullets' and linked these to **monoclonal antibodies** aimed at human colon cells growing in 'nude mice' (7).

"Tumor cell growth was significantly inhibited," researchers at the University of Washington said.

This was associated with changes in cancer cells' shape as well as other changes that indicate "the occurrence of butyrate-induced differentiation" (7).

While butyric acid therapy represents an exciting, nontoxic approach to cancer, there are several drawbacks. First, "the treatment requires the continuous presence of butyric salts in the target area," according to doctors at the Hôpital St. Vincent-de-Paul in France. This raises serious practical problems.

In 1991, French doctors bound butyric acid to certain natural carbohydrates (called monosaccharides). These new compounds retained most of the biological properties of butyric acid but broke down in the body much more slowly. This led to better effects in mice. "These butyric complexes thus seem potentially useful for therapeutic applications," the French doctors report (8).

In Israel, scientists have come up with a different derivative of butyric acid, AN-9. This is about ten times more concentrated than butyric acid. Once it is ensconced inside a cancer cell, AN-9 breaks down into butyric acid.

AN-9 increased the survival time of mice with lung cancer and "significantly decreased the number of lung lesions of the animals inoculated with highly metastatic cells." However, it did not affect overall life span. Short-term studies have shown that AN-9 "possesses low toxicity." Doctors at Beilinson Hospital in Petach Tikva, Israel call AN-9 a "potential antineoplastic agent" (9).

Negative: Rats with bowel tumors caused by a carcinogen were given one to two percent sodium butyrate dissolved in their drinking water. Rather than reducing the cancer, the sodium butyrate treatment seemed to actually enhance the development of colon cancer (10).

⊕ References

1.   Anger G, et al. [Treatment of multiple myeloma with a new cytostatic agent: gamma-l-methyl-5-bis-(beta-chlorethyl)-amino-benzimidazolyl-(2)-butyric acid hydrochloride]. Dtsch Med Wochenschr.1969;94:2495-500.

2.   Finklestein JZ, et al. Unorthodox therapy for murine neuroblastoma with 6-hydroxydopamine (NSC-233898), bretylium tosylate (NSC-62164), papaverine (NSC-35443), and butyric acid (NSC-8415). Cancer Chemother Rep.1975;59:571-4.

3.   Prasad KN and Sinha PK. Effect of sodium butyrate on mammalian cells in culture: a review. In Vitro.1976;12:125-32.

4.   Nordenberg J, et al. Growth inhibition of murine melanoma by butyric acid and dimethylsulfoxide. Exp Cell Res.1986;162:77-85.

5.   Nordenberg J, et al. Biochemical and ultrastructural alterations accompany the antiproliferative effect of butyrate on melanoma cells. Br J Cancer. 1987;55:493-7.

6.   Novogrodsky A, et al. Effect of polar organic compounds on leukemic cells. Butyrate-induced partial remission of acute myelogenous leukemia in a child. Cancer.1983;51:9-14.

7.   Otaka M, et al. Antibody-mediated targeting of differentiation inducers to tumor cells: inhibition of colonic cancer cell growth in vitro and in vivo. A preliminary note. Biochem Biophys Res Commun.1989;158:202-8.

8.   Pouillart P, et al. Butyric monosaccharide ester-induced cell differentiation and antitumor activity in mice. Importance of their prolonged biological effect for clinical applications in cancer therapy. Int J Cancer.1991;49:89-95.

9.   Rephaeli A, et al. Derivatives of butyric acid as potential antineoplastic agents. Int J Cancer.1991;49:66-72.

10.   Freeman HJ. Effects of differing concentrations of sodium butyrate on 1,2-dimethylhydrazine-induced rat intestinal neoplasia. Gastroenterology. 1986;91:596-602.

❧ *DMSO*

DMSO (dimethyl sulfoxide) is a solvent derived from coal, oil and lignin, the intercellular cement of trees. (Lignin is also the source of the artificial flavoring, vanillin.) DMSO is found in milk, fruits, vegetables and grains and is even normally present in small quantities in the human body.

This remarkable chemical was first isolated in Russia in 1866, then rediscovered in the 1960s by a Crown Zellerbach chemist looking for marketable byproducts of wood.

Stanley Jacob, MD, a scientist at the University of Oregon Medical School, then discovered DMSO's medical uses. Scores of articles and books have now been written about this compound. According to Jacob, "DMSO is the most significant new therapeutic principle presented to science in the last half of the twentieth century."

In the US, DMSO can only legally be prescribed for interstitial cystitis of the bladder. That is because studies of DMSO in the 1960s raised questions about possibly harmful changes in the eyes of some animals.

The FDA then all but banned DMSO, yet monkeys never developed any eye problems when they were given 30 times the average human dose for 18 months. In fact, after 25 years, there still has not been a single documented case of eye damage to humans caused by DMSO, despite its use worldwide. In 1980 the FDA somewhat relaxed its restrictions. But widescale testing and drug company sponsorship have never resumed.

DMSO indisputably has one adverse side effect: an overpowering garlic-like odor on the breath.

DMSO is like a liquid hypodermic needle, ferrying other substances with it through the skin right into the body. As early as 1968, it was mixed with other drugs in cancer therapy. At first it was used simply as a carrier. For example, an experimental drug hematoxylin (a dark yellow dye derived from logwood, *Haematoxylon campechianum*) was dissolved in DMSO as a novel way of administering it as cancer therapy (1,2).

In an article in the *Annals* of the New York Academy of Science, scientists showed that the continuous drinking of water that was 32 percent DMSO was not toxic but had no effect on the tumor. When both DMSO and an anticancer drug were added to drinking water, however, "it did increase antineoplastic potency" (3).

One of the hallmarks of a cancer cell is that it loses its ability to mature, or differentiate, like a normal cell. But in 1975 scientists found that leukemia cells in culture were forced to differentiate once again when they were treated with DMSO. (**Vitamin B$_{12}$** had a similar effect.)

Such differentiation lasted for several days when cells were recultured without DMSO. By safely transplanting them back into healthy mice, scientists then showed that these redifferentiated cells were no longer cancerous (4).

It is believed that DMSO works by making cancer cells benign rather than trying to kill them all off (5). Some leukemia cells are very resistant to such positive changes, however. Nor do they respond to **vitamin A** or another agent called azaCyd. But when all three were combined, such "resistance was completely reversed." Scientists still do not understand why (6).

DMSO also "significantly depresses" the energy levels of tumor cells. This "may explain the previously reported antineoplastic efficacy of this solvent."

Once again, DMSO worked better in combination with other agents than alone (7).

 A variety of standard drugs was tested in samples of 24 malignant ovarian tumors. In each case, a 10 percent solution of DMSO was added. There were 14 different responses that were better when DMSO was added to the chemotherapy than with chemotherapy alone. Seven of these responses were highly significant.

This is "strong evidence" that 10 percent DMSO really improves the performance of chemotherapy.

DMSO "may be useful in the treatment of certain ovarian cancers," scientists concluded in the *American Journal of Obstetrics and Gynecology (8)*. "Lower doses of antineoplastic agents might be delivered in DMSO, producing the same cytotoxic [cell-killing] effect as a full dose of drug without DMSO, but with less systemic toxicity," the same scientists wrote (9).

DMSO was also tested against cells from a rare cancer called rhabdomyosarcoma. Once again, exposure to DMSO and some other agents (including one called HMBA) significantly stopped the uncontrolled growth of cells. At the same time it increased their maturity, according to a study in the *British Journal of Cancer (10)*.

Chemotherapy for prostate cancer is often reserved for people who have not responded to standard treatment. "These patients generally are in poor health and tolerate chemotherapy poorly," doctors wrote in the journal, *Prostate*. If the dose of conventional chemotherapy could be decreased while preserving the same degree of activity, "then conventional chemotherapy could become an attractive treatment modality." They therefore investigated the use of DMSO with the conventional drugs cyclophosphamide, cisplatin and 5-FU in prostate cancer in rats. By itself, DMSO did not significantly retard these tumors. But used in combination, DMSO enabled doctors to use lower doses of these conventional agents (11).

Mitomycin-C is an antitumor antibiotic commonly used

for patients with advanced anal, breast, colorectal, gastric, lung or pancreatic cancers. It can cause severe injury and ulceration if it accidentally spills onto the skin as it is being injected. Local applications of heat, ice and common antidotes have failed to reduce such reactions.

Plastic surgery may even be required to stop the pain and overcome the loss of function. DMSO has been used to treat such chemotherapy burns. Although the *Journal of Oncology Nursing* reported on only two such cases, "the response to treatment in both patients was so pronounced," the authors said, "that others may find this useful in their practice" (12).

⊕ References

1. Tucker EJ and Carrizo A. Haematoxylon dissolved in dimethylsulfoxide used in recurrent neoplasms. Int Surg.1968;49:516-27.

2. Stjernvall L. Penetration of cytostaticum in DMSO into malignant cells. Naturwissenschaften.1969;56:465.

3. Thuning CA, et al. Mechanisms of the synergistic effect of oral dimethyl sulfoxide on antineoplastic therapy. Ann NY Acad Sci. 1983;411:150-60.

4. Sugano H, et al. Differentiation of Friend virus-induced leukemia cells. Bibl Haematol.1975;40:221-8.

5. Spremulli EN and Dexter DL. Polar solvents: a novel class of antineoplastic agents. J Clin Oncol.1984;2:227-41.

6. Schwartsmann G, et al. Resistance of HL-60 promyelocytic leukemia cells to induction of differentiation and its reversal by combination treatment. Eur J Cancer Clin Oncol.1987;23:739-43.

7. Arbeit JM, et al. Inhibition of tumor high-energy phosphate metabolism by insulin combined with rhodamine 123. Surgery.1988;104: 161-70.

8. Pommier RF, et al. Synergistic cytotoxicity between dimethyl sulfoxide and antineoplastic agents against ovarian cancer in vitro. Am J Obstet Gynecol.1988;159:848-52.

9. Pommier RF, et al. Cytotoxicity of dimethyl sulfoxide and antineoplastic combinations against human tumors. Am J Surg.1988;155:672-6.

10. Gerharz CD, et al. Heterogeneous response to differentiation induction with different polar compounds in a clonal rat rhabdomyosarcoma cell

line (BA-HAN- 1C). Br J Cancer.1989;60:578-84.

11. Mickey DD, et al. Conventional chemotherapeutic agents combined with DMSO or DFMO in treatment of rat prostate carcinoma. Prostate. 1989;15:221-32.

12. Alberts DS and Dorr RT. Case report: topical DMSO for mitomycin-C-induced skin ulceration. Oncol Nurs Forum.1991;18:693-5.

☙ *Ellagic Acid*

....

Ellagic acid is a natural substance (called a phenol) found in many nuts and berries. It inhibits cancer formation in a number of different experimental systems.

At the Medical College of Ohio at Toledo, scientists Gary D. Stoner and Elaine Daniel fed rats controlled diets containing, among other things, ellagic acid. Two weeks later, they gave them cancer. Tumor incidence was reduced 60 percent in the group receiving ellagic acid (1,2).

The Ohio scientists also tested ellagic acid's ability to inhibit esophageal cancer in rats. It "produced a significant (21 to 55 percent) decrease" in the number of such tumors, and also inhibited precancerous growths (3).

French Canadian scientists compared ellagic acid to the widely used food antioxidant, BHA, for their effects on cancer. Mice were given a carcinogenic tobacco derivative in their drinking water for seven weeks. Each developed on average 15 tumors in the lungs. Two weeks before the start of the experiment, however, some mice were fed either ellagic acid or food grade BHA. The treatment with ellagic acid cut the number of lung tumors in half. BHA, a powerful antioxidant, did even better, reducing tumors on average from 15 to less than 2 per mouse (4).

Cancer cells from the esophagus, trachea, colon, stomach and bladder of rats were put in the test tube with ellagic acid for 24 hours. Then the DNA from these tumors was extracted, purified and measured. California researchers found that ellagic acid bound to the DNA in all these samples. This suggested that ellagic acid may stop mutations (5) by latching onto DNA, "masking" sensitive sites on the genetic material that might otherwise be occupied by a harmful chemical (6).

However, scientists at Research Triangle Park, NC tested 28 compounds to see which prevented cancer in rat cells. Many substances proved successful, but ellagic acid was not one of them (7).

⊕ References

1. Daniel E. Quantitation and liberation of ellagic acid in dietary sources, and its effects, in combination with 13-cis retinoic acid, on the development of N-nitrosobenzylmethylamine-induced esophageal tumors in F344 rats [PhD dissertation]. Medical College of Ohio at Toledo, 1990.

2. Daniel E and Stoner G. The effects of ellagic acid and 13-cis-retinoic acid on N-nitrosobenzylmethylamine-induced esophageal tumorigenesis in rats. Cancer Letter (Ireland).1991;56:117-124.

3. Mandal S and Stoner G. Inhibition of N-nitrosobenzylmethylamine-induced esophageal tumorigenesis in rats by ellagic acid. Carcinogenesis (UK).1990;11:55-61.

4. Pepin P, et al. Inhibition of NNK-induced lung tumorigenesis in A/J mice by ellagic acid and butylated hydroxyanisole. Cancer J (France). 1990;3:266-273.

5. Terwel L, et al. Antimutagenic activity of some naturally occurring compounds towards cigarette-smoke condensate and benzo[a]pyrene in the Salmonella/microsome assay. Mutat Res.1985;152:1-4.

6. Teel R. Ellagic acid binding to DNA as a possible mechanism for its antimutagenic and anticarcinogenic action. Cancer Lett.1986; 30:329-336.

7. Steele VE, et al. Inhibition of transformation in cultured rat tracheal epithelial cells by potential chemopreventive agents. Cancer Res.1990;50: 2068-74.

❦ ℰNZYME 𝒯HERAPY

Enzymes are natural proteins that accelerate biological processes. The body's 'vocabulary' of 20,000 or more enzymes are all built up from an 'alphabet' of over 20 amino acids. Most of these enzymes are produced by the body itself out of these amino acids. Others are ingested in food, although these are generally broken down in the stomach before they can enter the bloodstream.

One enzyme used in conventional cancer therapy is L-asparaginase, which has been approved by the FDA for the treatment of acute lymphoblastic leukemia (ALL). Its discovery was a classic of serendipity. In 1953, a doctor happened to inject some guinea pig serum into rodents with tumors. Mysteriously, their cancers disappeared.

The substance in the blood that caused this remission turned out to be an enzyme called asparaginase. Aside from the South American steppe hare, or agouti, the guinea pig is the only animal which normally has a high concentration of asparaginase in its blood. The enzyme exerted its curative effect by depleting the necessary amino acid, asparagine, from leukemic blood cells.

At first, there were "dramatic clinical responses" to such therapy (1). Because of this, other enzymes that deplete a particular amino acid were also tried against cancer. But although L-asparaginase was highly effective in treating this one kind of leukemia, in general, the conventional use of such enzymes has been disappointing.

Andrew Weil, MD has written of enzymes, "There is no point in taking them as supplements. The reason is simple: enzymes that are ingested are simply broken down in the stomach and small intestine and digested like any other proteins" (*Natural Health, Natural Medicine,* Boston:

Houghton Mifflin Company, 1990). He warns against wasting money on such enzymes as **superoxide dismutase** (SOD) or any other food supplement ending in -ase (designating an enzyme).

The one exception, Weil says, are digestive enzymes made by the stomach and pancreas, which he prescribes for people with digestive problems. In alternative medicine, pancreatic enzymes have a long and controversial history in the treatment of cancer.

The idea behind such use is ancient. Native Americans used papaya (which contains the enzyme papain) to treat external tumors. In 1820, an American physician used stomach juice to treat skin lesions. In 1871, another applied the purified enzyme pepsin to ulcerated lesions. By the end of the nineteenth century, the pancreatic enzyme trypsin had been isolated and was being given intravenously.

The pancreatic enzyme treatment for cancer came to fruition with the work of John Beard, DSc (1858-1924), a comparative embryologist at the University of Edinburgh Medical School for over 30 years. In Beard's day there were only a few enzymes known, such as the pancreatic enzyme trypsin, and the amylases. Such preparations tended to be "grossly impure, antigenic, and a highly variable mixture of non-enzymatic factors," according to Dr. Ernst T. Krebs, Jr., the head of the John Beard Foundation, who has himself strongly advocated the use of purified pancreatic enzymes in the treatment of cancer for many years.

Beard's cancer theory was that trophoblast cells, which naturally enable the embryo to carve its niche in the uterine wall, become cancerous when they express themselves in the wrong place at the wrong time. And indeed if the trophoblast of pregnancy grows unchecked, it creates one of the most malignant of all cancers, choriocarcinoma (today treated successfully with chemotherapy).

Beard believed that pancreatic enzymes could form the basis of a rational therapeutics. He summarized his views in a book, *The Enzyme Treatment of Cancer.* But when crude pancreatic enzymes were injected into patients, these generally failed to cure cancer. Advocates contended that this failure was due to a lack of standards in manufacturing enzyme preparations. Enzyme therapy continued to develop, but slowly.

The most popular form of enzyme therapy has been the German Wobe Mugos (Mucos, GmbH, Gruenwald, Germany). These consist of protein-digesting extracts from the pancreas, calf thymus, peas, lentils and papaya.

Today, enzymes are incorporated into many unorthodox treatment modalities, often along with vitamins and other substances. For example, some doctors believe that cancer itself is a misfunctioning of the metabolism of protein which is brought on by the inadequate production of crucial enzymes. Dr. Nicholas Gonzalez of New York prescribes dozens of pancreatic enzyme pills for his patients to take every day (see **metabolic typing**).

More orthodox scientists are also looking at new uses for enzymes. They examined T-cells (a type of white blood cells) in cancer patients, compared to healthy people. T-cell counts in the middle-aged and older non-cancer patients were "significantly lower" than in healthy young adults. These scores were further reduced in the people with cancer.

The addition of a protein-digesting enzyme called brinase (obtained from a mold, *Aspergillus oryzae*) "increased the T-cell counts significantly in all groups." This was most marked in the older age groups and the patients with malignant disease, according to a report in the *British Journal of Cancer.* Another enzyme, streptokinase, has had similarly good effects (2,3).

⊕ References

1. Holcenberg JS. Enzyme therapy of cancer, future studies. Cancer Treat Rep.1981;4:61-5.
2. Holland PD, et al. The enhancing influence of proteolysis on E rosette forming lymphocytes (T cells) in vivo and in vitro. Br J Cancer. 1975;31:164-9.
3. Bube FW and Egenolf F. [Detection of fibrinolytic split products in patient collections with disordered hemostasis. I. In pathologically verified lung cancer. II. In thrombotic/embolic occurrences]. Folia Haematol (Leipz).1981;108:447-54.

☙ 𝓕LUTAMIDE

Flutamide (Eulexin®) is one of the first drugs approved by the FDA for the treatment of prostate cancer. Flutamide is generally used either with surgical or medical ablation of the testes (castration) or with another drug called leuprolide acetate (1). Some doctors consider it a treatment alternative by itself, however, "in patients with previously untreated advanced prostatic cancer who wish to preserve sexual potency" (2).

A study at NCI involving 617 patients showed that when used in patients with metastasized disease, flutamide extended their median survival by 27 percent (8). Other studies have shown 50 to 100 percent increases. The time to disease progression was also extended 19 percent in patients receiving Flutamide plus medical castration. Many doctors consider this improvement in survival rate is "not a huge advance but is a step in the right direction" (3).

Flutamide works by blocking the uptake of androgens, male hormones that play an important role in the progression of prostate cancer. Androgens originate in two places in the body and stimulate the growth of prostate cancer cells. Testosterone originates in the testes, while certain substances manufactured by the adrenal glands (adjacent to the kidneys) are processed by the prostate into a hormone called DHT (dihydrotestosterone). DHT is in fact the major stimulator of prostate cell growth.

Flutamide does not halt the production of these adrenal androgens. Rather, it competes with DHT and blocks its uptake by the prostate tumor.

In the past, doctors used surgical or medical castration, or radical removal of the prostate, as the sole way to treat prostate cancer. But castration stops production of testosterone alone and does nothing about DHT. In fact, DHT production increases after monotherapy.

Therapy with flutamide generally begins at least two hours before surgical removal of the testes in order to prevent the tumor from accelerating (tumor flare) immediately after the surgery.

In clinical trials at NCI, flutamide was relatively nontoxic. The most common side effect was mild diarrhea. Other side effects, such as hot flashes, impotence, loss of libido, growth of breast tissue in males, were no more common than with orchiectomy alone.

There were also some rare reports of liver function test abnormalities. No heart attacks or blood clots were associated with flutamide in the NCI tests. Rheumatologists at the E. Herriot Hospital in Lyon, France have reported on a case of a patient receiving flutamide who developed methemoglobinemia. This is a rare disease in which a harmful substance called methemoglobin is found in the circulating blood after poisoning. "Flutamide may be considered as a potential methemoglobin-inducing agent," they concluded (4).

Some doctors believe that hormonal therapy should only be used in cases of advanced prostate cancer. But other studies have recently shown that stage C patients benefit even more (8).

Scientists fear that by using flutamide patients will delay the surgical removal of their prostates. But studies have shown that once patients start combination therapy the disease progression halts, the prostate decreases in volume, and the PSA (Prostate Specific Antigen, a marker of cancer) decreases. Sometimes no sign of cancer can be found upon the surgical removal of the prostate. Patients also tend to have fewer complications after surgery.

Some patients have had regeneration of their bone marrow from taking flutamide (5).

In a trial at the National Cancer Institute of Mexico, it was found that after bilateral castration with flutamide pain disappeared or decreased in 83 percent of patients at three months, 62 percent of patients at 6 months, and 25 percent of patients at 12 months. They considered it a "safe and effective approach that increases survival and improves the quality of life of patients with advanced prostatic carcinoma" (6).

Flutamide is also used as a treatment for "hirsutism" (excess hairiness) in women (7).

Flutamide is given in two 125 milligram capsules taken orally three times a day at eight hour intervals. This totals 750 milligrams a day. Since it is a blocking agent, it must be in the body continually. In other countries, a larger 250 milligram capsule is used. It should not just be taken at mealtime, because that will leave long hours in which the hormone DHT will have a chance to do its work. Most flutamide clears from the body in several hours.

Flutamide was approved by the FDA in January, 1989, after a fierce struggle by US prostate cancer patients, who were importing it for their own use from Canada. It is generally covered by most insurance plans, but not by Medicare, since it is considered a self-administered medication.

⊕ References

1.   Benson RC. A rationale for the use of non-steroidal anti-androgens in the management of prostate cancer. Prostate.1992;4:85-90.

2.   Brogden RN, Chrisp P. Flutamide. A review of its pharmacodynamic and pharmacokinetic properties, and therapeutic use in advanced prostatic cancer. Drugs Aging.1991;1:104-15.

3.   Crawford ED and Nabors WL. Total androgen ablation: American experience. Urol Clin North Am.1991;18:55-63.

4.   Schott AM, et al. Flutamide-induced methemoglobinemia. Dicp. 1991 25:600-1.

5.   Berna L, et al. Bone marrow regeneration after hormonal therapy in patients with bone metastases from prostate carcinoma. J Nucl Med. 1991;32:2295-8.

6.   Mendoza VA, et al. The treatment of advanced prostatic carcinoma with total androgenic blockade using bilateral orchidectomy and flutamide: experience at the National Cancer Institute in Mexico. Semin Oncol.1991;18:19-20.

7.   Motta T, et al. Flutamide in the treatment of hirsutism. Int J Gynaecol Obstet.1991;36:155-7.

8.   Labrie F, et al. Long term treatment with luteinising hormone releasing hormone agonists and maintenance of serum testosterone to castration concentrations. Br Med J (Clin Res Ed). 1985;291:369-70.

❦ GOSSYPOL

Gossypol is a pigment isolated from cottonseed in 1937. Its name is derived from the plant's botanical name, *Gossypium L.* Gossypol reduces the sperm count and has gained attention as an oral contraceptive for men, widely used in China.

Because of this effect on sperm, gossypol has been studied as a possible control for cancers of the reproductive system, in women as well as men. And indeed, the drug has been found to have an "antiproliferative effect" on these related kinds of cancer cells. But scientists at the Dana-

Farber Cancer Institute in Boston have found that it also stops rapidly-dividing cells in general, cancerous as well as non-cancerous (1).

Gossypol does not alter the number of chromosomes or increase genetic abnormalities. But it causes a 60 percent decline in blood flow to pancreatic cancers in mice (2).

Even in low concentrations, gossypol inhibited the synthesis of DNA. The longer the exposure, the less genetic material synthesized. An electronmicroscopic study at Lafayette College in Easton, PA showed that gossypol actually punched holes in the surface of mouse leukemia cells, after only two days of treatment (3).

Gossypol has also been studied as an antitumor agent for breast cancer. It changed the rate of division (kinetics) of the cell, but this dose-dependent change was reversible after just four days. The cottonseed derivative was also found to have a "strong inhibitory effect" on the growth of breast cancer cells.

"This study may be of clinical significance in the treatment of breast cancer,"
French scientists said, "since gossypol shows strong antiproliferative properties" (4).

In the above study, the drug was only found to be toxic at the highest dose levels tested. (It was far more toxic in other studies.)

While it could render 66 percent of mice free of tumor cells in one test, the remaining 34 percent died of the drug's toxicity. At lower doses, most mice died of their tumors, while at higher doses all the animals died of toxicity. In other words, the drug was only effective within a very narrow range (5).

Dr. M.R. Flack and colleagues at NIH and Cellco Advanced Bioreactors, Inc. have studied the effect of gossypol on cancer of the adrenal cortex. According to a paper presented at the 81st annual meeting of the AACR, gossypol inhibits such cells in the test tube and in nude mice (*NCI Cancer Weekly*, 5/28/90).

NIH scientists then gave this drug, by mouth, to a single patient with adrenal cortex cancer, who also had multiple metastases to the liver and lungs. The patient had previously failed to respond to either **suramin** or the antibiotic, Adriamycin. After three weeks, CAT (computerized axial tomography) scans showed a complete resolution of lung metastases and a more than 50 percent decrease in the size of liver metastases.

There was also less abdominal pain, ascites (excess fluid) and better lung function. The Maryland scientists are therefore conducting a phase I clinical trial of gossypol for the treatment of metastatic cancer of the adrenal cortex. Although its toxicity in animal studies can be formidable, the above patient's side effects consisted mainly of fatigue, dryness of the mouth and tremors.

Gossypol might also be useful in treating a difficult disease called endometriosis, in which specialized cells from the lining of the uterus spread to other parts of a woman's body. Gossypol inhibited the prostaglandin content of such cells. "It is pertinent to ask," say Chinese scientists, "whether these drugs can be used to improve endometriosis-associated infertility or dysmenorrhea as well" (6).

⊕ References

1.   Band V, et al. Antiproliferative effect of gossypol and its optical isomers on human reproductive cancer cell lines. Gynecol Oncol.1989;32:273-7.

2.   Benz CC, et al. Gossypol effects on endothelial cells and tumor blood flow. Life Sci.1991;49:72.

3.   Majumdar SK, et al. Genotoxic effects of gossypol acetic acid on cultured murine erythroleukemia cells. Environ Mol Mutagen.1991;18:212-9.

4.   Thomas M, et al. Effects of gossypol on the cell cycle phases in T-47D human breast cancer cells. Anticancer Res.1991;11:1469-75.

5.   Rao PN, et al. Antitumor effects of gossypol on murine tumors. Cancer Chemother Pharmacol.1985;15:20-5.

6.   Huang HF and Wang M. [Effects of gossypol and GnRHa on the prostaglandins contents of endometriotic cell and in situ]. Chung Hsi I Chieh Ho Tsa Chih.1991;11:527-9.

❦ HYDRAZINE SULFATE

Hydrazine sulfate is a common industrial chemical, which was used as a component of rocket fuel during World War II. It was first proposed as a cancer treatment in the early 1970s by Joseph Gold, MD, of the Syracuse Cancer Research Institute, Syracuse, NY. Gold drew on the work of Nobel laureate Otto Warburg, who in the 1930s theorized that cancer derived its energy from anaerobic glycolysis (i.e., fermenting sugar) rather than respiring in the normal way. In 1968, Gold proposed using chemicals to control cancer's growth by exploiting this "Warburg effect."

In the early 1970s, Gold indicated that hydrazine sulfate could inhibit the growth of leukemia, lymphoma, melanoma and other cancers in rats (1,2). He suggested that by cutting off a tumor's supply of "new glucose" in the liver, the drug could help starve the tumor. This, in turn, would stop cancer from preferentially depleting the body's energy pools and put an end to cachexia, the terrible wasting process that appears in the final stages of the disease.

In fact, it is this wasting process that often kills the cancer patient. Some doctors believe that the answer to the weight loss in advanced cancer is to inject patients with all the nutrients they need through an intravenous drip. This is called total parenteral nutrition (TPN). However, carefully controlled studies have shown "no significant improvement in either response or survival" associated with TPN for most kinds of cancer. In fact, in two instances, TPN was associated with decreased survival (3).

Gold also showed that hydrazine sulfate could enhance the effect of such conventional drugs as Cytoxan, Mitomycin C, methotrexate and bleomycin in rats. He proposed that a "combination chemotherapy with hydrazine sulfate and a cytotoxic agent may be useful in the treatment of human cancer" (4).

Gold analyzed 84 terminally ill cancer patients who had been treated with hydrazine sulfate under a drug company's investigational new drug (IND) license. He found that 59 out of the 84, or 70 percent, improved subjectively while 14 out of the 84, or 17 percent, improved objectively. Subjective responses included increased appetite, weight gain or stoppage of weight loss, increased strength, improved performance status and decreased pain.

Objective responses included measurable tumor regression, disappearance of cancer-related medical problems and more than one year of stabilized condition. About half of the people who responded had no other cancer therapy while they were receiving hydrazine sulfate. Some patients relapsed quickly; other remissions were long-term (5).

In Gold's 1975 study, the side effects were mild, consisting for the most part of a few incidents of tingling in the fingers and toes, nausea, itching and drowsiness. There was no indication of bone marrow depression (5).

Hydrazine sulfate could be used alone or in combination with other drugs (6). In 1981, Gold showed that hydrazine sulfate treatment resulted in marked appetite improvement. In those patients receiving hydrazine sulfate alone, appetite improvement occurred in over 86 percent. In those who were also receiving conventional chemotherapy, it was almost 70 percent. Average weight gain for people receiving hydrazine sulfate alone was 8.2 lbs, while for those with other therapies it was only 0.6 lbs (7).

In the 1980s, Rowan Chlebowski, MD, PhD and colleagues at Harbor Hospital–UCLA studied 38 patients with advanced cancer and weight loss. Patients were placed in a carefully-controlled study to evaluate the influence of hydrazine sulfate on carbohydrate metabolism. They were given a standard dose of 60 milligram capsules three times a day for 30 days. Glucose tolerance was much better in patients who received hydrazine sulfate than in those who received a placebo ('sugar pill').

Side effects of hydrazine sulfate were minimal. In one study, over 70 percent of the patients reporting no toxic effects (8). The UCLA team concluded that "hydrazine sulfate can influence the abnormal carbohydrate metabolism associated with weight loss in patients with cancer" (9).

Hydrazine sulfate was also evaluated in 101 heavily pre-treated cancer patients who were suffering from weight loss. After one month, 83 percent of the hydrazine sulfate-treated patients, but only 53 percent of the controls, were able to maintain or increase their weight. In addition, UCLA scientists reported appetite improvement was more than twice as frequent in the hydrazine group. The hydrazine sulfate patients did not simply consume more calories, but utilized calories better than did the control patients (8).

Writing in the *Lancet*, UCLA researchers reported on 12 malnourished patients with lung cancer. They too received 60 milligrams three times a day for a month. There was less loss of the amino acid lysine in the hydrazine sulfate group than in those receiving the placebo. These too concluded that hydrazine sulfate reduced the "flux" of amino acids and could therefore favorably influence abnormalities in digestion among late-stage cancer patients (10).

In a larger study of lung cancer patients, the UCLA researchers reported on 65 patients with non-small-cell lung cancer which could not be operated on. All the patients received the same combination of standard chemotherapy (cisplatin, vinblastine and bleomycin) and the same dietary counseling. But patients who received hydrazine sulfate showed much greater intake of calories. Survival was somewhat greater in the hydrazine sulfate-treated group, especially those with less advanced cancers (11,12).

A team of 11 scientists at the N.N. Petrov Research Institute of Oncology, Leningrad (St. Petersburg) have been working on hydrazine sulfate since the 1970s. The Russians have had the greatest single clinical experience with hydrazine sulfate, having treated and evaluated over 740 patients (13).

The patients were of many kinds, including 200 with lung cancer, 138 with stomach cancer, 66 with breast, 63 with Hodgkin's disease and 31 with melanoma. Patients were treated for one month at a time. If their disease became stabilized, there was an interruption of two to six weeks. Then they were treated again for a month.

Nearly half the patients had less cachexia while on the treatment: 14 percent had pronounced and 33 percent had moderate benefits. In addition, 10 percent showed tumor regression. All had disease stabilization.

Thus, in the Russian, as in the Syracuse and UCLA studies, hydrazine sulfate did something few other treatments could do: it inhibited the wasting process. The best results were seen with desmosarcoma, neuroblastoma, laryngeal cancer, Hodgkin's disease and breast cancer (13).

Later studies showed:

**hydrazine sulfate increased appetite,
decreased pain, diminished anorexia, stabilized
tumor growth and promoted survival.
And it had few side effects (14).**

Hydrazine sulfate is inexpensive and accessible. In most studies, the treatment regimen was three 60 milligram tablets each day for a month. Then patients stop for two to six weeks, and take another course as needed.

In the Russian studies, such courses were repeated two or three times. In some cases (especially neuroblastoma) there were 10, 20 or even 40 repeated courses. For cancer of the esophagus or larynx, the drug was administered as a 0.4 percent solution (in which 15 milliliters equalled one 60 milligram tablet). Barbiturates and alcohol are strictly prohibited during the administration of hydrazine sulfate.

Hydrazine sulfate's use in cancer has always been controversial. After years of denigrating its use, NCI finally agreed to sponsor a phase III clinical trial at three medical centers. They are now under way.

⊕ References

1.   Gold J. Inhibition of Walker 256 intramuscular carcinoma in rats by administration of hydrazine sulfate. Oncology.1971;25:66-71.

2.   Gold J. Inhibition by hydrazine sulfate and various hydrazides, of in vivo growth of Walker 256 intramuscular carcinoma, B-16 melanoma, Murphy-Sturm lymphosarcoma and L-1210 solid leukemia. Oncology. 1973; 27:69-80.

3.   Chlebowski RT. Critical evaluation of the role of nutritional support with chemotherapy. Cancer.1985;55:268-72.

4.   Gold J. Enhancement by hydrazine sulfate of antitumor effectiveness of cytoxan, mitomycin C, methotrexate and bleomycin, in Walker 256 carcinosarcoma in rats. Oncology.1975;31:44-53.

5.   Gold J. Use of hydrazine sulfate in terminal and preterminal cancer

patients: results of investigational new drug (IND) study in 84 evaluable patients. Oncology.1975;32:1-10.

6.   Gold J. Potentiation by clofibrate of in-vivo tumor inhibition by hydrazine sulfate and cytotoxic agents, in Walker 256 carcinosarcoma. Cancer Biochem Biophys.1978;3:41-5.

7.   Gold J. Anabolic profiles in late-stage cancer patients responsive to hydrazine sulfate. Nutr Cancer.1981;3:13-9.

8.   Chlebowski RT, et al. Hydrazine sulfate in cancer patients with weight loss. A placebo-controlled clinical experience. Cancer.1987;59:406-10.

9.   Chlebowski RT, et al. Influence of hydrazine sulfate on abnormal carbohydrate metabolism in cancer patients with weight loss. Cancer Res. 1984;44:857-61.

10.   Tayek JA, et al. Effect of hydrazine sulphate on whole-body protein breakdown measured by 14C-lysine metabolism in lung cancer patients. Lancet.1987;2:241-4.

11.   Chlebowski RT, et al. Hydrazine sulfate influence on nutritional status and survival in non-small-cell lung cancer. J Clin Oncol.1990;8:9-15.

12.   Gold J. Hydrazine sulfate in non-small-cell lung cancer [letter; comment]. J Clin Oncol.1990;8:1117-8.

13.   Filov V, et al. Results of clinical evaluation of hydrazine sulfate. Vopr Onkol. 1990;36:721-726.

14.   Gold J. Hydrazine sulfate: a current perspective. Nutr Cancer. 1987;9:59-66.

❦*I*SCADOR

Iscador® is a fermented preparation of the European mistletoe (*Viscum album*), a parasitic plant that grows on deciduous trees. Mistletoe has long been used in European folk medicine. (Some people say such usage goes back to the tree-worshipping Druids.)

Since the 1920s followers of a spiritual-philosophical movement called Anthroposophical Medicine have claimed that this extract has a beneficial effect on life quality and survival of patients with most kinds of solid tumors. Iscador is given either as a single agent or as part of a broader immune-enhancing treatment. There are numerous clinical studies on Iscador, many of which show positive results, and some of which are summarized below.

There are a variety of mistletoe preparations, but the most widely known is Iscador, marketed by Weleda AG (of Switzerland and Germany). Fermented mistletoe is combined with tiny homeopathic doses of various metals such as silver, copper and mercury.

Iscador is approved for medical use in Germany and Switzerland. In northern Europe, Iscador is said to be "widely used in cancer chemotherapy" (1). Worldwide, about 40,000 people were taking Iscador in the 1980s.

Although its use has been condemned by the American Cancer Society, there is a great deal of scientific evidence (most of it in German) confirming Iscador's beneficial effects in enhancing immune function.

The Lucas Clinic in Arlesheim, Switzerland is the world center of Iscador studies. Scientists at the Laboratory of Immunology there believe one of its active ingredients is a lectin, a type of plant protein that mimics an antibody. This particular lectin is named "ML 1." Injection into rabbits resulted in a significant increase in natural killer cell activity, the levels of other white blood cells, and the scavenging activity of macrophages.

When Iscador was injected into cancer patients, there were similar immune-boosting effects. Writing in the American journal *Cancer Research*, scientists reported that they found these results encouraging and hoped to further explore such lectin-carbohydrate interactions (2).

In 1988, scientists at the Institute for Cancer Research, Norwegian Radium Hospital, Oslo, discovered a distinctly different lectin in Iscador (1).

The weight of the thymus gland, central to immunity, nearly doubled following six daily injections of the drug into rabbits. And rats treated with Iscador for 16 weeks showed a 78 percent average increase in the weight of their thymuses. This increased thymus weight was due to an increase in immune-related thymus cells.

Thymus cells of Iscador-treated animals were 29 times more responsive to a stimulant. Iscador also increased antibody production and had beneficial effects on blood-forming cells. It accelerated the recovery of bone marrow and spleens of irradiated animals. The scientists concluded "we believe that *V. album* (Iscador) preparations may be valuable" in stimulating the thymus in humans (3).

In 1988, scientists at the Amala Cancer Research Centre in Kerala, India identified yet another tumor-fighting factor in Iscador. It was a peptide that reduced the size of a solid lymphoma in mice (4).

In the following year, they found that mice with cancer produced a chemical that specifically binds with an anti-cancer portion of Iscador. This protein was mainly found in cancer cells responsive to Iscador, but not in cells that did not respond to the drug (5).

Iscador was also given to prevent recurrences of lung cancer. It prolonged survival time (6). Writing in *Oncology*, scientists reported on the treatment of over 160 cases of widespread lung cancer. These patients were given injections of Iscador directly into the chest. Results showed that "Iscador has two distinct activities." It directly killed cancer cells and also stimulated the immune system (7).

Immunologists at the Lucas Clinic studied the blood of breast cancer patients who received Iscador. They found "a significant enhancement" in the scavenger activity of white blood cells. After an initial drop, there was a significant increase in NK activity, as well as other types of immunity. Such responses, they said, were similar to treatment with the toxic immune agent, interferon-alfa (8).

Twenty-five women with primary cancers of the ovary (including 20 advanced cases) received treatment with

Iscador after surgery. Five-year survival rates with this combined treatment were 100 percent in stages I and II, 23 percent in stage III and 0 percent in stage IV. This group of patients was then compared to women who had received the standard drug Cytoval® after surgery.

Iscador patients had more advanced disease than the Cytoval group. Yet they survived on average 16.2 months, compared to 5.2 months in the Cytoval-treated group. Iscador-treated patients in stage III (with metastases outside the pelvis) survived 4.2 times longer than the Cytoval patients.

The scientists concluded that Iscador is a useful and effective treatment of carcinoma of the ovary, particularly since it usually does not cause serious and undesired side effects (9).

But not all tests have confirmed such activity. In 1975 German scientists reported no inhibition of the Walker carcinosarcoma in rats (10). In 1983, others reported testing Iscador in four animal models, involving some 300 rodents. Although they employed varying doses of the agent, no significant antitumor effect could be observed (11).

At the Finsen Institute in Copenhagen, Denmark, scientists studied 14 patients who were suffering from stage IV kidney cancer. Iscador had no measurable influence on these advanced patients (12).

In Europe, Iscador is often combined with a basically vegetarian diet, which bans mushrooms, hardened fats, refined sugar, new potatoes, tomatoes, as well as alcohol and tobacco.

Anthroposophical medicine also lays great stress on psychological factors (see **psychotherapy**), by encouraging artistic activities such as movement therapy (which they call eurhythmy), painting, light and color therapy, music, exercise, heat baths, oil baths and massage (13).

In controlled dosages, Iscador is generally agreed to be non-toxic. "Apart from local reactions around the injection sites and moderate fever on the day of injection," even the above-mentioned Danish scientists found "the treatment was well-tolerated with no major toxicities" (12).

But both European (*Viscum album*) and American (*Phoradendron flavescens*) mistletoe are poisonous, and one should not attempt to produce any home-made preparation from these plants. Large doses of mistletoe can have a detrimental effect on the heart, and the berries are particularly dangerous for children.

⊕ References

1.   Holtskog R, et al. Characterization of a toxic lectin in Iscador, a mistletoe preparation with alleged cancerostatic properties. Oncology. 1988;45:172-9.

2.   Hajto T, et al. Modulatory potency of the beta-galactoside-specific lectin from mistletoe extract (Iscador) on the host defense system in vivo in rabbits and patients. Cancer Res.1989;49:4803-8.

3.   Rentea R, et al. Biologic properties of iscador: a Viscum album preparation I. Hyperplasia of the thymic cortex and accelerated regeneration of hematopoietic cells following X-irradiation. Lab Invest. 1981; 44:43-8.

4.   Kuttan G, et al. Isolation and identification of a tumour reducing component from mistletoe extract (Iscador). Cancer Lett.1988;41:307-14.

5.   Kuttan G, et al. Presence of a receptor for the active component of Iscador in ascites fluid of tumour bearing mice. Cancer Lett.1989;48:223-7.

6.   Salzer G and Muller H. [Topical treatment of malignant pleural effusions with iscador, a mistletoe preparation (author's transl)]. Prax Klin Pneumol.1978;32:721-9.

7.   Salzer G. Pleura carcinosis. Cytomorphological findings with the mistletoe preparation iscador and other pharmaceuticals. Oncology.1986; 1:66-70.

8.   Hajto T. Immunomodulatory effects of iscador: a Viscum album preparation. Oncology.1986;1:51-65.

9.   Hassauer W, et al. [What prospects of success does Iscador therapy offer in advanced ovarian cancer?]. Onkologie.1979;2:28-36.

10.   Seitz W. [The effect of Iscador (Viscum praeparatum M.) on the

Walker carcinosarcoma of the rat (author's transl)]. Wien Klin Wochenschr.1975;87:131-2.

11. Berger M and Schmahl D. Studies on the tumor-inhibiting efficacy of Iscador in experimental animal tumors. J Cancer Res Clin Oncol.1983;105:262-5.

12. Kjaer M. Mistletoe (Iscador) therapy in stage IV renal adenocarcinoma. A phase II study in patients with measurable lung metastases. Acta Oncol.1989;28:489-94.

13. US Congress Office of Technology Assessment. Unconventional Cancer Treatments. Washington, DC: US Government Printing Office, 1990.

℞ MEGACE

••

Megace® (megestrol acetate) is a synthetic form of the hormone progesterone. It was patented by Searle in 1959 for use as an oral contraceptive. Megace has also been used as a palliative drug in the treatment of metastatic breast cancer. But doctors noticed that it seemed to produce weight gain in some of their patients. And so it is now among a handful of drugs being investigated as an anti-weight-loss (anticachexic) agent (1).

Weight loss is a severe problem in cancer, AIDS and other diseases. Cachexia produces "an ever-increasing spiral of anorexia, undernutrition, loss of tissue mass, muscle wasting, and increased susceptibility to infection and treatment toxicity" (2).

About one-quarter of the women with advanced breast cancer in a University of Maryland Cancer Center study gained weight with conventional doses of this drug and almost all (27 out of 28) with high doses (480 to 1600 milligrams per day). Almost all also had "subjective improvement in appetite." Nearly all those on high doses reported "an increased sense of well-being" (3). This weight gain was independent of pretreatment weight, extent of metastases or response to therapy, the Baltimore doctors said (4).

Weight gain occurred in 80 percent of all patients and in 90 percent of those patients who were treated for at least six weeks. The median weight gain was 5.5 kilograms (12 pounds). Some gained much more, and most of the women reported improvement in appetite, as well (2).

In 1990, NCI conducted a study of Megace in 133 cancer patients suffering from both anorexia and cachexia. Patients who got Megace reported improved appetite and food intake. Eleven out of 67 gained at least 15 pounds. Megace patients also reported significantly less nausea and vomiting. NCI scientists saw no "significant toxic reactions" that they could ascribe to Megace, except for mild swelling (edema). They concluded:

Megace "can stimulate appetite and food intake in patients with anorexia and cachexia associated with cancer, leading to significant weight gain in a proportion of such patients" (5).

After this, Chicago doctors decided to study the drug in people with AIDS. Twenty-two such people were given oral doses, four times a day. All had previously lost an average of 25 pounds over the course of their illness. In this study, 21 of the 22 gained weight, on average 16 pounds. Three people with AIDS who failed to gain weight at the ordinary dose did so at a higher dosage, and only one continued to lose weight even at a very high dose.

It took about 14 weeks to reach peak weight. Seven returned to within 2.2 pounds of their normal body weight. All patients were said to tolerate the drug well, but one patient developed a deep vein thrombosis. No patient developed edema or drug-related impotence. The improvement in appetite and weight gain seen in this initial experiment was encouraging, according to doctors at Northwestern University Medical School in Chicago (6).

In 1990, German doctors gave fairly high doses of Megace to 26 cancer patients for eight weeks. Twelve out of 26 gained weight, and those receiving higher doses responded more frequently, with greater weight gain. There was marked appetite improvement in all treatment groups, but due to its small size, the test was not statistically significant. Side effects were "mild," Hannover, Germany, doctors reported. Only in the high-dose group was there an increase in both fat and lean body mass (7).

These studies do not fully answer the question of how and why Megace helps patients gain weight, however. Is there a desirable increase in muscle, or is the gain mostly in retained water and/or fat?

Scientists at Aston University in Birmingham, UK studied the drug's effects in two animal systems: mice given tumor necrosis factor (TNF), a drug which induces weight loss; and mice with a tumor known to especially cause cachexia. Megace prevented weight loss in both situations. There was increased intake of both food and water. However, the major component of this increase was water, along with fat in some animals. Rats with the cachexia-inducing tumors also had a "significant increase in tumour weight" after Megace. "These results suggest that an increase in appetite and weight gain alone are not sufficient to justify the anticachectic effect of a particular agent," the UK scientists concluded (8).

⊕ References

1. Gorter R. Management of anorexia-cachexia associated with cancer and HIV infection. Oncology (Williston Park).1991;5:13-27.

2. Aisner J, et al. Studies of high-dose megestrol acetate: potential applications in cachexia. Semin Oncol.1988;15:68-75.

3. Tchekmedyian NS, et al. Appetite stimulation with megestrol acetate in cachectic cancer patients. Semin Oncol.1986;13:37-43.

4. Tchekmedyian NS, et al. High-dose megestrol acetate. A possible treatment for cachexia. JAMA.1987;257:1195-8.

5. Loprinzi CL, et al. Controlled trial of megestrol acetate for the treatment of cancer anorexia and cachexia [see comments]. J Natl Cancer Inst.1990;82:1127-32.

6. Von Roenn J, et al. Megestrol acetate for treatment of anorexia and cachexia associated with human immunodeficiency virus infection. Semin Oncol.1990;17:13-26.

7. Schmoll E, et al. Megestrol acetate in cancer cachexia. Semin Oncol.1991;18:32-34.

8. Beck SA and Tisdale MJ. Effect of megestrol acetate on weight loss induced by tumour necrosis factor alpha and a cachexia-inducing tumour (MAC16) in NMRI mice. Br J Cancer.1990;62:420-4.

❦ METHYLENE BLUE

Methylene blue is a synthetic dye discovered in the 1890s and widely used in biology as a standard stain. It comes as a dark green crystalline powder with a bronze luster, soluble in water or alcohol.

Methylene blue was the first synthetic dye to be used medicinally, as an antidote for various kinds of poisoning and as an antiseptic, especially for the urinary tract. *E. coli* bacteria can survive up to 25 minutes in a solution of methylene blue, but other microbes are more sensitive. It inhibits, rather than kills, bacteria (1).

Scientists at the Beijing Lung Tumor Research Institute, China, have found that methylene blue inhibits the growth of three standard kinds of animal cancer, Ehrlich ascites tumor, L1210 leukemia and P388 leukemia in mice. The average life span of the treated animals, they said, was "obviously longer" than that of controls. The dye was clearly superior to the antimetabolite 5-FU in the treatment of L1210 leukemia; two-thirds of the mice with P388 leukemia were healthy and survived for more than 60 days after they were given methylene blue.

When the conventional drug adriamycin was given to mice at the same time as methylene blue, its acute toxicity was decreased and survival time was prolonged.

Methylene blue is said to combine well with tissues, and high concentrations can be maintained for several hours. It can also easily pass through the blood-brain barrier (2), making it a potentially-useful experimental treatment in brain cancer.

Methylene blue may prove useful in **phototherapy**, as well. Six kinds of bladder cancer cells were studied in the test tube. Phototherapy worked within 60 minutes. But that time was cut in half if the cells were first stained with methylene blue. These results suggest that methylene blue and phototherapy "may be useful" as an adjuvant [helper] treatment for superficial bladder cancer (3).

Dr. Michael J. Kelner, a UCSD pathologist has also found that "methylene blue effectively inhibits" free radical activity. He adds that "as methylene blue is already approved for medicinal use in humans and is relatively nontoxic, the drug may have a role in reducing tissue injury..."(4).

⊕ References

1.   Goodman L and Gilman A. The pharmacological basis of therapeutics (3rd. ed.). New York: Macmillan, 1965.

2.   Lai BT. [Antitumor effect of methylene blue in vivo]. Chung Hua Chung Liu Tsa Chih.1989;11:98-100.

3.   Yu DS, et al. Photoinactivation of bladder tumor cells by methylene blue: study of a variety of tumor and normal cells. J Urol.1990;144:164-8.

4.   Kelner MJ, et al. Potential of methylene blue to block oxygen radical generation in reperfusion injury. Basic Life Sci.1988;49:895-8.

℣𝒩AFAZATROM

Nafazatrom, produced by Miles Laboratories of West Haven, CT, is an antithrombotic agent (i.e., it prevents blood clots). It has also been shown to also be a "potent inhibitor of tumor metastasis" (1). Initially there was a great deal of excitement about nafazatrom since it:

• inhibited the growth of experimental tumors;

• killed certain cancer cell lines;

• induced differentiation (restoration to normal) of at least three kinds of cancer; and

• caused no toxicity in either animals or humans (1).

However, nafazatrom did not turn out to be an effective anticancer agent per se. Forty-eight patients with various metastatic tumors (mostly breast, colon and kidney cancers as well as soft tissue sarcomas and melanoma) were tested. No objective remissions were observed but 12 patients remained stable for periods in excess of 8 weeks (2).

In another study, 30 patients with a wide variety of advanced cancers were treated for up to 638 days, but again "no tumor responses were seen." Nafazatrom was a safe and well-tolerated agent. Toxicity was mild, with just two cases of mild skin rashes, one of nausea and vomiting, and one of diarrhea. The scientists suggested that nafazatrom be tried as an antimetastatic agent and "that further efforts should proceed to identify the appropriate dose for such a trial" (1, 3).

However, nafazatrom may yet have value. Mice with tumors treated with nafazatrom showed a remarkable six-fold reduction in secondary growths (metastases) in their lungs compared to controls. The drug stopped a process of cellular breakdown that leads to metastases. "Thus the interference with this process appears to provide an explanation for the inhibition of malignant cell dissemination," scientists wrote in the *JNCI* (4).

⊕ References

1.   O'Donnell JF, et al. A clinical trial of nafazatrom (Bay g 6575) in advanced cancer. Am J Clin Oncol.1986;9:152-5.

2.   Hortobagyi GN, et al. Phase I clinical study of nafazatrom. Invest New Drugs.1986;4:251-5.

3.   Warrell RJ, et al. Clinical study of a new antimetastatic compound, Nafazatrom (Bay g 6575). Effects on platelet consumption and monocyte prostaglandin production in patients with advanced cancer. Cancer.1986; 57:1455-60.

4.   Maniglia CA, et al. Interference with tumor cell-induced degradation of endothelial matrix on the antimetastatic action of nafazatrom. J Natl Cancer Inst.1986;76:739-44.

⍦ ONCONASE

Onconase® is a purified antitumor protein derived from early stage embryos of the common North American Leopard frog (*Rana pipiens*). Even in high doses, this enzyme-like protein remains relatively non-toxic. It was developed in the early 1970s by Kuslima Shogen, then an undergraduate at Fairleigh Dickinson University, New Brunswick, NJ.

Shogen was studying the effects of such embryos on kidney tumors in frogs as well as on tumor cells of other species, including humans. Results were promising. In 1981, she founded the Alfacell company to develop such substances for the market. Onconase (formerly called P30 Protein) is the most advanced of the young company's products.

In 1984, the company developed an unpurified extract of leopard frog embryos. It was found to exert unique effects on cell lines. Toxicity studies showed that it did not cause organ damage in rats or dogs.

In 1987, it isolated a specific protein from embryos, purified it to 99.5 percent and compared it to over 10,000 defined substances in the Protein Identification Resource Center of Georgetown University, Washington, DC. Based on such comparisons, they found that Onconase is a unique compound, which, however, bears a striking resemblance to a well-known pancreatic **enzyme**, ribonuclease. Its enzyme-like activity "seems to be essential for its antiproliferative/cytotoxic effects" (1).

There was a "striking increase in survival" in mice bearing one type of cancer (Madison carcinoma), according to a study in the *JNCI*. Animals in the control group survived on average two weeks. But in one group of treated animals, one-third were actually cured of their tumors. Survival on average was more than 12 times that of the control group (2).

In rats and dogs, there was some central nervous system toxicity, muscle degeneration and alteration of body chemistry at very high doses. In patients, there was a cumulatively toxic effect. This mainly consisted of protein in the urine (a sign of possible kidney problems) and swelling, with or without fatigue (3). But such toxicity generally disappeared when smaller doses were given once a week.

In April 1989, the FDA approved early (Phase I) trials with Onconase. Three cancer centers began testing the drug against various types of cancer. In December 1990, after the company had demonstrated a lack of serious toxicity, the FDA approved Phase II trials. These are ongoing at two centers, the Thompson Cancer Survival Center in

Knoxville, TN and the New York Medical College in Valhalla, NY. By July 1991 the company had received two patents and a trademark on the name, Onconase.

Patients in the Phase I trials generally tolerated Onconase well. For example, with the daily administration of the drug, it was impossible to even reach the maximum tolerated dose. The second Phase I trial used a single large weekly intravenous administration of the drug. This was suggested by animal experiments, which showed that the drug yielded superior results when given on a weekly, rather than daily, schedule.

About 100 patients received the drug, and the maximum tolerated dose was finally reached. The third Phase I study employed a weekly dose of Onconase along with daily oral **Tamoxifen**. This was designed for the treatment of patients with advanced pancreatic cancer. Twenty patients have been treated so far, but definite results are not yet available.

Side effects in some patients included flushing, muscle pains, transient dizziness and decreased appetite. At high doses, two patients developed reversible low blood pressure, preceded by flushing. The maximum dose appears to be about sixteen times the effective dose.

There are no published reports yet on the drug's effectiveness in humans. However, there has been a mention in the literature of objective responses in non-small-cell lung, esophageal, pancreatic and colorectal cancer (3).

"We are most excited about this compound...," said Dr. John Costanzi, medical director of the Thompson center. "The fact that we are seeing responses in previously resistant patients is, in my view, extraordinary."

Ms. Shogen has assembled an impressive group of scientific collaborators, including Stanislaw M. Mikulski,

MD, a medical oncologist formerly of NCI, and currently professor at the University of Medicine and Dentistry of New Jersey; Zbigniew Darzynkiewicz, MD, PhD, professor, New York Medical College, Valhalla and director of its Cancer Research Institute; and Soldano Ferrone, MD, PhD, chairman of the Department of Microbiology and Immunology at the New York Medical College in Valhalla, NY, among others.

⊕ References

1.   Ardelt W, et al. Amino acid sequence of an antitumor protein from Rana pipiens oocytes and early embryos. Homology to pancreatic ribonucleases. J Biol Chem.1991;266:245-51.
2.   Mikulski SM, et al. Striking increase of survival of mice bearing M109 Madison carcinoma treated with a novel protein from amphibian embryos. J Natl Cancer Inst.1990;82:151-3.
3.   Costanzi JJ, et al. A phase I study of P-30 protein (PP) administered intravenously on a weekly schedule. American Society for Clinical Oncology. Houston: ASCO, 1991: Abstract #286.

⸙ SOD

SOD (superoxide dismutase) is a nontoxic substance with great promise in counteracting the side effects of radiation and chemotherapy. When injected, it also has anticancer effects of its own.

When oxygen passes through a cell, it is generally converted to water by enzymes. But about one percent of the molecules pick up an electron in the process. These come from enzymes, which "leak electrons like bad insulation on an electrical wire," according to Joe McCord, a biochemist at the University of South Alabama College of Medicine. A molecule that lacks electrons is called a 'free radical.'

Such free radicals must then attempt to filch electrons from other molecules. This is not always unhealthy. For example, when a white blood cell kills bacteria "it kills it by exposing it to a free radical," according to McCord, quoted in MIT's *Technology Review* (11/12/88). But the loss of an electron usually triggers a harmful chain reaction.

Radicals have a special affinity for the lipids that make up the outer membrane of a cell. These are damaged by the same process that causes butter to become rancid. **Vitamin E, vitamin C, beta-carotene** and uric acid are all effective free radical scavengers. Another effective free radical scavenger is superoxide dismutase (SOD). It was developed by McCord's mentor, Dr. Irwin Fridovich of Duke University, in the late 1960s.

SOD is a naturally-occurring enzyme that absorbs free radicals and converts them to hydrogen peroxide. Other enzymes then harmlessly break that down to water and oxygen.

The presence of SOD may explain why some women's breast cancer cells are more susceptible to carcinogens than others. Scientists have found that the more susceptible the cell to carcinogens, the less SOD it contained. Conversely, the more SOD, the less such vulnerability (1).

Researchers at many universities and drug companies are now testing SOD against a variety of illnesses, such as adult respiratory distress syndrome, a severe irritation of lung tissue. Companies such as Upjohn, Chiron and Bio-Technology General are experimenting with genetically-engineered forms of SOD. (Frederick R. Adler, a director of MSKCC, told *Business Week*, 9/9/85, that German doctors used SOD to ease his own joint pain. He was so impressed, he founded Bio-Technology.)

Free radical scavengers are of interest to cancer therapists, not least because they might counter the free radical damage that is the result of radiation therapy.

In China, scientists measured SOD activity in the blood of cancer patients. They divided 151 cancer patients into five groups: those with lung, digestive tract, breast, gynecological and other cancers. SOD levels in the blood of each group were higher than in healthy adult controls. This seemed to show that SOD was actively fighting their cancers. But 31 patients had low SOD levels. This may have been due to the radiation or chemotherapy they received just before the tests were taken, according to doctors at the Liaoning Tumor Institute in Shenyang (2).

Lung cancer cells were also "significantly inhibited" by SOD. Scientists concluded that "SOD plays an important role" in the destruction of such cells (3).

SOD comes in different varieties, depending on the type of trace mineral with which it is combined. Chinese scientists looked at the levels of copper-zinc SOD in lung cancer. Again, such patients had higher levels of this type of SOD in their blood, which seemed to indicate that the body was mobilizing it to fight the cancer. Measuring SOD may be "helpful in the diagnosis of lung cancer," they said (4).

Two new forms of copper-containing SOD had a pronounced anticancer effect in rats. Just 4 doses resulted in a remarkable 75 percent total remissions. "Sixty percent of the animals recovered totally" from a kind of cancer called carcinosarcoma, when SOD was given intravenously, said scientists at the University of Tubingen, Germany (5).

Lowered amounts of a manganese-containing SOD have been found in many tumor samples, scientists wrote in *Cancer Research*. Diminished amounts of copper and zinc-containing SOD have been found in many, but not all, tumors. Reduced enzyme activity, they suggest, along with free radical production, could explain some of the characteristics of cancer cells (6).

A copper-containing SOD (called CuDIPS) also retarded

the growth of cancer cells in mice. It penetrated cell membranes, scavenging the free radicals inside. Scientists saw a reduction in tumor size, a delay in the appearance of metastases and a significant increase in survival, they reported in the *JNCI* (7). The compound seemed to work by generating hydrogen peroxide inside the cancer cell (8).

Higher manganese-SOD levels have been found in patients with ovarian cancer, according to biochemists at Osaka University Medical School in Japan. They called it a good marker for detecting and monitoring this type of cancer (9).

One of the key problems with SOD in general has been the short period it remains effective in the body. In 1991, DDI Pharmaceuticals of Mountain View, CA received a US patent on a long-lasting form of SOD, called Orgotein®. But this US company can only sell its drug abroad, because its product is not yet approved by the FDA. Company officials claim it is the best treatment available to relieve pain and stiffness in certain types of arthritis, where it is injected directly into affected joints.

Orgotein injections can also be used "safely and effectively to ameliorate or prevent the side effects due to high-energy radiation therapy" of bladder tumors, without interfering with the cancer-killing effects of radiation or chemotherapy. Orgotein reduced the signs and symptoms in both the bladder and the bowel, showing that it actually prevented side effects (10).

One common side effect of radiation therapy is the development of fibrosis, tough painful tissue that interferes with health and comfort. French scientists have also shown that injections with a form of SOD called Lipsod® can be successfully used to treat long-established fibrosis caused by radiation therapy. After just three weeks of intramuscular injection, fibrosis was reduced on average by one-third and significant softening occurred in 82 percent of the cases. It did not matter how old the fibrosis was at the time of SOD treatment.

"Complete regression" was seen in some cases of long-standing prefibrotic inflammations. SOD also prevented fibrosis from developing in people undergoing radiation therapy.

This finding was made at Hôpital Necker in Paris (11).

These results were repeated by Necker scientists in 1989. In just three weeks, the volume of 45 fibroses decreased on average by 32 percent. A "marked or moderate softening was observed in 80 percent of the fibroses."

This was accompanied by "functional improvement in 75 percent of the patients." Decreases in the volume and hardness of the fibroses remained stable during a follow-up of 5 to 24 months. No other effective therapy currently exists to treat radiation-caused fibrosis (12).

Tumor necrosis factor (TNF) is a promising, but sometimes toxic, form of cancer therapy. Pretreating mice with SOD before they received TNF "increased survival rates" by up to 79 percent. And protection from TNF's toxicity was not associated with any reduction in the therapeutic effectiveness of TNF. In fact, cure rates were more than double in the mice that received SOD as well. TNF's toxicity—but not its effectiveness—appears to be caused by the release of powerful oxygen free radicals, precisely the kind that SOD fights against, according to NCI scientists (13).

But while injected SOD appears to be an effective new medicine, some doctors discourage the use of oral SOD as a treatment for anything. "Enzymes injected intravenously or directly into tissues might be effective, but those taken by mouth cannot be," according to Dr. Andrew Weil. This is because, he says, such enzymes are too easily destroyed in the stomach.

⊕ References

1. Werts ED and Gould MN. Relationships between cellular superoxide dismutase and susceptibility to chemically induced cancer in the rat mammary gland. Carcinogenesis.1986;7:1197-201.

2. Dai R. [Determination of superoxide dismutase (SOD) in serum of cancer patients by microchemical luminescence]. Chung Hua Chung Liu Tsa Chih.1989;11:272-4.

3. Glaves D. Intravascular death of disseminated cancer cells mediated by superoxide anion. Invasion Metastasis.1986;6:101-11.

4. Zhou D, et al. [Immunologic changes in serum CuZn-containing superoxide dismutase in patients with lung cancer]. Chung Hua Nei Ko Tsa Chih.1989;28:421-2.

5. Miesel R and Weser U. Anticarcinogenic reactivity of copper-dischiffbases with superoxide dismutase-like activity. Free Radic Res Commun.1990;11:39-51.

6. Oberley LW and Buettner GR. Role of superoxide dismutase in cancer: a review. Cancer Res.1979;39:1141-9.

7. Leuthauser SW, et al. Antitumor effect of a copper coordination compound with superoxide dismutase-like activity. J Natl Cancer Inst.1981;66:1077-81.

8. Oberley LW, et al. Possible role of glutathione in the antitumor effect of a copper-containing synthetic superoxide dismutase in mice. J Natl Cancer Inst.1983;71:1089-94.

9. Taniguchi N. [Superoxide dismutases: significances in aging, diabetes, ischemia and cancer]. Rinsho Byori.1990;38:876-81.

10. Menander-Huber K, et al. Orgotein (superoxide dismutase): a drug for the amelioration of radiation-induced side effects. A double-blind, placebo-controlled study in patients with bladder tumours. Urol Res.1978;6:255-7.

11. Baillet F, et al. Treatment of radiofibrosis with liposomal superoxide dismutase. Preliminary results of 50 cases. Free Radic Res Commun.1986;1:387-94.

12. Housset M, et al. [Action of liposomal superoxide dismutase on measurable radiation-induced fibrosis]. Ann Med Interne (Paris).1989;140:365-7.

13. Hauser GJ, et al. Manipulation of oxygen radical-scavenging capacity in mice alters host sensitivity to tumor necrosis factor toxicity but does not interfere with its antitumor efficacy. Cancer Res.1990;50:3503-8.

❧ SULINDAC

Sulindac is a common prescription item, classified as a non-steroidal anti-inflammatory drug (NSAID). While it was originally marketed to fight arthritis, gout and other rheumatic disorders (1), it is now believed to exercise a beneficial role against precancerous conditions and possibly against cancer itself.

Similar in many ways to fellow NSAIDs such as **aspirin** and indomethacin, sulindac was marketed as Clinoril® in 1971 by Merck. But starting in the early 1980s, there has been a remarkable new development. In 1983, a surgeon named William R. Waddell announced in a cancer journal that sulindac could be used to eliminate polyps in cases of hereditary diseases of the bowel, such as Gardner's syndrome or familial polyposis (2). Such wart-like growths almost always progress to malignancy; they represent about one percent of all colon cancer cases in the US.

Conventional treatment for such conditions is the surgical removal of part of the colon or, occasionally, high doses of radiation. Such surgery can have serious drawbacks. In addition to losing part of the colon, the patient faces a one-in-five chance of developing "postoperative fibrous dysplasia." This serious complication can lead to a mechanical blockage of the small intestine or ureters. And sometimes, paradoxically, surgery for colon polyps is followed by an explosive, life-threatening regrowth of polyps.

Sulindac therapy has the possibility of sparing thousands of people the pain and expense of radical intestinal surgery, with its potentially fatal complications. It also holds promise for the treatment of other kinds of premalignant conditions of the gastrointestinal tract and perhaps (this is untested) of colon cancer itself.

Gardner's disease is one such hereditary condition in which people develop a plethora of non-malignant warty growths in their colon. Eleven patients with this condition were treated with sulindac. Seven had previously had parts of their colons removed, while another four had not yet had any treatment. "All polyps were eliminated," surgeons at the University of Colorado in Denver said, "except for a few that arose in the rectal mucosa and the anal canal." And no cancers developed in the colon patients when they were reexamined (3).

A 1990 French study assessed sulindac's effectiveness in eradicating small polyps in eight patients with familial polyposis, another hereditary condition that often progresses to cancer. These patients had undergone removal of parts of their intestines years before, but small polyps remained in the rectum. Between 200 and 300 milligrams of sulindac were given daily. In these seven patients "eradication of micropolyps was obtained within 3.4 months" on average.

After discontinuing sulindac, there was a recurrence within three to four months of small polyps in four out of the seven patients. "A new eradication of micropolyps was obtained in these four patients with a second sulindac cure within three months," gastroenterologists in Angers, France reported (4).

"Three patients with Gardner's syndrome and multiple colonic polyps had complete regression of polyps after two to three months of sulindac therapy," scientists at the University of Washington School of Medicine reported. They called the idea that sulindac could prevent colorectal cancer in such cases, thereby eliminating the need for preventative surgery "intriguing," but not yet proven (5).

In this paper, Dr. William G. Friend, director of colon and rectal surgery training at Seattle's Swedish Hospital Medical Center, gave several remarkable case histories of sulindac therapy:

• A 47-year-old woman with a family history of Gardner's syndrome referred herself for partial removal of the colon. A barium enema showed a great number of polyps in her ascending colon. She agreed to postpone surgery and try sulindac. "Three months later, no polyps were seen," he wrote.

• A 12-year-old boy with Gardner's syndrome had dozens of polyps in his rectum. His father had had part of his own colon removed when he was 12, for the same condition. Instead of surgery, the son was placed on sulindac pills. Within six weeks, all rectal polyps had disappeared. The boy now takes a quarter-dose of sulindac every other day, and only a few small polyps have recurred at this dosage.

• A 42-year-old woman with Gardner's syndrome had had part of her colon removed 16 years earlier. Since that time, she had been seen at six-month intervals. Each time, the doctors usually found a few dozen small polyps in her rectum. This time the woman agreed to take sulindac for three months. At the end of this time, not a single polyps was evident on examination. She is currently on a maintenance dose of sulindac and has not had a recurrence (5).

Ten patients with rectal polyps who had been previously treated with surgery were given sulindac. Patients received either 300 milligrams a day of sulindac or a placebo for two four-month periods separated by a one-month rest. (One patient didn't follow the doctors' orders and was asked to leave the study.) With sulindac, there was a complete regression in six patients and an almost complete regression in the remaining three. Five of the six placebo patients had an increase in polyps, two had no change and the remaining two showed a decrease in the number of polyps, according to doctors at the Centre Hospitalier Louise Michel, Evry, France (6).

Desmoid tumors are slow-growing sarcomas that some-times invade local tissue but rarely spread to distant parts of the body, according to William R. Waddell and Wolff M. Kirsch of the Department of Surgery, University of Ari-zona. Sometimes these occur spontaneously, but more often they are associated with Gardner's syndrome, in which about 55 percent of the patients develop such growths.

Smaller growths can be removed but large tumors—for example those found in the abdomen, neck, pelvis, thigh or shoulder—often cannot be excised. These scientists have spent 17 years treating this kind of tumor with various agents. Their conclusion is that almost all cases can now be controlled by a combination of sulindac and other drugs such as indomethacin (another NSAID), **warfarin** with **vitamin K$_1$, tamoxifen** and the hormone, testolactone. (The latter interferes with estrogen, which appears to nurture the growth of desmoid tumors.) Sulindac (and indomethacin) may work by inhibiting the hormone prostaglandin, Tucson scientists said (3).

Sulindac is not without its side effects. These are essentially similar to those of aspirin. For example, gastrointestinal pain occurs in ten percent of the patients. Other GI effects can include indigestion, nausea, diarrhea, constipation, gas, anorexia and cramps in three to nine percent. Between three and nine percent of patients also experience rashes, dizziness and headache. About one to three percent have ringing in the ears and swelling.

As with many prescription drugs, there can be unexpected and serious reactions to substances that may be well-tolerated by most people. A reduction in dosage is believed to decrease the risk of these side effects with sulindac. Furthermore, a new drug called misoprostol (Cytotec®) has been approved by the FDA for use in preventing gastric ulcers in patients taking NSAIDs.

But the FDA has not yet approved sulindac for the treatment of hereditary polyps. In fact, in 1989, just as scientific reports were showing that this drug could eliminate the need for many operations, the FDA issued a warning about sulindac's side effects (7). Sulindac is of course easy to receive by prescription. And according to FDA's Personal Use Policy, doctors may prescribe and patients may use a prescription drug such as sulindac in their personal battle against cancer.

⊕ References

1.   Huskisson E and Franchimont P. Clinoril in the treatment of rheumatic disorders. New York: Raven Press, 1976.

2.   Waddell W and Loughry R. Sulindac for polyposis of the colon. J Surg Oncol.1983;24:83-7.

3.   Waddell WR, et al. Sulindac for polyposis of the colon. Am J Surg. 1989;157:175-9.

4.   Charneau J, et al. [Rectal micropolyps after total colectomy in familial polyposis. Efficacy of sulindac]. Gastroenterol Clin Biol.1990;14:153-7.

5.   Friend W. Sulindac suppression of colorectal polyps in Gardner's Syndrome. American Family Physician.1990;41:89-93.

6.   Labayle D, et al. Sulindac causes regression of rectal polyps in familial adenomatous polyposis. Gastroenterology.1991;101:635-9.

7.   Food and Drug Administration. Labeling revisions for NSAIDs. FDA Drug Bull.1989;19:3-4.

❦ SURAMIN

A derivative of urea, suramin sodium was discovered by German scientists in 1917 as a treatment for parasitic infections, such as African sleeping sickness. Suramin also has antiviral properties (1). Because it blocks the activity of enzymes and growth factors in different cellular systems (2), suramin is being considered as an anticancer agent. It has been called "an anticancer drug with a unique mechanism of action" (3). It has also been shown to be useful in treating patients with metastatic cancers that do not respond to other treatments.

To understand suramin's effect on prostate cancer, for example, NCI scientists studied its interaction with adrenal hormones. Five patients treated with suramin showed a 40 percent decrease in hormone levels. In the test tube, the drug inhibited cancer cells at doses that could be achieved in people without much toxicity. It also directly stopped the growth of prostate cancer cells (4).

Suramin builds up in the prostate cell. Two standard tests for the progression of prostate cancer, PAP and PSA, both fell as suramin levels increased. NCI researchers concluded that suramin, besides decreasing male hormones, also can inhibit the growth of prostate cancer cells (4).

In Germany, suramin has been used in the treatment of advanced cancers. A 45-year-old with a huge kidney tumor had failed to respond to all conventional treatments. Administration of suramin was begun in August 1987. After six weeks "the lung metastases regressed almost completely," according to doctors at the University Clinic of Cologne. But tumors returned in January 1988 while the patient was on a low-dose maintenance regimen. Increasing the dose stopped further growth, but did not make the metastases go away. The patient unexpectedly died a few months later of acute circulatory failure (5).

NCI scientists gave suramin to 15 patients with metastatic cancer. There were no complete responses, but four partial and two minimal responses. The partial responses were in cancers of the adrenal cortex, kidney and an adult leukemia-lymphoma. Scientists concluded that suramin is an active agent in the treatment of metastatic cancer, but that further work is necessary to define its scope of action (3). Suramin is undergoing clinical trials for advanced prostate cancer at NCI.

In 1992, French scientists reported that the drug was effective in the treatment of breast cancer, especially in women whose tumors did not have receptors to hormones, and therefore were unresponsive to antihormonal medication. Suramin prevented cell proliferation caused by various growth factors and hormones. It also drastically decreased a certain enzyme (cathepsin D) that has been shown to be associated with a high risk of metastasis. Effectiveness increased with the dose.

Scientists at the National Institute for Medical Research in Montpelier, France concluded that

---

"suramin might be a helpful additional therapeutic tool for breast cancer patients, especially for patients with estrogen receptor-negative tumors" (6).

Suramin has also been studied in combination with **tumor necrosis factor** (TNF) and/or interferon-gamma on prostate cells that are not responding to chemotherapy. At levels readily achievable in humans, TNF caused an approximately 50 percent inhibition in growth. And the combination of suramin plus TNF induced an even "greater inhibition of growth than did either agent alone," according to researchers in NCI. However, combining interferon with suramin provided less cell-killing benefit than did interferon alone. The researchers suggested "clinical trials employing the combination of TNF plus suramin in patients with advanced prostate carcinoma" (7).

Suramin is not without its side effects. In the aforementioned kidney cancer patient, the side effects were a reduction in one kind of white blood cell, problems with coagulation and a moderate amount of protein in the urine. At NCI, toxicity included protein in the urine in 14 out of 15 patients, reversible liver abnormalities, adrenal gland insufficiency and rarely a few other conditions (3).

Suramin was also investigated as a potential AIDS drug. In the test tube, it showed inhibition of HIV replication. However, in 1987 a controlled test showed no clinical benefit from suramin, and the drug is no longer being tested in US AIDS patients. It also failed to have an effect in an Amsterdam study. No clinical trials of suramin for Americans with AIDS are currently underway.

⊕ References

1.   Lane HC and Fauci AS. Immunologic reconstitution in the acquired immunodeficiency syndrome. Ann Intern Med.1985; 103:714-8.

2.   Klijn JG, et al. Growth factor-receptor pathway interfering treatment by somatostatin analogs and suramin: preclinical and clinical studies. J Steroid Biochem Mol Biol.1990;37:1089-95.

3.   Stein CA, et al. Suramin: an anticancer drug with a unique mechanism of action. J Clin Oncol.1989;7:499-508.

4.   La Rocca R, et al. Effect of suramin on human prostate cancer cells in vitro. J Urol.1991;145:393-8.

5.   Allolio B, et al. [Treatment of metastatic adrenal carcinoma with suramin]. Dtsch Med Wochenschr.1989;114:381-4.

6.   Vignon F, et al. Inhibition of breast cancer growth by suramin [see comments]. J Natl Cancer Inst.1992;84:38-42.

7.   Liu S, et al. The effect of suramin, tumor necrosis factor and interferon gamma on human prostate carcinoma. J Urol.1991; 145:389-92.

❦ TAGAMET

Tagamet® (cimetidine) is a prescription drug that inhibits the formation of stomach acid. Because of this property, it is used in the treatment of duodenal ulcers. It is in fact one of the most widely-used drugs in the world, with annual sales topping one billion dollars. Side effects are generally mild. These include diarrhea in 1 percent of the patients; headaches in 3.5 percent; and small possibilities of allergies as well as kidney and cardiovascular problems.

It may have immune-stimulating activity, as well. In fact, in 1985 a scientist called Tagamet one of "the most promising developments in this field to date" (1).

Early indications included a test tube study in 1978, in which it was found that tumor cell growth could be inhibited by treating animals with Tagamet (2). In 1982, scientists found that it delayed the appearance of tumors in animals but "with no significant change in the final survival rate" (3). On the other hand, it did prolong the survival of mice with lymphoma (4). In another animal study, Tagamet was fed to a group of mice for 70 days, during which time they also received skin-cancer-producing ultraviolet radiation five times a week. Scientists at the University of Sydney, Australia concluded that giving mice Tagamet "protected them against the later development of skin tumors" (5). The drug increases the number of white blood cells and their ability to incorporate the minerals **magnesium** and **zinc** (6) and increase Natural Killer cell activity (7).

In a Chinese study of primary liver carcinoma, the authors treated 30 patients with standard chemotherapy in combination with an immune booster called "Bai Nian Le" as well as **levamisole** and Tagamet. Natural Killer cell activity was "significantly elevated," as were other beneficial parameters of the immune system. "Expansion of the tumor mass was checked," Chinese scientists wrote, and "clinical conditions obviously improved" (8).

The search for AIDS remedies has led to a screening of Tagamet in its capacity as an immune stimulant. Human studies in 33 people with AIDS Related Complex (ARC) were carried out at the University of Essen and the University of Kiel in Germany.

After three months, researchers saw significant improvement in many aspects of the immune system. There was improvement in the patients' performance status, the way they rated their own health, their body weight and fever reduction. Diarrhea lessened and lymph nodes were significantly decreased in size. When Tagamet was stopped, these effects disappeared (9).

In a 1985 clinical trial, Tagamet had no appreciable effect on the immune system (10). But another, more advanced study is being conducted with people with AIDS who have a type of skin cancer known as Kaposi's sarcoma. The principal investigator is Thomas J. Smith at the Medical College of Virginia School of Medicine, Richmond, VA. His goals are to find out if Tagamet has beneficial effects on the immune system and Kaposi's sarcoma in particular.

While millions of people take Tagamet without serious side effects, there are a number of potential dangers for cancer patients. Because of its unusual effect on the immune system, Tagamet may be harmful to patients who have had organ transplants or suffer from auto-immune disorders. According to scientists at Michigan State University in East Lansing, Tagamet should be used as an immune booster "on an experimental basis only" (11).

TAMOXIFEN

References

1. Drews J. The experimental and clinical use of immune-modulating drugs in the prophylaxis and treatment of infections. Infection. 1985;13:S241-50.

2. Tutton PJ and Barkla DH. Cell proliferation in dimethylhydrazine-induced colonic adenocarcinomata following cytotoxic drug treatment. Virchows Arch [b].1978;28:151-6.

3. Cerutti I and Chany C. Coordinated therapeutic effects of immune modulators and interferon. Infect Immun.1983;42:728-32.

4. Strejcek J, et al. Further evidence of immunomodulatory effects of cimetidine. Allerg Immunol (Leipz).1984;30:117-22.

5. Matheson MJ and Reeve VE. The effect of the antihistamine cimetidine on ultraviolet-radiation-induced tumorigenesis in the hairless mouse. Photochem Photobiol.1991;53:639-42.

6. Brockmeyer NH, et al. Cimetidine and the immuno-response in healthy volunteers. J Invest Dermatol.1989;93:757-61.

7. Hast R, et al. Cimetidine as an immune response modifier. Med Oncol Tumor Pharmacother.1989;6:111-3.

8. Ling HY, et al. [Preliminary study of traditional Chinese medicine-Western medicine treatment of patients with primary liver carcinoma]. Chung Hsi I Chieh Ho Tsa Chih.1989;9:348-9.

9. Brockmeyer NH, et al. Immunomodulatory properties of cimetidine in ARC patients. Clin Immunol Immunopathol.1988;48:50-60.

10. Maguire LC, et al. Failure of cimetidine as an immunomodulator in cancer patients and normal subjects. South Med J.1985;78:1078-80.

11. Kumar A. Cimetidine: an immunomodulator. Dicp. 1990; 24: 289-95.

❦ TAMOXIFEN

Tamoxifen is a synthetic hormone (technically, a non-steroidal antiestrogen) derived from the carcinogenic hormone DES. It is sold in the US as Nolvadex® by ICI Pharmaceuticals. Tamoxifen was synthesized in 1964 and first marketed in 1977 as a treatment for advanced breast cancer. By the late 1980s it was shown that tamoxifen could

351

prevent breast cancer as well. (As a side benefit, it also seems to cut cholesterol levels.) This led to wild enthusiasm in the media for this adjuvant therapy.

Today, it has become common for women with breast cancer to be given tamoxifen after cancer surgery. A large-scale study is planned to see if tamoxifen can reduce the incidence of cancer in women who have a family history of the disease but who have not gotten it yet themselves. However, serious questions are being raised about tamoxifen's long-term safety.

Tamoxifen is called an "anti-estrogen" because it was originally thought to exert its effects by blocking the female sex hormone, estrogen. Now, however, it is believed that the drug has many unusual side effects in the body. Some of them, ironically, are similar in effect to estrogen, which promotes some tumors. Doctors are even considering using tamoxifen as a form of hormone replacement therapy. In fact, it is becoming routine for doctors to give tamoxifen to women whose tumors are "estrogen receptor positive" and chemotherapy for those who are "estrogen receptor negative."

Tamoxifen may become the conventional treatment of choice for elderly women with breast cancer. Between 1977 and 1983, 100 elderly Scottish breast cancer patients were treated with tamoxifen as their primary therapy. (Scotland, incidentally, has one of the highest cancer rates in the world.) Sixty-eight of the women "responded" to this therapy, with 40 complete and 28 partial responses. The median length of the responses was 47 months for the complete responders and 26 months for the partials. Twenty-two patients had their disease stabilized, while the tumors of the remaining 10 continued to grow. About a third died of breast cancer, while 22 percent remained free of recurrences at the end of ten years.

Tamoxifen is therefore considered a practical primary

therapy for breast cancer in elderly and frail women. It does away with the need for surgery in a high proportion of such cases, according to doctors at the Western General Hospital in Edinburgh (1).

In a study of women with Stage II breast cancer, women were given L-PAM and 5-FU either with or without tamoxifen. In women over 50 who had four or more positive nodes, there was said to be significant improvement in survival in the tamoxifen group. In addition, in all patients over 50 receiving tamoxifen there was improvement in disease-free survival. A Consensus Panel of the NIH recently advised that in Stage II, receptor-positive, postmenopausal women (who are entered into other studies), tamoxifen alone should be used as adjuvant therapy (2).

In a large study from the Institute of Cancer Epidemiology in Copenhagen, the incidence of new primary cancers was studied in over 3,500 post-menopausal women who had already had surgery for breast cancer. Of these patients, about half who had a low risk of recurrence received no further treatment. But high-risk patients were given either radiotherapy or radiotherapy plus tamoxifen. After about eight years, the scientists looked at the cancer incidence in these women.

All three groups had more cancer than the general population, mainly in the other breast or in the colon or rectum (for the high risk group). The risk of leukemia was increased among the women who received radiotherapy. But there was no difference in cancer incidence in the high-risk group that also received tamoxifen compared to those who just received radiotherapy. Nor was there any protective effect of tamoxifen on the opposite breast. However, "a tendency to an elevated risk of endometrial cancer was observed," the Danish scientists reported in the *Journal of the National Cancer Institute.*

In a slightly ominous note, they remarked in 1991 that

"continued and careful follow-up of women treated with tamoxifen is necessary to clarify the potential cancer-suppressive or cancer-promoting effects of this drug" (3).

A carcinogen can either initiate or promote the formation of a tumor. At the McArdle Laboratory for Cancer Research of the University of Wisconsin a novel cancer model was used to test the possibility that tamoxifen causes cancer. The drug was found not to initiate the formation of cancer at the dose tested. But when other groups of animals were first "initiated" with a small dose of chemicals, and then were fed tamoxifen, "the livers of these animals showed an increase in the size and number of altered hepatic [i.e., liver] lesions compared with those animals that were initiated but not exposed to tamoxifen."

The Madison researchers concluded: "This indicates that tamoxifen acts as a tumor promoter in the rat liver." Tamoxifen's strength as a tumor promoter can be judged by the fact that it was "four times that of phenobarbital, an agent commonly employed as a representative promoting agent in experimental carcinogenesis."

The scientists warned that long-term use of tamoxifen "should therefore be limited by the potential carcinogenic risk of this agent as an effective tumor promoter" (4). A study at Johns Hopkins also found that tamoxifen "paradoxically" is a promoter of liver cancer (5).

Tamoxifen is now being used as a second-line treatment for cancer of the endometrium (the lining of the uterus). But, ironically, in 1991 scientists at the Karolinska Hospital in Sweden reported "an increased incidence of endometrial cancer associated with long-term adjuvant tamoxifen." This follows reports that tamoxifen stimulates the female genital tract and has a "mainly estrogenic effect" on these tissues.

"An increased incidence of endometrial cancer may limit the usefulness of tamoxifen for benign indications," the

Swedish scientists reported in the *Annals* of the New York Academy of Science. In their opinion, the improvement in both recurrence-free survival and overall survival in early breast cancer "probably outweighs" the increased frequency of uterine tumors. However, they warn that the possibility of stimulating the growth of hidden groups of cancer cells "should be considered when tamoxifen is used in the treatment of endometrial cancer" (6).

To investigate the link between tamoxifen and endometrial cancer, doctors at Maimonides Medical Center in Brooklyn screened their breast cancer patients who had received tamoxifen for at least 12 months. Seventy such patients were interviewed and endometrial biopsies were obtained from 38. Seven (18 percent) had hyperplastic (i.e., pre-cancerous) changes.

A small prospective study was also conducted. After breast surgery but before the beginning of tamoxifen therapy, the doctors took a sample of endometrial tissue. After tamoxifen therapy was begun, such biopsies were repeated every four to six months as long as the patients remained asymptomatic. New hyperplastic changes were found in 3 out of 11 patients tested (27 percent). The preliminary results of this small study indicate that tamoxifen "may have some neoplastic effect on the endometrium of postmenopausal patients with breast cancer" (7).

A test was conducted at the Mayo Clinic to determine if therapy with tamoxifen plus fluoxymesterone (Halotestine®) was more effective than tamoxifen alone in the treatment of postmenopausal women whose breast cancer had already spread. While there were more "objective responses" in the group receiving both drugs and it took longer for the disease to progress, the "duration of response and survival were similar" in both groups. It was only among the senior patients who were positive for estrogen receptors that "there were highly significant advantages" for treatment with both agents, including a survival advantage. These preliminary data suggested that there was a substantive therapeutic advantage for tamoxifen plus fluoxymesterone over tamoxifen alone only in some elderly women (8).

It has become common to give women without any signs of cancer after breast surgery—so called "node-negative" women—adjuvant treatment with either tamoxifen or chemotherapy. These have demonstrated a "moderate reduction" in the risk of recurrence, but so far "overall survival has not improved with use of adjuvant therapy," according to other doctors at the Mayo Clinic's satellite clinic in Scottsdale, AZ (9).

Caution: "Further data are needed to support the case that hormone replacement with tamoxifen in healthy postmenopausal women would provide overall health benefits," according to a leading expert on the topic. Specifically, scientists need further data on "risk factors for cardiovascular disease, on bone, on the liver, on the uterus, and on the coagulation system" (10).

The records of over 2,600 patients in the Eastern Cooperative Oncology Group studies showed that postmenopausal women who received chemotherapy and tamoxifen had more circulatory-type "complications" than those receiving chemotherapy alone (11).

Sixty patients with metastatic kidney cancer were given the anticancer drug lonidamine with high dose tamoxifen for over six months. The results at the Hannover University Medical School in Germany suggest that lonidamine and high-dose tamoxifen do not cure this disease but are "moderately effective" in widespread kidney cancer if the "treatment intention is palliative" (12).

Side Effects: Major textbooks state that tamoxifen has "minimal side effects" (2). But this is only true in comparison with toxic chemotherapy. Studies show that tamoxifen may have to be taken for the rest of a woman's life. That being the case, compliance with long-term use largely depends "on the nature and severity of tamoxifen's side effects," according to Reuven R. Love of the University of Wisconsin Clinical Cancer Center and a leading tamoxifen researcher.

Love and his Madison colleagues evaluated the symptoms associated with tamoxifen therapy in 140 postmenopausal women, whose breast cancers were in remission. Drug recipients complained of either moderate or severe vasomotor (relating to nerves that control the size of blood vessels) symptoms up to 17 percent more frequently than those receiving an inert substance, and of gynecologic symptoms up to 4 percent more frequently.

More importantly, nearly half (48 percent) of tamoxifen recipients complained of "persistent vasomotor, gynecologic, or other major side effects." These carefully collected data show that there is a "significant 'cost' of tamoxifen therapy," that is "likely to compromise long-term compliance" (10, 13, 14).

In addition, there have been disturbing reports of possibly permanent eye damage from the use of tamoxifen. An article in the *Annals of Ophthalmology* detailed toxicity to the cornea, retina and optic nerve (15). Although this damage did not increase once the drug was stopped, it could not be repaired.

Other reports have shown that 6.3 percent of women receiving the conventional 20 milligrams of tamoxifen a day developed a "battery of visual problems" on the drug, although they were said to have generally resolved when the women went off the drug (*Science News*, 7/4/92).

⊕ References

1. Akhtar SS, et al. A 10-year experience of tamoxifen as primary treatment of breast cancer in 100 elderly and frail patients. Eur J Surg Oncol.1991;17:30-5.

2. Wittes R [Ed.]. Manual of oncologic therapeutics 1991/1992. Philadelphia: J.B. Lippincott, 1991, p. 478.

3. Andersson M, et al. Incidence of new primary cancers after adjuvant tamoxifen therapy and radiotherapy for early breast cancer. J Natl Cancer Inst.1991;83:1013-7.

4. Dragan YP, et al. Tumor promotion as a target for estrogen/antiestrogen effects in rat hepatocarcinogenesis. Prev Med.1991;20:15-26.

5. Yager JD and Shi YE. Synthetic estrogens and tamoxifen as promoters of hepatocarcinogenesis. Prev Med.1991;20:27-37.

6. Fornander T, et al. Effects of tamoxifen on the female genital tract. Ann NY Acad Sci.1991;622:469-76.

7. Gal D, et al. Oncogenic potential of tamoxifen on endometria of postmenopausal women with breast cancer—preliminary report. Gynecol Oncol.1991;42:120-3.

8. Ingle JN, et al. Combination hormonal therapy with tamoxifen plus fluoxymesterone versus tamoxifen alone in postmenopausal women with metastatic breast cancer. An updated analysis. Cancer.1991;67:886-91.

9. Hartmann LC, et al. Systemic adjuvant therapy in women with resected node-negative breast cancer. Mayo Clin Proc.1991;66:805-13.

10. Love RR. Antiestrogen chemoprevention of breast cancer: critical issues and research. Prev Med.1991;20:64-78.

11. Saphner T, et al. Venous and arterial thrombosis in patients who received adjuvant therapy for breast cancer. J Clin Oncol.1991;9:286-94.

12. Stahl M, et al. Lonidamine versus high-dose tamoxifen in progressive, advanced renal cell carcinoma: results of an ongoing randomized phase II study. Semin Oncol.1991;18:33-7.

13. Love RR, et al. Effects of tamoxifen on cardiovascular risk factors in postmenopausal women. Ann Intern Med.1991;115:860-4.

14. Love RR, et al. Symptoms associated with tamoxifen treatment in postmenopausal women. Arch Intern Med.1991;151:1842-7.

15. Gerner EW. Ocular toxicity of tamoxifen. Annals of Ophthalmology 1989;21:420-3.

❦ *T*HIOPROLINE

Thioproline (also known as timonacic or, in France, as Hépalidine) is a simple compound, prepared by combining formaldehyde and the amino acid cysteine. First discovered in 1937, it came into clinical use for treating liver disorders in the 1960s. Since 1980, thioproline has also been used experimentally in the treatment of cancer.

Experiments showed that thioproline could reduce cancer incidence. Mice given a carcinogen received two weeks of pretreatment with thioproline, followed by a maintenance dose for half a year. This reduced tumor incidence by 60 percent. But if the drug was given for only six weeks after the carcinogenic implant, it failed to alter the rate at which cancer developed (1).

In an experiment on small animals with cancer, encouraging results were seen. Thioproline was administered over 16 weeks to 23 dogs and one cat, half of whom had solid tumors, while the other half had incompletely removed malignancies. "Acute partial responses were observed in 3 of the 12 animals with solid tumors," the scientists wrote. In a case of breast cancer and one of mouth cancer, at first there was tumor enlargement but this was followed by a partial regression. The drug appeared to interfere with the tumor's blood supply.

Tumor progression occurred in 11 of the 12 other animals who had incompletely excised tumors. Four out of five of the dogs who had tumors of the nose were alive and relatively free of signs of cancer, nine months or more after surgery. But the scientists noted that there was no microscopic evidence of the reversal of cancer cells into normal cells, such as had been seen in earlier experiments. There also appeared to be a significant amount of pain from the injection and from the formation of abscesses that formed at the injection site (2).

In China, nearly 100 hamsters were first given precancerous growths. After six weeks, half were then given thioproline. Half of these precancers turned back into normal tissue, whereas 100 percent of the untreated animals went on to develop full-blown carcinoma (3).

There was great excitement when doctors in Madrid obtained four out of four remissions in skin cancer that had spread to the lungs using thioproline. These exciting results were supposedly due to the drug's ability to:

• hamper DNA formation in cancer cells;

• soak up nitrites, precursors of carcinogens; and

• form cyclic AMP, which can make cancer cells normal.

Unfortunately, two subsequent studies did not reproduce such effects. Scientists suggested that patients in the first study may have been taking other drugs that inadvertently enhanced the effect of thioproline (4).

⊕ References

1.   Parks RC, et al. Thioproline: an inhibitor of chemical carcinogenesis. Neoplasma.1982;29:535-7.

2.   Grier RL, et al. Pilot study on the treatment with thioproline of 24 small animals with tumors. Am J Vet Res.1984;45:2162-6.

3.   Xie JF. [The blocking effect of topically subepithelial injected thioproline on experimental oral premalignant lesions]. Chung Hua Kou Chiang Hsueh Tsa Chih.1989;24:224-7.

4.   Gosalvez M. On the irreproducibility of thioproline. Biomed Pharmacother.1982;36:387-8.

❦ UREA

Urine has been used in medicine almost since the beginning of history. Today, it is employed in diagnosis, prevention and even therapy. A number of very useful drugs are derived from it, such as the anticoagulant urokinase (Abbokinase®), the sex hormone Premarin® (originally from *pregnant mare's urine*) and the experimental cancer treatment **antineoplastons.**

Other than water, the most abundant chemical found in urine is urea. This is the chief end-product of nitrogen metabolism in mammals. About one ounce is excreted in human urine every day. Solid, it is a colorless or white crystal, and contrary to expectations, without odor.

Urea has been used in conventional medicine as a diuretic (to dispel water), in kidney function tests and for various skin disorders. It is also used with the papaya enzyme, papain, in a skin ointment (Panafil®) and as a treatment for the crises of sickle cell anemia, in doses ten times that given to the cancer patients in the studies cited below.

In cancer, at least, urine-derived products have always been surrounded by controversy. During World War II, there was a battle royal in England over a urinary product called "H11," which had been isolated at the Hosa Research Laboratories, Sunbury-on-Thames. The British scientists, headed by one J. H. Thompson, had discovered a growth-retarding factor in the parathyroid gland of animals. They then turned to urine as a cheaper and more accessible source of the same factor. These scientists claimed to see "definite evidence of inhibitory effects on cancerous tissue" (1).

This report from a relatively obscure laboratory caused

controversy, and, as a result, a review of 243 patient records was made by E. Cronin Lowe, the pathologist of Southport Infirmary (2). He found the following:

Extent of inhibition	Number of cases	% of cases
Partial or complete response	96	40
Temporary retardation	69	28
No inhibition	78	32

This "substantiates the primary claim" that H11 provides or stimulates some "growth inhibiting factor," he said (2).

Such claims led to a bitter exchange between Dr. Thompson and the director of the prestigious Imperial Cancer Research Fund (ICRF), Mill Hill, London. The ICRF concluded that "the preparations have no effect on the growth of malignant cells" (3).

Thompson claimed, however, that the ICRF had not given H 11 enough time to work. For instance, he stated that just 12 days after obtaining the drug the ICRF director wrote him that it did not work. But Thompson had previously written the director that "in the mouse tumour there is a steady increase in size up to about the 8th to 12th day" (4). Despite published reports of benefit, the treatment died out in the late forties (5).

But the idea of urine-derived therapy did not die. In the 1960s, Evangelos D. Danopoulos, MD of Athens, Greece wrote many articles about the use of urea, one of the simplest, least expensive and least toxic substances ever proposed for the treatment of cancer. Many of these peer-reviewed articles appeared in the *Lancet* (6-20).

Danopoulos was a professor at the Medical School of Athens University and a member of the governing board of the Hellenic Anti-Cancer Institute. His medical specialty was cancer of the eye.

Danopoulos said that with urea, "the smaller the tumor, the shorter the duration of treatment. Small lesions can be cured within one to two years, whereas in cases of more extensive tumors, the treatment has to be continued for longer periods, or even for life" (*Townsend Letter for Doctors*, Feb.-March, 1988).

Eight patients with cancer of the eye were successfully treated with urea, Danopoulos reported in 1975. One of them had a malignant melanoma, one Kaposi's sarcoma, and six had squamous cell carcinomas. At least four out of these eight patients would have been subjected to removal of their eyeball as the standard treatment (13).

In another study, 46 out of 47 people with large cancers in or around the eye were treated with local urea injections combined with thorough surgical removal of the growth (curettage). This combination treatment was effective in 100 percent of the cases, Danopoulos claimed.

"The full recovery of the skin which had been destroyed by the cancer, without any remnants of scar or other disfigurement, is a very remarkable phenomenon,"

---

he wrote in the journal *Ophthalmologica*. The eyelids remained functional, as well. Cure by conventional methods is very difficult or almost impossible to achieve in such tumors, he said. By adding urea, he reported unprecedented results with no side effects (15).

Nine people with extensive cancers of the conjunctiva (the mucous membrane on the inside of the eyelid) were treated by Danopoulos with a local application of urea. Five of these cases also had cancer impinging on the cornea of the eye. Eight out of the nine patients were cured. In the ninth patient, who also had a very extensive conjunctivitis (inflammation of the conjunctiva), the treatment was ineffective. Urea treatment, Danopoulos repeated, "is very simple and without any complications, apart from a transient opacity of the cornea."

Recurrences are easily and effectively re-treated. But if the eyeball has been destroyed, he cautioned, re-treatment is impossible. At least five of these patients would have had their eyeball removed if it hadn't been for the urea treatment (16).

Danopoulos also treated 30 instances of lip cancer in 28 patients, 23 of which were extensive or very extensive, using local urea injections combined with curettage. Twenty six out of the 30 cases were squamous cell carcinomas, three were basal cell carcinomas and one was an adenocarcinoma of the lip.

The treatment was effective in all of these patients but recurrences appeared in four. These were easily treated using the same method in three of four patients who returned for treatment. In three cases metastases appeared in the lymph nodes of the neck, which were then surgically removed (19).

While there has been surprisingly little reduplication of Danopoulos's work, indirect support for his position has come from scientists at the University of Illinois Medical Center. In *Clinical Oncology*, Bernard Ecanow and colleagues wrote that daily injections of urea directly into the tumor mass and into the area surrounding the growth were successful in "regressing and eradicating well-established malignant melanomas in hamsters" (21).

They ascribed this to the fact that urea breaks through the "structured water system" with which tumors surround themselves. **Heat therapy** also has this effect, and the authors employed both treatments concurrently (21).

Indian scientists found that urea could be used to successfully treat cancers of the cervix and the penis (22). And at an experimental biology meeting in Jerusalem, several scientists showed that urea could greatly inhibit the growth of cancer cells in the test tube (23).

Urea was the first organic chemical to be synthesized and has been used in medicine for over a century. According to Dr. Danopoulos, it is "by no means toxic." But according to the Chicago researchers, when urea is used with hyperthermia, while this enhances its anticancer effect, "it is also associated with an increase in the toxic potential of urea." Such toxicity can be controlled by adjusting the dosage of the drug. "It is our experience," they wrote, "that when injection is the method of administration, solutions of the drug should not exceed a 40 percent concentration" (21).

According to Danopoulos, urea taken orally goes to the liver and thus gives a "concentration of urea in the liver that has a greatly beneficial anticancer effect." Danopoulos has also said that if the liver is more than 30 percent involved with cancer, urea treatment will have no effect. if the liver is not more than 30 percent involved, then urea can be an effective therapy.

Small metastatic lesions of the lung can also be cured with oral urea treatments, he says. That is because, after passing through the liver, urea travels to the lungs. However, by the time it enters the general circulation its concentration is too low to be effective in other organs.

Danopoulos has attempted to remedy this problem by combining urea with orally-administered creatine hydrate (creatine is a chemical normally found in muscular tissue). This tends to distribute urea to other parts of the body.

⊕ References

1. Thompson J, et al. Antigrowth substances in the treatment of cancer. The Medical Press and Circular.1941;334-342.

2. Lowe E. A review of 243 cancer cases treated with H11 therapy. Medical World.1944:540-548.

3. Gye W. H 11 for cancer [letter]. British Medical Journal.1943; 149-150.

4. Thompson J. H11 for cancer [letter]. British Medical Journal. 1943; 149-50.

5. Ollerenshaw G. Observations on dosage of H11 extract. Medical World.1946;72-76.

6. Angelopoulos B, et al. Electrophoretic analysis of serum proteins, glucoproteins and lipoproteins in acute infectious diseases in infants and children. Med Pharmacol Exp Int J Exp Med.1966;14:517-27.

7. Angelopoulos B, et al. Transferrin variants in Greeks. J Med Genet. 1967;4:31-2.

8. Melissinos K, et al. [Hemolytic-uremic syndrome in an adult]. Med Welt.1971;45:1795-7.

9. Danopoulos ED and Danopoulou IE. Urea treatment of skin malignancies [letter]. Lancet.1974;1:1161.

10. Danopoulos ED and Danopoulou IE. Urea treatment of skin malignancies [letter]. Lancet.1974;1:115-9.

11. Danopoulos ED and Danopoulou IE. Urea treatment of skin malignancies [letter]. Lancet.1974;1:560-1.

12. Danopoulos ED and Danopoulou IE. Regression of liver cancer with oral urea [letter]. Lancet.1974;1:132.

13. Danopoulos ED, et al. Urea in the treatment of epibulbar malignancies. Br J Ophthalmol.1975;59:282-7.

14. Danopoulos ED and Danopoulou IE. The results of urea-treatment in liver malignancies. Clin Oncol.1975;1:341-50.

15. Danopoulos ED and Danopoulou IE. Effects of urea treatment in combination with curettage in extensive periophthalmic malignancies. Ophthalmologica.1979;179:52-61.

16. Danopoulos ED, et al. Effects of urea treatment in malignancies of the conjunctiva and cornea. Ophthalmologica.1979;178:198-203.

17. Danopoulos ED and Danopoulou IE. Eleven years experience of oral urea treatment in liver malignancies. Clin Oncol.1981;7:281-9.

18. Danopoulos ED and Danopoulou IE. Urea—treatment of liver metastases [letter]. Clin Oncol.1981;7:385-7.

19. Danopoulos ED, et al. The effects of urea treatment in combination

with curettage in extensive lip cancers. J Surg Oncol.1982;19:127-31.

20. Danopoulos ED and Danopoulou IE. Anticancer activity in urea [letter]. Clin Oncol.1983;9:89-91.

21. Ecanow B, et al. Tumor matrix destruction by the use of hydrophobic bond breakers: a preliminary report. Clinical Oncology.1977;3:319-320.

22. Gandhi G, et al. Urea management of advanced malignancies (preliminary report). Journal of Surgical Oncology.1977;9:139.

23. Glinos A, et al. Cell-cycle inhibitory effects of urea on HeLa cells in culture. Abstracts of the 13th FEBS Meeting. Jerusalem: , 1980: p. 256.

☀ Resources

Amygdalin: Apricot kernels are sometimes available in health food or Asian markets. Although they have been widely used, these are potentially toxic taken orally. For information on amygdalin therapy in combination with other treatments, contact: American Biologics-Mexico, S.A. Medical Center, International Admissions Office, 1180 Walnut Avenue, Chula Vista, CA 91911. Phone: 800-227-4458. International Phone Number: 619-429-8200. They sell one-pound bags of apricot kernels for $4.75 each.

Anticoagulants: Leo R. Zacharski, MD has conducted research on the use of anticoagulants in cancer for over a decade. He has achieved prolongation of survival in patients with small cell carcinoma of the lung. He has two addresses. 1) Research Department, North Hartland Road, White River Junction, VT 05009. Phone: 802-296-5149 Fax: 802-296-5173. 2) Dartmouth-Hitchcock Medical Center, 1 Medical Center Drive, Lebanon, NH 03756. Phone: 603-650-5527 General Fax: 603-650-8208.

There are a number of common substances which can thin the blood and inhibit coagulation and platelet aggregation. Some of these are aspirin, onions and garlic. A tasty alternative is the Chinese black tree fungus, called 'mo-ehr' or 'mu-er.' This is a common ingredient in such Chinese dishes as hot and sour soup. (In some restaurants this fungus is inaccurately referred to as a mushroom.) Mu-er is available at Chinese markets such as Wah Yin Hong Enterprises, 232 Canal Street, New York, NY 10013. Phone: 212-941-8954. $2.95 for a six-ounce package of dried mu-er, imported from China.

Antineoplastons: Only available in Texas under a court-ordered agreement with the FDA. For information, one can contact the Burzynski Research Institute, Outpatient Department, 6221 Corporate Drive, Houston, Texas. Phone: 713-777-8233. Fax: 713-777-3958. The Research Institute is at 12707 Trinity Drive, Stafford, Texas 77477. Phone: 713-240-5227.

Arginine: Many amino acids are available in purified form in health food stores. It is said that, when using an amino acid as a medicine, one should take it on an empty stomach, to avoid competing with other amino acids for absorption. Jo Mar Laboratories, 251 East Hacienda Avenue, Campbell, CA 95008, sells 150 grams of L-arginine powder for $9.50. Phone: 800-538-4545.

Aspirin: "Enteric coated" aspirins aid in protecting the stomach against injuries that can occur as a result of ingesting aspirin. Two over-the-counter brands are: Ecotrin Enteric Coated Aspirin® and Therapy Bayer Enteric Aspirin Caplets®.

Benzaldehyde: One can obtain natural benzaldehyde by eating figs or, indirectly, as a breakdown product of apple seeds, peach or apricot kernels. An excess of such products can be poisonous. All supermarkets sell Almond Extract, which normally contains 90 milligrams of benzaldehyde per teaspoon. The Essential Oil Source sells this and other such products. Half an ounce of benzaldehyde sells for $8.50. Phone: 800-289-8427.

Doctors studying benzaldehyde in cancer include:

• Dr. Michael Wick, Dana-Farber Cancer Institute, Department of Dermatology, Harvard Medical School, 44 Binney Street, Boston, MA 02115. Phone: 617-732-3670. The general phone number for Dana-Farber Cancer Institute is 617-732-3000; for Harvard Medical School: 617-432-1000.

• Dr. E. Kano, Department of Experimental Radiology and Health Physics, Fukyi Medical University, Japan.

• Dr. Hans Nieper. Outpatient office: Sedan Strasse 21, 3000 Hannover 1, Germany, 011-49-511-348-08-08. Fax: 011-49-511-318417. His publications can be obtained from the Brewer Science Library, Richland Center, WI 53581. Phone: 608-647-6513.

Butyric acid: Available from ProBiologic, Inc. West Willows Technoloy Ctr., 14714 NE 87th Street, Redmond, WA 98052. Phone: 800-678-8218. At the present time they only sell to health care professionals.

There is also a product called ButyrEn,® an enteric-coated extended shelf life nutritional formulation of calcium and magnesium salts of butyric acid, designed for delayed release in the gastrointestinal tract. From Allergy Research Group, 400 Preda Street, San Leandro, CA 94577. Phone: 800-545-9960.

DMSO is available through many health food outlets. It is widely used by many alternative clinics. See *Third Opinion*. For example,

• The American Biologics-Mexico S.A. Medical Center, Tijuana, Mexico. Phone: 800-227-4458.

• Natural Health Center, PO Box N-8941, Third Terrace, Collins Avenue, Nassau, Bahamas. Phone: 809-326-6565.

• Michael B. Schachter, MD, PC, and Associates, Two Executive Boulevard, Suite 202, Suffern, NY 10901. Phone: 914-368-4700. Fax: 914-368-4727. Ask for new-patient educators.

It is manufactured as Rimso-50® by Research Industries Corporation, Pharmaceutical Division, 6864 South 300 West, Midvale, UT 84047 but is only approved by FDA for interstitial cystitis.

Ellagic acid: A good food source is the Brazil nut, which also contains selenium. Ellagic acid is also found in raspberries, blackberries, strawberries, walnuts, pecans and cranberries.

Enzyme Therapy: For further information on the Beardian theory, Ernst T. Krebs, Jr., DSc, John Beard Memorial Foundation, PO Box 685, San Francisco, CA 94101. Phone: 415-824-1067. A videotape of enzyme pioneer, Karl Ransberger, PhD, speaking at the Cancer Control Society's 1991 annual meeting is available for $30, plus $5 postage and handling from Malibu Video, PO Box 6328, Malibu, CA 90265. Phone: 213-456-5186. Nicholas Gonzalez, MD, uses enzymes extensively in his practice. 730 Park Avenue, New York, NY 10021. Phone: 212-535-3993. His patients frequently obtain their enzymes and other supplies from:

Mr. David Sauder, Nutri Supplies, 1020 Stony Battery Road
Lancaster, PA 17601. Phone: 800-999-2700

NutriCology, Inc., Allergy Research Group, PO Box 489
San Leandro, CA 94577-0489. Phone: 800-782-4274

Treatment with enzymes, including Wobe Mugos:
Wolfgang Scheef, MD, c/o Robert Janker Clinic
Fauchklinik fur Tumorerkrankenungen, Baumschulallee 12-14
5300 Bonn 1, Germany. Phone: 011-49-7291-0

Janker Clinic (of Mexico), Eduardo Gallegos, MD
1527 Blvd. Sanchez Taboada & Mission San Diego, Suite 101
Zone Del Rio, Tijuana, Mexico 22320. Phone: 011-52-66-842200/157

Wakunaga of America Ltd., 2305 Madero, Mission Viejo, CA 92691. Phone: 714-855-2776. Makes Kyolic® Super Formula 102, which contains an enzyme complex in addition to aged garlic extract powder.

Flutamide: For an information packet on the use of flutamide, write or call: Patient Advocates for Advanced Cancer Treatments, Inc.
1143 Parmalee NW, Grand Rapids, MI 49504. Phone: 616-453-1477.

Gossypol: Not approved by the FDA, but widely used elsewhere as a male contraceptive. Merck Index 4435.

Hydrazine sulfate: Doctors and researchers can receive scientific information on hydrazine sulfate from Dr. Joseph Gold, Syracuse Research Institute, 600 East Genesee Street, Syracuse, NY 13202. Phone: 315-472-6616. Dr. Gold does not treat cancer patients nor is he involved in the marketing or distribution of this product. Hydrazine sulfate is available to the general public through Ms. Donna Schuster, Great Lakes Metabolics, 1724 Hiawatha Court, NE, Rochester, MN 55904. Phone: 507-288-2348. The cost of hydrazine sulfate is approximately $30-40 per 100 tablets, or about a dollar a day.

Iscador: For information on the availability of Iscador, contact the Society for Cancer Research (Swiss Anthroposophic organization) in Arlesheim, Switzerland. In the US, one can contact the Rudolf Steiner Fellowship Foundation, 241 Hungry Hollow Road, Spring Valley, NY 10977. Phone: 914-356-8494/914-425-6835. The Lukas Klinik in Arlesheim is devoted to Iscador research. Its address is CH-4144 Arlesheim, Switzerland. Phone: 011-41-61-72-3333. In Germany, research is taking place on two other mistletoe preparations. The first is Helixor, made without fermentation from a sap extract. The other is ABNOVAviscum, made from fresh mistletoe leaves in the absence of oxygen. This extract contains proteins, lipoproteins and lectins. For information on ABNOVA, one can contact Dr. H.B. von Laue, Klinik Oschelbronn, Am Eichhof, 7532 Niefern-Oschelbronn 2, Germany. Phone: 0 72 33 6 80. Fax: 0 72 33 6 81 10.

Megace: Dr. Jamie H. von Roenn, Department of Hematology/Oncology, Northwestern University Medical School, 233 East Erie, Room 700, Chicago, IL 60611. Phone: 312-908-5284. Dr. Roenn has done research on megace in cancer and HIV infection in humans.

Dr. Patricia A. Johnson, MD, Carle Clinic, University of Illinois, 602 West University, Urbana, IL 61801. Phone: 217-383-3010. Dr. Johnson has researched the use of megace as an "effective" primary hormonal therapy for advanced breast cancer.

Methylene blue: This dye is available by prescription in a number of preparations for relief of discomfort of the lower urinary tract. Star Pharmaceuticals, 1990 N.W. 44th Street, Pompano Beach, FL, 33064, produces an FDA-approved "Urolene Blue®" containing 65 mg of methylene blue, available by prescription. Phone: 304-971-9704. "Urised®," manufactured by Webcon Pharmaceuticals, PO Box 6380, Fort Worth, TX 76115, contains methylene blue and other substances. Phone: 817-293-0450.

Health Enhancement Services, Inc. 30 West Mashta Drive, Key Biscayne, FL 33149. Phone: 305-365-9000. Offers methylene blue as part of an unconventional approach to cancer and other diseases featuring electroacupuncture according to Voll (EAV) diagnosis. A minimum stay of 21 days is required. Some of their other recommendations include adrenal cortex extract; glutathione supplements; Vitamin C; B_{12} cyanocobalamin; biotin (a B vitamin); Vitamin B_2; and potassium chloride. This facility is operated by a licensed acupuncturist, not a physician.

Nafazatrom: Manufactured by Miles Inc. Pharmaceutical Division, 400 Morgan Lane, West Haven, CT. 06516. Phone: 800-468-0894.

Onconase: Clinical studies are now underway at two medical centers with Onconase. Treatment is free, although travelling and living expenses are not covered. To find out if a patient qualifies, contact:

New York Medical College, Department of Oncology, Munger Pavilion, Room 250, Valhalla, NY, 10595
Patient Contact: Dr. Mittleman or Dr. Chun.
Phone: 914-285-8374 Fax: 914-993-4420

LESS TOXIC RESOURCES

The Thompson Cancer Survival Center, Knoxville, TN
Principal Investigator: Dr. John Costanzi
Patient Contact: Jan Miller. Phone: 615-541-4966

For general information on Onconase:, Alfacell Corporation, 225 Belleville Avenue, Bloomfield, NJ 07003. Phone: 201-748-0882. Fax: 201-748-1355

SOD: Superoxide Dismutase is widely available in health food stores. Choice Metabolics, 1180 Walnut Avenue, Chula Vista, CA 92100 offers Oxy-5000 Forte which includes 5000 units of SOD, as well as other enzymes, minerals, amino acids and vitamins. $22.00 for 90 tablets. Phone: 800-227-4473.

Sulindac: Available as a prescription drug as Clinoril Tablets (Merck Sharp & Dohme) or as Sulindac Tablets from Lederle or Warner Chilcott. For polyps, doctors generally recommend a starting dosage of 150 milligram once a day for adult patients. When the polyps have disappeared, the dosage is usually reduced to a daily dose of 75 milligrams. Patients are usually re-evaluated for growths at six-month intervals.

Research on Sulindac:

William G. Friend, MD, Colon and Rectal Clinic, 1221 Madison, Suite 1220 Seattle, WA 98104 Phone: 206-622-4745. Dr. Friend is an attending surgeon at: Swedish Hospital Medical Center, 747 Summit Avenue, Seattle, WA 98104 Phone: 206-386-6000

William R. Waddell, MD and Wolff M. Kirsch, MD of the Department of Surgery, University of Arizona Medical Center, 1501 North Campbell Avenue, Tucson, AZ 85724. Phone: 602-694-0111.

Suramin is also known as germanin, sodium suramin, suraminum natricum, Bayer 205, Fourneau 309, Naganium, and Naganol. It is manufactured by Bayer Pharmaceuticals, West Haven, CT. It is not approved by the FDA. Patients can contact NCI through the Cancer Information Service. Phone: 800-4-CANCER, to learn of availability, if any, of suramin trials.

Tagamet: Manufactured by SmithKline Beecham Pharmaceuticals, 1 Franklin Plaza, PO Box 7929, Phildelphia, PA 19101. Phone: 215-751-4000. Clinical research has been conducted by Thomas J. Smith, MD, MCV Station, PO Box 230, Richmond, VA 23298. Phone: 804-786-9641. He works at the Medical College of Virginia, School of Medicine, Sanger Hall, 1101 East Marshall St., Richmond, VA 23219. Phone: 804-786-9793.

Tamoxifen: Widely used in the treatment of breast cancer.
For information on current studies, call the National Cancer Institute. Phone: 800-4-CANCER.

Urea: US doctors using urea therapy include:
David Steenblock, DO, 22821 Lake Forest Drive, Suite 114,
El Toro, CA 92630. Phone: 714- 770-9616

Vincent Speckhart, MD, 902 Graydon Avenue, Suite 2, Norfolk, VA
23507. Phone: 804-622-0014. If no answer, call: 804-622-5333
Urea is potentially an inexpensive treatment for cancer. Pharmaceutical
grade urea runs around $28 per pound from standard supply houses
(although most such companies will not sell it for medical uses).

Bio-Tech of Fayetteville, AR sells both urea and creatine hydrate. Their
address is P.O. Box 1992, Fayetteville, AR 72702. Phone: 800-345-1199 or
501-443-9148. Bio-Tech sells only to doctors, health professionals or pharmacies, but will ship directly to the patients, if a doctor so directs.

A product called "Carbatine" contains urea and creatine mixed together
in a palatable form. Each container is reconstituted. One adds 28 ounces
of purified water to the four ounces of concentrate in a provided mixer for
a total volume of 32 ozs. Shake the bottle so that all the creatine sediment
is emptied into the mixer. Each quart is then divided into six or seven
doses. A 30 day supply (30 four ounce concentrates plus the mixer) is sold
for $310.00. A 60 day supply is $585.00 from: Pharmaceuticals International, 539 Telegraph Canyon Road #227,Chula Vista, CA 92010. Phone:
800-365-3698.

Dr. Evangelos D. Danopoulos: Now in his eighties, Dr. Danopoulos
(12 Rigillis Str, 106-74 Athens, Greece. Phone: 011-301-721-5318) is
retired. His daughter, Dr. Iphigenia E. Danopoulos, is a dermatologist in
Athens. Dr. Danopoulos's latest protocol published in *The Townsend Letter for Doctors*, consists of 28 grams of urea dissolved in a quart of water.
This quart is then divided into seven equal portions. One portion is taken
every one and a half hours throughout the waking day. At the same time,
3.5 grams of creatine hydrate are taken seven times a day, along with the
urea. Every seven to ten days, a test is done for serum urea. In treating
far-advanced liver cancer, he says, one should decrease the dosage of urea
to two grams and that of creatine hydrate to 3 grams, both seven times a
day. The creatine hydrate should be put into something like peanut butter
to mask its unpleasant taste.

$\mathcal{E}$LECTROMAGNETISM

In this section are gathered a rather diverse group of therapies, all of which share utilization of some part of the electromagnetic spectrum. This includes light, heat and magnetism. Such 'energy medicine' has been controversial since the time of Franz Mesmer (1734-1815), the German doctor who enthralled Paris with his displays of 'animal magnetism.'

Mesmer was debunked by a blue ribbon panel of experts, including Benjamin Franklin. This has tended to give such ventures a bad name for two hundred years.

Interest in such questions has been rekindled by a newfound respect for Asian medicine. When the first Chinese acupuncturist got tired of twirling the needles and attached a small electric current to it instead, he or she triggered a revolution in energy medicine. The field of electroacupuncture was born. This has branched off in two directions. In conventional medicine, it has largely evolved into TENS (transcutaneous electrical nerve stimulation), a fairly standard application for controlling pain.

But it has also spawned a variety of electroacupuncture-like devices for diagnosing and treating illnesses of all sorts. Use of these devices (such as EAV, electroacupuncture according to Voll) are often banned by official medicine and hence scientific evaluation of their claims is extremely difficult. One gets the impression that the official use of acupuncture in the West only scratches the surface of the potential of such methods in the understanding and treatment of cancer.

In at least one hospital, electroacupuncture has been

used as an effective method of reducing the side effects of chemotherapy. This modern technique is based on the ancient Chinese practices. Scientists at the Northern Ireland Radiotherapy and Oncology Centre of Queen's University found that a small current applied for five minutes to one particular acupuncture point was a very effective antinausea treatment for patients receiving a variety of anticancer drugs.

The Belfast study involved 130 patients with a history of "distressing sickness" after previous treatment. On the basis of previous experience, nearly all of them could be expected to get sick, given further conventional treatment. But when they were given electroacupuncture treatment, "sickness was either completely absent or reduced considerably in 97 percent of patients and no side effects were encountered."

Acupuncture depends on stimulating certain precisely delineated sections on the skin, called acupoints. When a "dummy" acupoint was electrically stimulated, as a test, the patients experienced no beneficial effects.

The problem with electroacupuncture, however, is that its effects tend to wear off rather quickly (1).

The same Irish scientists found that beneficial effects could be obtained through the use of TENS at the P6 antiemetic acupuncture point. They studied TENS in over 100 patients for whom chemotherapy-induced sickness was not adequately controlled by antiemetic (antivomiting) drugs. Although they said the results were not quite as good as with acupuncture, more than 75 percent of the patients did achieve "considerable benefit" from this nontoxic procedure. Best results were achieved when the patients themselves were asked to administer five minutes of TENS every two hours (2-3).

⊕ References

1.   Dundee JW, et al. Acupuncture prophylaxis of cancer chemotherapy-induced sickness. J R Soc Med.1989;82:268-71.

2.   Dundee JW and Yang J. Prolongation of the antiemetic action of P6 acupuncture by acupressure in patients having cancer chemotherapy. J R Soc Med. 1990;83:360-2.

3.   Dundee JW, et al. Non-invasive stimulation of the P6 (Neigun) antiemetic acupuncture point in cancer chemotherapy. J R Soc Med. 1991;84:210-2.

ϙ *Ε*LECTRIC *Τ*HERAPY

Since the time of Pasteur, biologists have generally focused on the cellular level of life. Meanwhile, other important influences on health have tended to be neglected. These include the effects of electricity. Everyone knows in a general way that the body runs on electricity. The brain and the nervous system could never function without the steady flow of electrical impulses. These facts are indisputable, yet the electrical dimension is only superficially taught in medical schools and mentioned in standard textbooks. In truth, electricity can powerfully influence both health and disease. Eastern medicine, approaching the body from a different point of view, has taken a more active interest in this subtle question.

In the West, a few pioneers have done outstanding work in this field (1). In America, for example, Robert Becker, MD, a professor at the Upstate Medical Center, Syracuse, New York, and author of a popular book, *The Body Electric*, has pioneered research into this topic. In Europe, a prominent Swedish scientist Bjorn Nordenstrom, MD has explored the use of electricity, with and without concurrent drug treatment, to affect the growth of cancer.

Nordenstrom has reported results of electrical treatment on lung metastases in three patients whose tumors originated elsewhere. One breast cancer metastasis completely disappeared after treatment with an electrode. Two large uterine metastases regressed when attached to an electrical field but progressed when attached to the opposite kind of field. Different tumors showed variable responses to different electromagnetic fields. A metastasis from a bladder cancer proved resistant to two kinds of electrical fields (2).

Fourteen patients with incurable cancer, who no longer responded to conventional methods, showed benefit from a combination of electrochemical treatment and the standard drug Adriamycin. The use of this combined approach enabled scientists to reduce the total dose and many unwanted side effects of the drug. An intravenous infusion of "charged Adriamycin" was able to hone in on the cancer, which had been charged in an opposite direction (3).

This science is in its infancy and electrical stimulation occasionally has the effect of promoting the tumor, as well.

⊕ References

1.   Dihel LE, et al. Effects of an extremely low frequency electromagnetic field on the cell division rate and plasma membrane of Paramecium tetraurelia. Bioelectromagnetics.1985;6:61-71.

2.   Nordenstrom B. Electrochemical treatment of cancer. I. Variable response to anodic and cathodic fields. American Journal of Clinical Oncology.1989;12:530-536.

3.   Nordenstrom B. Electrochemical treatment of cancer. II. Effect of electrophoretic influence on adriamycin. American Journal of Clinical Oncology.1990;13:75-88.

ᔆ*H*EAT *T*HERAPY

Hyperthermia is the scientific use of heat for the treatment of cancer (or other diseases). In the body, externally applied heat acts like an artificially-induced fever (1). Some doctors are coming to believe that fever is a natural healing mechanism of the body, stimulating the immune system, while disarming microbes and cancer cells. Raising the temperature of the tumor has been called an "exploitable Achilles heel."

This is because solid tumors have bizarrely-organized blood supplies. These consist of normal blood vessels that have been "parasitized" by the cancer, as well as new vessels that have been induced to grow by hormone-like chemicals released by the tumor itself. "These vessels are inadequate in many respects, being tortuous, thin-walled, chaotically arranged, lacking innervation [nerves] and with no predetermined direction of flow," wrote scientists at the Mount Vernon Hospital, Northwood, Middlesex, UK (2).

Hyperthermia is one of the most promising ways to exploit this weakness, said Dr. Mijenki V. Pilepich:

"Recurrent cancers untreatable by conventional forms of treatment can melt away permanently," the Michigan scientist has said.

For many types of cancer, heat therapy increases the chances of controlling the disease by 25 to 35 percent. For example, promising results have been obtained in cancers of the brain, breast, head and neck area and skin (*NCI Cancer Weekly*, 5/29/89).

Heat has been used therapeutically since the time of the

Pharaohs and is mentioned in Hippocrates and other ancient medical writers. In 1866, a doctor named Busch reported the "spontaneous" cure of a sarcoma in a middle-aged women, after she suffered a bout of the fever-inducing skin infection erysipelas (3). This experiment of nature was rediscovered, repeated and then systematically developed into a full-scale therapy called **Coley's toxins** by Dr. William B. Coley of Memorial Hospital, New York. Ironically, many scientists only began to take the effects of heat on cancer seriously after concerns were raised about the negative effects of "everyday electrical appliances, wiring in the home, and power transmission lines" (5).

At Indiana University radiation oncologists applied microwave heat (just 2° Celsius, or 3.5° Fahrenheit, above the body's normal temperature) to a series of patients once a week. Laboratory studies of their blood showed that "by inducing a fever-like condition, the immunological responses are enhanced" (4).

Some scientists have called for a reintegration of fever into conventional therapy. They recognize that prolonged, natural fever enhances the effects of natural body defense proteins (6). Steps are being taken in that direction. For example, doctors at the University of Massachusetts, Amherst are adding interferon-gamma and **TNF** to improve the results of whole body hyperthermia (7).

Today, hyperthermia is used all over the world in many different ways and thousands of papers have been written on the topic. Enhanced temperatures are usually created artificially with different kinds of electromagnetic waves (8). Hyperthermia is generally used in combination with standard therapies, such as chemotherapy and especially radiation (9).

In one experiment, cancer cells were implanted in the brains of 28 rabbits, which were then divided into four groups of seven each. The first group got hyperthermia, by means of a needle into the tumor maintained at 45° C. for half an hour. The second group received chemotherapy. In the third group, 10 minutes after the chemotherapy injection, hyperthermia was induced. The fourth group received no treatment.

The animals receiving hyperthermia lived longer. Japanese scientists concluded that in "this rabbit brain tumor model, hyperthermia alone was significantly superior to no treatment." However,

---

"Combined treatment with hyperthermia and chemotherapy was more effective than either treatment alone" (10).

How hot is hot? Recommendations differ from 104° F (40° C) all the way up to 120° F (48.8° C). In one experiment, for example, raising the temperature from 98.6° F (37° C) to 104° F (40° C) significantly increased white blood cell activity. The strength of this reaction was more noticeable in healthy people than in cancer patients, suggesting that "immunotherapy should be initiated early in patients with malignant disease before there is systemic involvement from an increasing tumor burden" (11).

Many types of cancer cells are selectively damaged at temperatures of 107° to 109.4° F (42 to 43° C) (1). In Madison, WI, doctors used a radiant heat system to raise the whole body to 107° F (41.8° C). They called this "a safe and effective method...suitable for combination therapy" (12).

Heating tumors to 107° F (42° C) or more leads to their self-destruction. This temperature slows down the malignant cells and their oxygen respiration. Heat accumulates selectively in the cancer tissue at 107° to 111° F (42° to 44° C). This is probably related to the defective blood supply within the tumor (13). Some scientists are striving to raise the temperature of tumors as high as 122° F (50° C) without harming the patient (1).

Tumors on or near the skin surface are obviously easy to reach with the heat treatment. But reaching deep-seated tumors, without also seriously injuring internal organs, is a challenge. It requires accurate measurements of just how hot internal organs actually get (3).

One attendant problem is that accurately monitoring the heat of internal organs is sometimes more difficult and dangerous than the procedure itself. Sometimes it involves sticking a probe into the liver, for example. "Invasive monitoring is imperfect and somewhat risky when used in deeply seated tumors," according to Dr. F. L. Moffat (3). This need is lessened when lower temperatures are used. Some doctors warn that the act of measurement, as required by governmental regulations, should not become a goal in itself, hindering progress in hyperthermia.

Another technique has been to administer drugs along with the heat therapy. For example, Flagyl® caused an increase in tumor temperature above that achieved by hyperthermia alone. Radiofrequency hyperthermia, in combination with chemotherapy, produced "objective evidence of tumor repression in 30 to 50 per cent of the patients with metastatic cancer," according to Dr. Rudy Falk of Toronto (14). Others have noted that when the main tumor regresses, the secondary growths (metastases) sometimes also regress. This has been seen especially with recurrent melanomas and sarcomas of the limbs.

The danger of heat to other organs can also be overcome by using laser light transmitted through thin flexible fibers. Laser energy was delivered directly into the center of a tumor via needles. Ultrasound was then used to locate the tumor and study the effects. Five patients were so treated (including those with cancer of the breast, pancreas and liver). In one, a liver tumor had not increased over 10 months, and afterwards the patient showed no sign of cancer (15).

"This simple technique can be applied safely and effectively to common tumors in humans," according to scientists at University College, London.

Radio waves are another means of delivering heat to tumors. At the Micro-Radio Frequency Hyperthermia Clinic in Forlì, Italy the results have been "definitely encouraging, even in cases apparently with no hope" (16).

When heat is used as an addition to radiation therapy, it "can increase tumor regression significantly," said oncologists at the University of Wisconsin Clinical Cancer Center in Madison.

Two of the techniques used there to treat brain tumors are Scan Focused Ultrasound and Interstitial Ferromagnetic Seed Implants. These techniques employ the "most sophisticated use of diagnostic radiology methods." (8).

Ninety patients were also treated with a new microwave heating system called HTS-100, at Tokyo Metropolitan Komagome Hospital, Kyoto University and Aichi Cancer Center in Japan. Even large tumors were satisfactorily heated to temperatures above 107° F (42° C). Two-third of the tumors either partially or completely regressed.

There were over 60 percent remissions in patients with large and deep tumors (17). Results were so good that in 1991 Japanese scientists concluded that this system "can be expected to play an important role in clinical cancer hyperthermia" (18).

Side effects of HTS-100 treatment included pain in 15.6 percent; unpleasant sensations in 6.3 percent; and burns in 3.6 percent. But most such side effects were transient and slight. There was a higher frequency of pain than with conventional microwave heating, but this was attributable to an expansion of the heating area (17).

In St. Louis, 60 cancer patients were treated with radiation and microwave heat therapy. The overall local control rate was 50 percent, but there had to be at least one session in which the temperature went to 109.4° F (43° C) for half an hour, according to scientists at Washington University School of Medicine (19).

In another test, 45 tumors were given a combination of radiation and heat therapy. Initially, there were 69 percent complete responses, 22 percent partial responses and 9 percent without any change. Over the long term, there was 90 percent local control and 10 percent recurrences. Acute side-effects occurred in a third, according to scientists at Hahnemann University in Philadelphia (20).

A scanned focused ultrasound hyperthermia system was used to treat 71 patients who had a total of 87 tumors. Most of these patients also received conventional radiation therapy. There was a 62 percent "overall response rate" and 22 percent of the tumors completely disappeared. There was also "dramatic local pain reduction" in 42 percent. Tolerance of the treatment was good, with chronic skin blisters and burns in only two patients (21).

At Stanford University, six prostate cancer patients underwent radiotherapy after tumor recurrence. Four also received hyperthermia from an electromagnetic system. Three of the six are free from disease; two had recurrences and one died, presumably of his disease (22).

Duke University Cancer Center is treating ovarian cancer patients with a combination of chemotherapy and heat. The conventional drug Cisplatin is infused by catheter into the abdominal cavity. The woman is then given hyperthermia (to 41.5° C) directly to the area where the drug is given. Overall body temperature is maintained at 100.4° F (38° C), similar to a low-grade fever.

"It feels like a heating blanket at a high setting," one of the doctors says. The treatment consists of microwaves that travel through a water-filled bag, which then radiates heat to the patient.

Patients chosen for this study were no longer responding to conventional therapy. Cisplatin is considered the most effective standard drug for ovarian cancer but Duke scientists say they have increased its effectiveness several-fold by combining it with heat therapy. The hyperthermia team at Duke is one of the largest in the country, and includes 35 specialists, including physicians, and biomedical and electrical engineers.

⊕ References

1.   Dickson JA. Hyperthermia in the treatment of cancer. Lancet.1979; 1:202-5.

2.   Denekamp J. Vascular attack as a therapeutic strategy for cancer. Cancer Metastasis Rev.1990;9:267-82.

3.   Moffat FL, et al. Hyperthermia for cancer: a practical perspective. Semin Surg Oncol.1985;1:200-19.

4.   Park MM, et al. The effect of whole body hyperthermia on the immune cell activity of cancer patients. Lymphokine Res.1990;9:213-23.

5.   Wilkening GM and Sutton CH. Health effects of nonionizing radiation. Med Clin North Am.1990;74:489-507.

6.   Keen AR and Frelick RW. Response of tumors to thermodynamic stimulation of the immune system. Del Med J.1990;62:1155-6.

7.   Rosen P. The synergism of gamma-interferon and tumor necrosis factor in whole body hyperthermia. Med Hypotheses.1990;33:173-4.

8.   Hynynen K and Lulu BA. Hyperthermia in cancer treatment. Invest Radiol.1990;25:824-34.

9.   Robins HI. Combined modality clinical trials for favorable B-cell neoplasms: lonidamine plus whole body hyperthermia and/or total body irradiation. Semin Oncol.1991;18:23-7.

10.   Tanaka T, et al. Effect of combined treatment with magnetic induction hyperthermia and chemotherapy in a rabbit brain tumor model. Neurol Med Chir (Tokyo).1989;29:377-81.

11.   Goldsmith HS and Stettiner L. Thermal influence on the lymphocytic

response of cancer patients. Am J Surg.1979;138:668-71.

12. Robins HI and Cohen JD. Radiant heat systemic hyperthermia clinical trials. Adv Exp Med Biol.1990;267:189-96.

13. Dreznik A, et al. Hyperthermia as a treatment for neoplasia. Can J Surg.1982;25:603-8.

14. Falk RE, et al. The effect of radiofrequency hyperthermia and chemotherapy upon human neoplasms when used with adjuvant metronidazole. Surg Gynecol Obstet.1983;157:505-12.

15. Steger AC, et al. Interstitial laser hyperthermia: a new approach to local destruction of tumours [see comments]. BMJ.1989;299:362-5.

16. Bazzocchi G, et al. Centred radio-frequency hyperthermia in solid tumours. Adv Exp Med Biol.1990;267:405-10.

17. Matsuda T, et al. [Clinical research on hyperthermia of cancer using microwave heating equipment of lens applicator type]. Nippon Gan Chiryo Gakkai Shi.1990;25:1635-47.

18. Matsuda T, et al. Clinical research into hyperthermia treatment of cancer using a 430 MHz microwave heating system with a lens applicator. Int J Hyperthermia.1991;7:425-40.

19. Myerson RJ, et al. Tumor control in long-term survivors following superficial hyperthermia. Int J Radiat Oncol Biol Phys.1990;18:1123-9.

20. Phromratanapongse P, et al. Initial results of phase I/II interstitial thermoradiotherapy for primary advanced and local recurrent tumors. Am J Clin Oncol.1990;13:259-68.

21. Harari PM, et al. Development of scanned focussed ultrasound hyperthermia: clinical response evaluation. Int J Radiat Oncol Biol Phys. 1991;21:831-40.

22. Kaplan I, et al. Secondary external-beam radiotherapy and hyperthermia for local recurrence after 125-iodine implantation in adenocarcinoma of the prostate. Int J Radiat Oncol Biol Phys.1991;20:551-4.

℁ℳICROCAPSULES

In order to deliver anticancer drugs, such as the antibiotic mitomycin C, in a precisely targeted way, scientists are putting them into tiny magnetic 'bullets' called microcapsules and then directing them to their target with magnets. The basic purpose of this method is to deliver drugs to the cancer while keep them away from the sensitive bone marrow (1). Several kinds have now been created.

One, called the outer type, has the drug as its core, with zinc ferrite on the outside. The other, inner type has both the drug and zinc ferrite as the core. Either type is a kind of "sustained release chemotherapy," directed to its target via magnetism.

"Animal studies showed that magnetic microcapsules could be magnetically controlled in the artery and urinary bladder," Japanese scientists wrote. Tumors in a rabbit's limbs and bladder were successfully treated through such magnetic control. Microcapsules "markedly enhanced" the drug's absorption into the surrounding tissues for a prolonged period of time.

These results show that magnetic microcapsules can be effective as a drug delivery system (2). Russian scientists claim that microcapsules made of an iron compound make the best drug carriers (3).

Another way of using magnetism against cancer is the "pulsing magnetic field" (PMF). This can also be combined with the conventional antitumor drug, mitomycin C. The combination was applied to two experimental tumors, a fibrosarcoma and a liver cancer in rats. The pulsing magnetic field was generated by a solenoid coil. One week after tumors were implanted into the thighs of rats, the animals were given mitomycin C injections, immediately followed by applications of 200 Hz of magnetism for one hour. Three months afterwards, survival of the rats was as follows:

Treatment	Number Survived	% Survived
No Treatment	0 out of 10	0
Mitomycin C	4 out of 12	34
PMF	6 out of 13	47
Mitomycin + PMF	10 out of 13	77

Scientists at Hokkaido University School of Medicine in Sapporo concluded that pulsed magnetic fields "exhibited a potentiation of the antitumor effect of mitomycin C" (4).

⊕ References

1.   Gupta PK and Hung CT. Magnetically controlled targeted micro-carrier systems. Life Sci.1989;44:175-86.

2.   Kato T, et al. Magnetic microcapsules for targeted delivery of anti-cancer drugs. Appl Biochem Biotechnol.1984;10:199-211.

3.   Ternovoi KS and Derzhavin AE. [Distribution and removal of magnetic microcarriers of antineoplastic agents from the body]. Eksp Onkol.1984;6:66-9.

4.   Omote Y, et al. Treatment of experimental tumors with a combination of a pulsing magnetic field and an antitumor drug. Jpn J Cancer Res.1990;81:956-61.

⚕ PHOTOTHERAPY

Phototherapy (also called photodynamic therapy or photochemotherapy) is the use of light in the treatment of diseases such as cancer. Phototherapy causes the destruction of tumors through the administration of a "photosensitizing agent" that is retained in tumors. This relatively harmless substance is then activated by shining a light on the tumor in order to generate cell-killing agents on the spot.

Since 1975, phototherapy has been reported to be effective in treating head and neck tumors that had failed to respond to conventional treatment, including surgery, cryotherapy (cold treatment), chemotherapy, hyperthermia or radiation (1).

The use of light as a therapy goes back to ancient Egypt,

India and Greece. A surprisingly sophisticated system was used on the Nile between 2,000 to 1,200 BC. The sun provided the energy and the reactive agents were derived from plants such as the Nile weed, *Ammi majus*, which contains a chemical known as a psoralen. This early Egyptian form of phototherapy was used to treat vitiligo and other skin diseases.

This ingenious treatment eventually died out. But the principle was rediscovered at the beginning of the twentieth century through the work of two Germans, Oscar Raab and Herman von Tappeiner. A brilliant and eccentric Danish scientist, Niels R. Finsen, won the 1903 Nobel prize for his discovery that skin lesions of tuberculosis could be eliminated after being exposed to ultraviolet light. The discovery of antibiotics led medicine in different directions, however.

The first modern studies on phototherapy, with the drug 8-MOP were done, appropriately enough, by Abdel M. El Mofty of the University of Cairo in the 1940s.

In 1937, German scientists had developed a drug called hemoporphyrin (also called hematoporphyrin), a deep red, almost purple, crystal derived from the breakup of red blood cells. This colorful agent showed a special ability to hone in on cancer cells. When light was directed at such cells, they died. Thus was born the modern age of phototherapy, which has been called "a promising tool in modern cancer treatment" (2). Today, such therapy is central to the treatment of psoriasis, acne and some kinds of jaundice in newborns.

"Light-activated drugs" were the subject of an excellent article by Richard L. Edelson in the *Scientific American* (8/1988). Dr. Edelson calls current methods "harbingers of an entirely new class of therapeutic agents." He explains how light plus 8-MOP are now being used to treat cutaneous T-cell lymphoma (CTLC), a white blood cell malignancy which previously had a poor prognosis. The original work on this was done by Barbara Gilchrest at the Harvard Medical School and has been extended by Edelson and his colleagues (3-5).

Scientists took a variety of artificially-created cell lines which had been prepared by fusing mouse with human leukemia cells. They then joined antibodies against such cells to hematoporphyrin (HP) and tested them for their ability to bind to such hybrids. Under fluorescent light it was clear that this compound had indeed linked up with these hybrid cells. It was also shown that the HP-containing compound would kill large numbers of cells, even when concentrations were very low, whereas HP or antibody alone would not kill cancer cells unless concentrations were over one hundred times higher, it was reported in *Cancer Research* (6).

Ovary cells from the Chinese hamster were incubated with a form of HP and then exposed to red light at different dose rates. A total of five different dose rates were examined following a one-hour incubation with the drug. Similar levels of cell kill were obtained for the different dose rates.

Albino mice were then given injections of hematoporphyrin. Twenty-four hours later, each mouse's right hind leg was bathed in red light. There was acute skin damage induced by this combination of drug and light. Again, comparable levels of damage were induced, regardless of the dose of light. Therefore, the photosensitizing efficiency of this therapy is not affected by the dose of light delivered (7).

In a variation on this procedure, scientists are using other tumor-targeting dyes and lasers. Many new dyes, other than just HP, and various laser wavelengths are being tested in an attempt to improve drug uptake into the tumor. They also are trying to increase drug retention and lower toxicity.

Magnetic resonance imaging (MRI) "may now provide an extremely sensitive way to detect and monitor laser-tissue effects," surgeons at the UCLA School of Medicine reported (8). It also allows access to deep and sometimes inaccessible tumors. Attempts are also being made to combine dyes with monoclonal antibodies to better home in on the cancer (6).

Truly selective destruction of cancer cells can be produced in experimental colon cancers with a complete sparing of normal colon tissue.

In addition, this procedure does not interfere with the "mechanical strength of the colon," even when tissue is damaged or killed in some normal areas (9).

In contrast, laser by itself can seriously weaken the wall of the colon and may even perforate it. This is because the "submucosal collagen layer" is preserved after phototherapy, but is destroyed by the usual laser therapy. An initial clinical trial was carried out on 10 patients at the Walton Hospital in Liverpool, UK. All had inoperable tumors, with metastatic disease or severe medical problems. Phototherapy was shown to be safe (9).

All patients were given the HP-derivative 48 hours before starting phototherapy. Up to four parts of the tumor were treated with red laser light delivered through a flexible fiberoptic tube inserted into the tumor. Two patients had their small lesions "totally eradicated" and they remained tumor-free for 20 and 28 months, respectively, after the start of phototherapy. However, one patient with an advanced tumor had a serious hemorrhage that may have been the result of the therapy.

Liverpool scientists concluded that phototherapy:

"may be most suitable for the treatment of small tumors or for small areas of persistent tumor where the bulk has been removed by alternative techniques" (10).

They also found that the treatment works better with a smaller dose of another photosensitizer (11). They called this therapy, coupled with other cancer treatments, "very intriguing."

In addition, the investigation of phototherapy in viral disease is "just being opened to clinical investigation," according to surgeons at the University of Utah in Salt Lake City. They expect that the field will blossom with improvements in laser technology and greater familiarity with the photosensitizers (12).

Surgeons in Holland are exploring the use of phototherapy in the treatment of papillomas, a kind of benign tumor. Their model is the skin of the Dutch Belted rabbit. Using two photosensitizing agents called Photofrin II and Chlorin, in conjunction with lasers, they were able to produce regression of these warty growths. Total regression without any recurrences was achieved with Photofrin II and a gold laser at all light dosages, scientists at the University Hospital of Maastricht said (13).

In Vienna, scientists encouraged by success in treating various kinds of cancer involving T-cells (white blood cells), decided to try what is called extracorporeal (outside the body) phototherapy against a leukemia of the opposite type of cells, the B cells. Three such patients were treated for a year. Two of them showed stabilization of disease with a desired reduction of white blood cell count. The lymph nodes of another were normalized. One patient did not respond to this experimental therapy.

"No significant side effects" were observed, dermatologists at the University of Vienna reported. This treatment "may have a positive effect on the course" of B-cell leukemia in selected patients. The Austrian doctors called for further clinical trials (14).

In another experiment, Japanese researchers were able to make tumors regress four days after a single application of phototherapy. (Microwave heat therapy worked about as well.) However, a major problem was that "all the tumors treated with these single modalities regrew within four weeks after the treatments," the Fukui Medical School doctors noted. They therefore combined phototherapy with hyperthermia. At high doses, this combination was highly effective and "no tumor regrowth occurred for 45 days" (15).

Scientists at the Beckman Laser Institute and Medical Clinic at UC Irvine have been examining the same combination. They used multiple combinations of photosensitizing drugs and various wavelengths. With some combinations they "achieved a cure rate of up to 100 percent." This was as much as 40 percent better than using a single drug or wavelength. Smaller amounts of drug were needed, lowering the chances of side effects (16).

UC Irvine scientists also tried this therapy on a variety of pets—10 cats, 2 dogs and 3 snakes—which had differing tumor types. A new sensitizing drug called CASPc was utilized. Some of the larger tumors were first surgically debulked. No significant toxicity was seen in any animal. Beckman doctors reported that "tumor responses were comparable to those seen with conventional" treatments, including cryotherapy, hyperthermia and surgery:

Degree of response	Number	%
Complete	12	67
Partial	4	22
No response	2	11

Since the overall tumor response was considered very good, and sensitivity to the light was practically nonexistent, it is expected that using this therapy (technically called CASPc-PDT) "to eradicate human tumors would also yield comparable results" (17).

And in fact at the Henry Ford Hospital in Detroit, complete and/or partial remissions were obtained in 11 out of 12 patients with a variety of head and neck cancers, including not just carcinomas of the nasopharynx, palate and uvula, but also AIDS-related Kaposi's sarcoma in the mouth, head and neck (1).

In China, cancer of the nose and pharynx (upper portion of the digestive tube) is extremely common. There is therefore a great interest in finding new treatments. Specialists at the First Affiliated Hospital in Changsha are investigating the use of phototherapy for this type of cancer. In animals, they found that combination therapy inhibited cancers up to 70 percent. They then tried it on 20 patients.

Eight patients had complete responses while ten experienced "significant remission."

**Doctors in the Hunan port city achieved
"an overall response rate of 90 percent"
—a remarkable result.**

The blood picture remained stable after the therapy.

Only three patients developed mild skin reactions, but this did not affect subsequent treatments. In addition, there was no immunosuppression (18).

In recent years, Japanese doctors report seeing more patients with multiple primary cancers in their lungs. Since 1980, 145 lung cancer patients were treated with phototherapy at Tokyo Medical College. Thirteen of these had multiple primary lung cancers, three of whom were treated with phototherapy alone.

In the other ten cases, surgery was the main treatment, but phototherapy was used to mop up smaller tumors. The mean survival after phototherapy, alone or in combination with surgery, was 38 months. Seven of the patients remained alive as of 1991. Japanese surgeons concluded that phototherapy is useful for "improving the prognosis of patients with multiple primary" lung cancers (19).

One new way in which phototherapy can be utilized is by treating blood outside the body in a process called "photopheresis." In this process, blood cells are removed from the body, then passed through tiny tubes between two high-intensity ultraviolet A sources. In each treatment, about half a liter of blood (the amount in a single blood donation) is passed by the lights.

In a multi-center trial at Yale, Columbia, Vienna, and other universities, of 37 patients who were unresponsive to standard therapy 27 responded, a remarkable result. There were minimal side effects. This procedure has now been approved by the FDA for this form of cancer.

One of the advantages of this treatment is that the drugs used (psoralens) are relatively non-toxic agents. But when they are exposed to ultraviolet A they become highly active for a few millionths of a second, just "long enough for a chemical reaction but brief enough so that when the radiation is turned off, the drug reverts immediately to the inert form," according to Prof. Edelson.

While there is much that is new in phototherapy, 'sun-worshippers' will hardly be surprised by the health benefits of light. One innovative researcher, John Ott, has long maintained that full spectrum light is essential to health. Light, he says, serves a dual function, to see by, of course, but also to activate crucial hormones within the brain. Ott has long advocated the use of full spectrum light bulbs, so that people could avoid the allegedly debilitating effects of fluorescent bulbs. His work has received little attention from the orthodox medical community, although he has published in peer-reviewed journals (20-23).

⊕ References

1.   Schweitzer VG. Photodynamic therapy for treatment of head and neck cancer. Otolaryngol Head Neck Surg.1990;102:225-32.

2.   Daniell MD and Hill JS. A history of photodynamic therapy. Aust N Z J Surg.1991;61:340-8.

3.   Gasparro FP, et al. Effect of monochromatic UVA light and 8-methoxypsoralen on human lymphocyte response to mitogen. Photodermatol.1984;1:10-7.

4.   Gasparro FP, et al. Phototherapy and photopharmacology. Yale J Biol Med.1985;58:519-34.

5.   Santella RM, et al. Monoclonal antibodies to DNA modified by 8-methoxypsoralen and ultraviolet A light. Nucleic Acids Res.1985;13:2533-44.

6.   Mew D, et al. Ability of specific monoclonal antibodies and conventional antisera conjugated to hematoporphyrin to label and kill selected cell lines subsequent to light activation. Cancer Res.1985;45:4380-6.

7.   Gomer CJ, et al. In vitro and in vivo light dose rate effects related to hematoporphyrin derivative photodynamic therapy. Cancer Res.1985; 45: 1973-7.

8.   Castro DJ, et al. Future directions of laser phototherapy for diagnosis and treatment of malignancies: fantasy, fallacy, or reality? Laryngoscope.1991;101:1-10.

9.   Barr H, et al. Photodynamic therapy for colorectal disease. Int J Colorectal Dis.1989;4:15-9.

10.   Barr H, et al. Photodynamic therapy for colorectal cancer: a quantitative pilot study. Br J Surg.1990;77:93-6.

11.   Barr H, et al. Selective necrosis in dimethylhydrazine-induced rat colon tumors using phthalocyanine photodynamic therapy. Gastroenterology.1990;98:1532-7.

12.   Davis RK. Photodynamic therapy in otolaryngology-head and neck surgery. Otolaryngol Clin North Am.1990;23:107-19.

13.   Go PM, et al. Laser photodynamic therapy for papilloma viral lesions. Arch Otolaryngol Head Neck Surg.1990;116:1177-80.

14.   Knobler RM, et al. Experimental treatment of chronic lymphocytic leukemia with extracorporeal photochemotherapy. Initial observations. Blut.1990;60:215-8.

15.   Matsumoto N, et al. Combination effect of hyperthermia and photo-

dynamic therapy on carcinoma. Arch Otolaryngol Head Neck Surg. 1990;116:824-9.

16. Nelson JS, et al. Use of multiple photosensitizers and wavelengths during photodynamic therapy: a new approach to enhance tumor eradication. J Natl Cancer Inst.1990;82:868-73.

17. Roberts WG, et al. Photodynamic therapy of spontaneous cancers in felines, canines, and snakes with chloro-aluminum sulfonated phthalocyanine. J Natl Cancer Inst.1991;83:18-23.

18. Zhao SP, et al. Photoradiation therapy of animal tumors and nasopharyngeal carcinoma. Ann Otol Rhinol Laryngol.1990;:454-60.

19. Okunaka T, et al. Photodynamic therapy for multiple primary bronchogenic carcinoma. Cancer.1991;68:253-8.

20. Ott J. The eyes' dual function. I. Eye Ear Nose Throat Mon.1974;53:276-7.

21. Ott J. The eyes' dual function. II. Eye Ear Nose Throat Mon.1974;53:309-16.

22. Ott J. The eyes' dual function. III. Eye Ear Nose Throat Mon. 1974;53: 465-9.

23. Ott J. The influence of light on the retinal hypothalamic endocrine system. Ann Dent.1968;27:10-6.

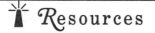

Resources

For basic research on electricity and cancer:

Dr. Bjorn E.W. Nordenstrom, Department of Diagnostic Radiology Karolinska Hospital, Box 60500, S-104 01, Stockholm, Sweden

On the general subject of electricity and life, two useful books are:

1). Robert O. Becker and Gary Selden. *The Body Electric: Electromagnetism and the Foundation of Life* (New York: Morrow, 1985) and Richard Gerber, *Vibrational Medicine* (Santa Fe, NM: Bear & Co., 1988) which is one of the best introductions to new age medicine.

Electroacupuncture: For scientific information about EAV one can write to the *American Journal of Acupuncture*, PO Box 610, Capitola, CA 95010, (408) 475-1700. Attn: Deborah Salisbury. They offer a special "Voll" issue of the *Journal* for $20. EAV is available from a growing number of alternative practitioners, including Health Enhancement Services, Inc., 30 West Mashta Drive, Key Biscayne, FL 33149. Phone: 305-365-9000 and Fuller Royal, MD, Nevada Clinic, 6105 West Tropicana, Las Vegas, NV 89103. Phone: 800-641-6661 or 702-871-2700.

CANCER THERAPY

Heat Therapy: This is now used at scores of medical centers.

HI Robins, MD, PhD, Director of Medical Oncology
University of Wisconsin Clinical Cancer Center,
800 Highland Avenue, Madison, WI 53792-0001. Phone: 608-263-1416.

Haim I. Bicher, MD, Director, Valley Cancer Institute
Contact Stan Smith, Public Affairs, 12099 W. Washington Blvd, Suite 304,
Los Angeles, CA 90066. Phone: 310-398-0013, Fax: 310-398-4470.

Duke University Cancer Center, PO Box 3843 Medical Center, Durham,
NC 27710. Dr. James Oleson, professor of radiation oncology. Phone: 919-
684-3742 and Dr. Daniel Clarke-Pearson, chief of gynecologic oncology.
Phone: 919-684-3765. They specialize in ovarian tumors.

Catherine McAuley Health Center, Department of Radiation Oncology,
St. Joseph Mercy Hospital, 5301 East Huron River Drive, Ann Arbor, MI.
48106. Phone: 313-572-3596. Fax: 313-572-5344. Dr. Mijenki V. Pilepich.

Department of Radiation Oncology, Stanford University School of
Medicine, Stanford, CA 94305. Phone: 415-723-6939 or 415-723-6442. Fax:
415-723-7382 or 415-725-8231. Dr. George M. Hahn, PhD and Dr. Daniel
Kapp, PhD. Mainly treats breast cancer, with radiation and heat therapy.

John S. Stehlin, Jr., MD, Scientific Director of Stehlin Foundation for
Cancer Research, 1315 Calhoun, Suite 1818, Houston, TX 77002. Phone:
713-652-3161. Fax: 713-659-1503. Specializes in melanoma.

Radiation Oncology Center, Mallinckrodt Institute of Radiology,
Washington University School of Medicine, 4939 Children's Place,
5th Floor, St. Louis, MO 63310. Phone: 314-362-8510. Fax: 314-362-8521.
Dr. Robert Myerson, oncologist.

Holistic Medical Clinic offers advanced cancer patients hyperthermia induced by immune boosters, ginseng, vitamins, an herbal medicine called
Sun Advance® and plasma exchange. Treatment takes 3 to 6 months. 1-
18-11 KY Bldg., #6F, Kita-oostsuka, Toshima-ku, Tokyo 170 Japan.
Phone: 03-3940-8071. Fax: 03-3917-9753. Tsuneo Kobayashi, MD, director.

Magnetic Microcapsules information:
Dr. Y. Omote, Laboratory of Pathology
Hokkaido University School of Medicine, Sapporo, Japan

Photodynamic Therapy information:
W.G. Roberts, Department of Cell Biology, Beckman Laser Institute,
University of California, Irvine, CA 92714. Phone: 714-856-6996

IMMUNE BOOSTERS

'Immune booster' is a name often given to substances that optimize the performance of white blood cells. The name is not quite accurate, since some of these substances are capable of decreasing, when necessary, an overcharged immune response. Thus, technically it might be more correct to call such agents 'immunomodulators.'

Scientists sometimes also call them 'biological response modifiers' (BRMs), since they modify the way the body responds to foreign substances and cancer.

There are basically two kinds of immune boosters:

• Hormone-like substances called cytokines produced by white blood cells to either destroy invaders or stimulate other cells. The most prominent of these for cancer are interferons, interleukins and tumor necrosis factor (TNF).

• Various substances, such as herbs or vaccines, which when ingested or injected stimulate the production of such cytokines in the body. These immune stimulants include BCG, bestatin, C. Parvum, Coley's toxins, levamisole, etc.

One cytokine, interferon, was discovered in the late 1950s, but a lack of supply limited research. Over the last decade or so, it has become possible to isolate small quantities of these substances, and then mass produce them through the marvels of genetic engineering. Many of the cytokines are now being cloned, patented, commercially manufactured and aggressively marketed.

A new world of immune function has opened up. It is clear for instance that these chemicals not only have important effects on health and disease, but affect one another in intricate, overlapping ways. Some influence the control of cancer. Using biological response modifiers, scientists have achieved a few dramatic complete remissions of otherwise intractable cancers.

Combinations of such agents, with or without conventional therapies, are now being used experimentally at many cancer centers. Some "limited successes" have been reported; but very often their curative powers have been hampered by extreme toxicity when they are injected in purified form into the human body (1). Sometimes, in fact, these treatments have been more toxic than the chemotherapy they were intended to replace. As University of Chicago Medical Center scientists said, "quite unexpected and unpredictable toxicities have been noted" (2).

Scientists are feeling a "cautious optimism" about the future of cytokine research based on the limited progress that has already occurred.

One problem has been that cytokines are very specific: they seem to work in small subsets of patients, rather than across broad categories. This individuality may have dissuaded some investigators, especially those affiliated with drug companies, who prefer therapies that are predictable across-the-board.

Scientists at Smith Kline & French Laboratories in King of Prussia, PA, for example, hope to create look-alike versions of cytokines ("appropriate analogs"), through the use of cloning and gene splicing technology. They hope these will be effective in broader categories of patients (3).

Because of their often severe toxicity, there will no extended discussion of such cytokines as interferon and interleukin in this book. Instead, we will concentrate on the natural products which stimulate the production of such proteins without the harsh and self-limiting side effects seen with the purified products.

⊕ References

1.   Keen AR and Frelick RW. Response of tumors to thermodynamic stimulation of the immune system. Del Med J.1990;62:1155-6.

2.   Gilewski TA and Golomb HM. Design of combination biotherapy studies: future goals and challenges. Semin Oncol.1990;17:3-10; disc. 38-41.

3.   Talmadge JE. Development of immunotherapeutic strategies for the treatment of malignant neoplasia. Pathol Immunopathol Res.1989;8:250-75

❦ BCG

BCG (*Bacillus Calmette-Guerin*) is a weakened strain of the microbe *Mycobacterium bovis*, which is used worldwide as a vaccine for tuberculosis.

BCG was among the first immune boosters used in cancer therapy, but its mechanism of action is still poorly understood. Basically, it stimulates the white blood cells, particularly the lymphocytes and macrophages, to attack cancer cells in a nonspecific way (1). This may be by provoking them to produce cytokines such as those mentioned above.

Although there have been many studies of BCG, there is still no consensus about its effectiveness. One reason is that since BCG is made from living organisms, various preparations differ in strength, and it is difficult to reproduce studies or accurately compare the results.

BCG seemed effective in several experimental models of leukemia (2, 3). The strongest effects seem to come when BCG is brought into direct contact with cancer cells, through local administration. In one study, for example, the disease-free interval for early stage lung cancer was significantly prolonged in patients who received a single injection of the vaccine into their lung space.

Melanoma is the best-studied type of cancer treated with BCG: there have been numerous studies showing that injections into and around a lesion can lead to regression.

BCG has also successfully been used to treat urinary tumors by directly instilling it into the bladder, with a significant reduction in recurrences. The disease-free interval was also increased. One BCG preparation (Thera-Cys® from Connaught Laboratories, Ltd., Ontario, Canada) has been approved by the FDA for use in bladder cancer.

Side Effects: In its use against bladder cancer, side effects were seen in over 50 percent of cases. This included a burning sensation and increased frequency and urgency, as well as some bleeding, upon urination. Fever and a flu-like malaise are commonly described. Irritation of the prostate has also occurred.

When BCG is injected locally, as for melanoma, pustules may arise, as well as local ulcerations and swollen glands. When injected directly into a tumor, there has been inflammation and hardening, leading to ulcers and the destruction of tissues. Acute fevers may also occur. Occasionally, patients have gone into anaphylactic (allergic-type) shock.

⊕ References

1.   Bruley RM, et al. In vivo and in vitro macrophage activation by systemic adjuvants. Agents Actions.1976;51:594-607.

2.   Verloes, R., et al. Influence of micrococcus, BCG and related polysaccharides on the proliferation of the L1210 leukaemia. Br J Cancer.1978;38:599-605.

3.   Verloes R, et al. Successful immunotherapy with micrococcus, BCG or related polysaccharides on L1210 leukaemia after BCNU chemotherapy. Br J Cancer.1981;43:201-9.

❦ BESTATIN

••

Bestatin® (also known as ubenimex or UBX) is a powerful immune stimulant discovered by Japanese scientists in 1976. Like some other anticancer agents (such as **Coley's toxins**) it was isolated from a broth of the 'strep' organism, in this case *Streptomyces olivoreticuli*. But unlike many other strep compounds, Bestatin is hardly toxic, even after long-term oral administration (1).

Bestatin is a simple peptide, just two amino acids which inhibit a pair of enzymes that are normally found in the membranes of cells. Bestatin, given orally, has shown anti-cancer effects against colon cancer and leukemia in rodents. Mice with colon cancer who received bestatin along with standard chemotherapy, such as 5-FU, lived longer than those that just received toxic drugs.

Bestatin stimulates T lymphocyte cells, activates the scavenger macrophages, and stimulates certain blood-producing cells in the bone marrow called erythroid pro-genitors (2) as well as other parts of the blood renewal system (3). Studies have shown that the drug concentrates in the kidney, in macrophages around solid tumors, in the spleen, the thymus, the liver and in some lymph nodes (4).

The invasiveness of two kinds of cancer (melanoma and lung cancer) was slowed in the presence of Bestatin. Immunologists at Hokkaido University, Sapporo felt that this ability was related to its activity as an enzyme inhibitor (5).

The level of certain T-cells, commonly depressed in cancer patients, was brought back to normal through administration of Bestatin. In the test tube, the release of interleukin-1 and -2, was enhanced by Bestatin. In a preliminary clinical study in Japan, the optimal dose was set at

10 to 100 milligrams, two to three times weekly. Sometimes, however, it was administered daily (6).

In a larger clinical trial, Bestatin prolonged the survival of patients with acute non-lymphocytic leukemia. It was used alongside conventional chemotherapy to induce complete remissions. Japanese scientists noted "minimal side effects" (6).

Other Japanese researchers have studied Bestatin's antitumor effects on the spleens of animals. Given seven days after tumor inoculation, Bestatin inhibited the growth of carcinoma. "Spleen cells taken from these mice showed a marked suppression of the tumor growth," they wrote. Bestatin appears to work by stimulating T-cells and Natural Killer cells.

Significantly, the "antitumor effect of [Bestastin] was not observed in X-ray-irradiated" mice, showing that conventional treatments can sometimes destroy any chance of success with immunotherapy (7, 8).

In a study of acute nonlymphocytic leukemia in adults, the length of remissions was prolonged when patients got Bestatin in addition to standard chemotherapy. This was especially true of elderly patients. Controlled studies were also performed in patients with solid tumors, including malignant melanoma, carcinoma of the lung, stomach, bladder, head/neck and esophagus.

Some benefit was definitely seen for some of the above-mentioned cancers but the scientists at Nagoya Memorial Hospital in Japan suggest that Bestatin needs to be further investigated in larger-scale controlled studies in order to confirm its effectiveness (1).

Bestatin has also generally yielded positive results in the treatment of blood diseases. For example, most of the patients with myelodysplastic syndrome (MDS), a condition marked by malfunction of the blood-forming cells, showed an increase in platelet and neutrophil (white blood cell) counts. "Great improvement" was seen in some refractory kinds of anemia (9).

Ten patients with chronic myelocytic leukemia (CML) were treated with Bestatin as well as conventional therapy. Six of the ten experienced partial remissions within three months. However "one case showed a marked increase in white cell count and blast count," an adverse sign in this type of cancer. From such findings hematologists at Osaka City University Medical School in Japan concluded that Bestatin could be used in either of these blood diseases, if the patient were unable to stand stronger chemotherapy (9).

Not surprisingly, both Natural Killer (NK) and Lymphocyte Activated Killer (LAK) cell levels were significantly lowered in patients with cancers of the blood. But both of these cell populations normalized when Bestatin was administered (10). Doctors at Toyama Medical and Pharmaceutical University said:

"Bestatin is a powerful immunomodulator that augments or restores some immune functions in patients with hematological [blood-based] malignancies."

The well-known French immunologist George Mathé has shown great interest in Bestatin and similar compounds. In 1979, he attempted to slow the effects of aging in mice by the long-term administration of either high or low doses of the drug. Weekly injections for six months resulted in mixed effects, depending on the dose. Macrophage (scavenger) cells only became activated at high doses.

While even continuous treatment with the drug did not prevent the appearance of certain harmful suppressor cells induced by aging, there was a significant reduction in the incidence of spontaneous tumors in mice given repeated high doses (11).

When combined with another immune booster, **levamisole,** "a significant reduction of spontaneous tumors and prolongation of median survival was observed in mice given repeated injections," the French doctors noted (12).

In 1986, 30 patients with cancer and 4 with AIDS-related complex (ARC) who had severe T-cell defects or imbalances were treated with Bestatin. "The drug has no toxicity of any kind," Dr. Mathé reported, and there was a "significant improvement of the absolute number of CD_4 cells in peripheral blood." CD_8 subsets were normalized. Both of these were positive signs for patients.

Mathé concluded that "Bestatin appears to have immunomodulating properties which might be useful in cancer patients" (13).

Bestatin stimulated both interleukin-1 and -2 production in mice, and enhanced T-cell, B-cell and macrophage reactions. In a clinical trial of 41 patients with Hodgkin's disease, non-Hodgkin's lymphoma and solid tumors, Bestatin corrected problems in various kinds of T-cells.

In the same study, a **zinc** compound also had a stimulatory effect on some lymphocytes. Oral administration of zinc gluconate corrected deficiencies in patients with severe T-cell deficiencies. These were admittedly only short-term studies. No attempt was made to see whether the treatment affected the underlying disease (14).

In France, Bestatin has also been used together with other immune boosting agents, such as zinc, levamisole, muramyl dipeptide (MDP), and a simple but effective agent called tuftsin.

Tuftsin is another naturally-occurring peptide made of four amino acids. It was discovered in 1970 during studies of the familiar blood constituent gamma globulin. It is normally found in that part of gamma globulin called leucokinin, and can be spontaneously released by the action of two enzymes.

Treatment with immune boosters can sometimes have unusual or even contradictory results. For example, both tuftsin and MDP can be used to activate macrophages. But "a stimulation as well as an inhibition of tumor cell growth can result from macrophage activation depending on the timing and dose injected," French scientists cautioned.

Repeated applications of tuftsin generally resulted in a repair of certain powers of macrophages that generally decrease with aging (15).

Scientists are also experimenting with look-alike forms of tuftsin, in which one or more of its four amino acids is exchanged for some other. Some of these new forms have stronger immune boosting effects than tuftsin itself (16).

Bestatin also stops the breakdown of natural chemicals called "enkephalins," which are pain relievers produced by the body itself. Mathé finds it encouraging "to study its analgesic action" of this simple drug (17).

Tuftsin, administered once a week for six months to old, immuno-depressed mice, restored the activity of various kinds of white blood cells (macrophages and T-cells). At this dosage level, tuftsin prevented spontaneous tumor development. The drug was also well-tolerated in preliminary studies and increased white blood cells, especially the T-4 cells (crucial in AIDS).

Mathé concluded that tuftsin and Bestatin together "constitute a biopharmacologic system" that can be developed to influence and control the immune system in patients with cancer and AIDS, as well as in the elderly (18).

Negative: Radiologists at the Karolinska Hospital in Stockholm studied the effects of Bestatin on a group of patients with cancer of the bladder. Half the patients who received full-dose bladder irradiation were also given

Bestatin orally. Doctors found no difference in the overall survival of those who got Bestatin as opposed to those who simply received radiation (19).

⊕ References

1. Ota K. Review of ubenimex (Bestatin): clinical research. Biomed Pharmacother.1991;45:55-60.

2. Aoki I, et al. Effects of ubenimex on erythroid progenitors (CFU-E and BFU-E) in human bone marrow. Exp Hematol.1991;19:893-8.

3. Blazsek I, et al. Modulation of bone marrow cell functions in vitro by bestatin (ubenimex). Biomed Pharmacother.1991;45:81-6.

4. Yamashita T, et al. Autoradiographic study of tissue distribution of [3H]ubenimex in IMC carcinoma-bearing mice. Int J Immunopharmacol. 1990;12:755-60.

5. Saiki I, et al. Inhibition of tumor cell invasion by ubenimex (bestatin) in vitro. Jpn J Cancer Res.1989; 80:873-8.

6. Tsukagoshi S. [A new antitumor drug with immunomodulating activity, ubenimex (bestatin)]. Gan To Kagaku Ryoho.1987;14:2385-91.

7. Ishizuka M, et al. Antitumor cells found in tumor-bearing mice given ubenimex. J Antibiot (Tokyo).1987;40:697-701.

8. Shibuya K, et al. Enhancement of interleukin 1 and interleukin 2 releases by ubenimex. J Antibiot (Tokyo).1987;40:363-9.

9. Tatsumi N, et al. Effects of ubenimex, a biological response modifier, on myelodysplastic syndrome and chronic leukemia. Biomed Pharmacother.1991;45:95-103.

10. Yamazaki T, Sugiyama KIchihara K. Effect of ubenimex on the immune system of patients with hematological malignancies. Biomed Pharmacother.1991;45:105-12.

11. Bruley RM, et al. Restoration of impaired immune functions of aged animals by chronic bestatin treatment. Immunology.1979;38:75-83.

12. Bruley RM, et al. Correction of immuno-deficiency in aged mice by levamisole and bestatin administration. Recent Results Cancer Res.1980; 75:139-46.

13. Mathe G, et al. Immunomodulating properties of bestatin in cancer patients. A phase II trial. Biomed Pharmacother.1986;40:379-82.

14. Mathe G, et al. From experimental to clinical attempts in immunorestoration with bestatin and zinc. Comp Immunol Microbiol Infect Dis.1986;9:241-52.

15. Bruley RM, et al. Macrophage activation by tuftsin and muramyldipeptide. Mol Cell Biochem.1981;41:113-8.

16. Florentin I, et al. In vivo immunopharmacological properties of tuftsin (Thr-Lys-Pro-Arg) and some analogues. Methods Find Exp Clin Pharmacol.1986;8:73-80.

17. Mathe G. Bestatin, an aminopeptidase inhibitor with a multi-pharmacological function. Biomed Pharmacother.1991;45:49-54.

18. Mathe G. Do tuftsin and bestatin constitute a biopharmacological immunoregulatory system? Cancer Detect Prev Suppl.1987;1:445-55.

19. Blomgren H, et al. Adjuvant bestatin (Ubenimex) treatment following full-dose local irradiation for bladder carcinoma. Acta Oncol.1990; 29:809-12.

❦ COLEY'S TOXINS

One of the most remarkable developments in the history of cancer therapy was the discovery by William B. Coley, MD in the late 19th century of an all-natural method of treating and even curing cancer. As chief bone surgeon at Memorial Hospital (now MSKCC), Coley initiated a forty-year experiment in the use of bacterial toxins (mixed bacterial vaccine) in the treatment of cancer.

Coley's toxins are the starting point of all modern immunotherapy. They are the byproducts of two common bacteria, *Streptococcus pyogenes* and *Serratia marcescens*. In 1943, a National Cancer Institute scientist, M. J. Shear, discovered that a biologically active substance in Coley's toxins was lipopolysaccharide (LPS, also called endotoxin), which occurs in the cell wall of certain bacteria. It was by injecting LPS into mice previously treated with the **BCG** vaccine that Dr. Lloyd Old and colleagues at Coley's alma mater, MSKCC, discovered tumor necrosis factor in 1975.

The toxins cause profound, if transient, biological effects. This can include a rise in temperature from 0.5 to 6 degrees, a pulse of 100 to 106, chills, tremblings and headaches. Unlike conventional chemotherapy such side effects, while unpleasant for the patient, are not emblematic of an immunity-destroying process. Quite the opposite: they are the result of pushing the immune function to the limit of excitability. The increase in bodily temperature, for example, seems to function as a biological form of **heat therapy.**

How effective was Coley's approach? According to Dr. Lloyd Old, member and former vice president of Sloan-Kettering Institute:

"Those who have scrutinized Dr. Coley's records have little doubt that the bacterial products that came to be known as Coley's toxins were in some instances highly effective" (1).

The results of approximately 1,000 cases treated by Coley's toxins have been evaluated by Dr. Coley's daughter, Mrs. Helen Coley Nauts. Patients with inoperable tumors of various kinds had 45 percent five-year survival, while those with operable tumors had 50 percent.

The best results were seen in giant cell bone tumors where 15 out of 19 (or 79 percent) of inoperable patients and 33 out of 38 (or 87 percent) of the operable ones were cured (five-year survival). These were not only outstanding results for their time, but compare favorably with results achieved today.

In breast cancer, the results were equally impressive. Thirteen of 20 of the inoperable (65 percent) and 13 out of 13 of the operable patients had five-year survival. Comparable results were seen in other types of cancer (for example, 67 percent in Hodgkin's disease, 67 percent in inoperable ovarian cancer, 60 percent in inoperable malignant melanoma) (2-5).

There is considerable historical and recent evidence

showing the antagonisms between acute bacterial infections or their toxins and cancer and other diseases. Publication of Mrs. Nauts's data has created renewed interest among scientists in many countries to study mixed bacterial vaccines (3-5).

For over 30 years, Dr. Frances Havas, professor (emeritus) of the Department of Microbiology and Immunology, Temple University School of Medicine, Philadelphia studied the effects of Coley's toxins in mice and humans (6-9). The results of her studies were generally favorable, even in the advanced patients.

Havas says, however, that the clinical benefits of Coley's toxins today are less dramatic than they were 100 years ago for two main reasons. First: people today have received so many antibiotics that their immune system does not react to immunological products as strongly as they did in the prepenicillin era.

Second: usually, patients treated with experimental methods such as Coley's toxins have already been treated with conventional treatments that decimate the immune system. Nevertheless, Havas remains optimistic about the value of the toxins in cancer. Unfortunately, the money for her study ran out and she herself has retired.

Temple doctors found that when the toxins were injected into the muscle (as opposed to the veins) there was much less fever and fewer other side effects. Havas claims the immunological results were the same.

Her opinion is not shared by all. Scientists at Du Pont, for instance, have made the case that immune boosters are likely to have an effect "in the presence of a naturally-produced fever than [through] treatment from just one lymphokine" (10).

A spiking fever is often characteristic of biological treatments, but this is generally treated as an unwanted side effect and "there has been no obvious effort to relate the extent of the fever to any tumor responses." In fact, most of the scientific literature has focused on the destructive effects of temperature per se on tumor cells, rather than as "part of an immune response to control tumor growth." Yet there is much clinical experience showing that an increase in temperature "can enhance the results of radiotherapy and chemotherapy in some situations."

The Du Pont scientists consider it "logical" to test the deliberate employment of fever in the clinical situation. However, "it is surprising that the combined effect of fever and lymphokine stimulation has not been reported aside from Coley's work...." LPS is a widely known fever-causing agent, but "more effective and more available pyrogens" (i.e., fever-producers) could be developed, if there were demand for such (10).

In the late 1980s there was an attempt to use a product derived from the weaker half of the Coley formula, *Serratia marcescens*, to treat cancer. ImuVert® was manufactured from the ribosomes and natural membrane vesicles of the microbe (11). Studies at New York Hospital showed that it increased Natural Killer cell activity in a number of cell systems.

Other studies showed that the abnormal Natural Killer cell activity of patients infected with the HIV virus was "significantly augmented" in the test tube by ImuVert, which also strongly stimulated one kind of interferon production and worked together with interleukin to produce more interferon than either of them could by itself (11). ImuVert also was able to block the development of a kind of leukemia in rats (12,15).

In 1991, K. F. Kölmel and colleagues in Göttingen, Germany reported on the treatment of advanced malignant melanoma through the use of Coley's toxins. Fifteen patients were given intravenous injections of Coley's toxins (which the scientists called "pyrogenic [fever-producing] bacterial lysate.") The scientists wrote:

"In three cases with skin metastases, this kind of treatment resulted in a total and long lasting remission. In another case...a five month period of stability was achieved" (13).

Side effects included fever, nausea, headache, back pain and, occasionally, cold sores (herpes labialis). Laboratory studies revealed a "marked increase" in the monocyte type of white blood cells. During bouts of fever, **TNF** levels increased.

Coley's toxins are now used not just in Germany but at a number of centers in China, including a new Coley's hospital there. Scientists at the Beijing Children's Hospital have told how they were astounded by a complete and lasting "spontaneous remission" of an enormous sarcoma in a seven-month-old boy. Like many such 'spontaneous remissions,' the cure was not really spontaneous, but followed an acute 'staph' infection, in this case in the biopsy wound of the boy's thigh. Ten years later the boy was still alive and well.

This led Chinese doctors to investigate deliberately inducing such infections as a method of treating cancer. Further inquiries led them to Coley's daughter, Helen Coley Nauts, in New York City.

Between 1985 and 1988, the toxins (or mixed bacterial vaccine, as they are now frequently called) were used as part of a combination treatment for liver cancer. Thirty-eight patients who were receiving conventional therapy (surgery, radiation, cisplatin, etc.) were randomized to receive, or not receive, Coley's toxins. In every case, survival rates were better for the group also receiving toxins compared to those receiving only conventional therapy.

The Chinese scientists wrote that Coley's toxins "could also prevent such immunosuppression as decrease of macrophage activity caused by radiotherapy" (14).

Japanese researchers have also isolated fever-producing LPS from various natural substances. They have investigated the use of LPS in cancer but found that its "strong toxicity" made it difficult to use. In order to induce the same anticancer effect but without toxicity, LPS and its components were placed on tiny polystyrene beads. Spleen cells were then activated by contact with these beads. There was little toxicity when LPS was administered in this way.

Activated spleen cells were then injected into the tumors of mice. Tumor growth was suppressed and the mice lived longer. Activated spleen cells were also injected intravenously into rats with advanced cancer. The scientists reported that "lung metastasis almost vanished" (17).

References

1. Old L and Boyse E. Current enigmas in cancer research. In: The Harvey Lecture, vol 67. New York: Academic Press, 1973.

2. Nauts H. Immunotherapy of cancer by bacterial vaccines. International Symposium on Detection and Prevention of Cancer. New York, 1976.

3. Nauts H. Bacterial vaccine therapy of cancer. Dev Biol Stand. 1977; 38:487-94.

4. Nauts H. Bacterial pyrogens: beneficial effects on cancer patients. Prog Clin Biol Res.1982;107:687-96.

5. Nauts H. Bacteria and cancer—antagonisms and benefits. Cancer Surv.1989;8:713-23.

6. Havas H, et al. Mixed bacterial toxins in the treatment of tumors. I. Methods of preparation and effects on normal or Sarcoma 37-bearing mice. Cancer Res.1958;18:141-148.

7. Havas H, et al. Mixed bacterial toxins in the treatment of tumors. III. Effect of tumor removal on the toxicity and mortality rates in mice.

Cancer Res.1960;20:393-396.

8. Havas H and Donnelly A. Mixed bacterial toxins in the treatment of tumors. IV. Response of methylcholanthrene-induced, spontaneous, and transplanted tumors in mice. Cancer Res.1961;21:17-25.

9. Havas H, et al. The effect of a bacterial vaccine on tumors and the immune response of ICR/Ha mice. J Biol Res Mod.1990;9:194-204.

10. Keen AR and Frelick RW. Response of tumors to thermodynamic stimulation of the immune system. Del Med J.1990;62:1155-6.

11. Cunningham RS and Pearson FC. ImuVert activation of natural killer cytotoxicity and interferon gamma production via CD16 triggering. Int J Immunopharmacol.1990;12:589-98.

12. Jimenez JJ, et al. Treatment with Imuvert aborts development of chloroleukemia in newborn rats. J Biol Response Mod.1990;9:300-4.

13. Kölmel K, et al. Treatment of advanced malignant melanoma by a pyrogenic bacterial lysate. A pilot study. Onkologie.1991;14:411-417.

14. Zhao YT, et al. Preliminary result of mixed bacterial vaccine as adjuvant treatment of hepatocellular carcinoma. Med Oncol & Tumor Pharmacother.1991;8:23-28.

15. Cress NB, et al. ImuVert therapy in the treatment of recurrent malignant astrocytomas: nursing implications. J Neurosci Nurs. 1991;23:29-33.

16. Jaeckle KA, et al. Phase II trial of Serratia marcescens extract in recurrent malignant astrocytoma. J Clin Oncol. 1990;8:1408-18.

17. Abe H. [Antitumor effect of LPS immobilized beads]. Nippon Geka Gakkai Zasshi.1991;92:627-35.

❧ *C*SF

Colony Stimulating Factors (CSF) are hormone-like chemicals responsible for healthy blood development. They include:

• Erythropoietin, or EPO, the major stimulator of red blood cell production;

• G-CSF, or granulocyte colony stimulating factor, which stimulates one kind of white blood cell, the neutrophil granulocyte;

• GM-CSF, or granulocyte-macrophage colony stimulating factor, which increases the production of a number of important white blood cells, called neutrophils and eosinophils; and

• M-CSF, or macrophage colony stimulating factor, which as its name implies, stimulates macrophage production.

The development of high-tech recombinant DNA technology has made large quantities of these once-scarce factors available for clinical trials and other experiments. Some are now being aggressively marketed and used in hospitals.

For example, a recombinant form of EPO has been approved by the FDA for the treatment of anemia due to kidney disease. This can sometimes reduce the need for transfusions in such patients. This could also have obvious uses in cancer and AIDS patients, as well. G-CSF is being marketed under the name Neupogen® (Amgen).

Patients with a variety of cancers have been experimentally treated with both G-CSF and GM-CSF. The goal has been to overcome blood problems created either by the cancer itself or by chemotherapy; reduce infections; and make immature cells in blood-related cancers mature. Both agents seem fairly effective in accomplishing these important aims. Blood counts have improved.

In a small group of patients with hairy cell leukemia there were no significant changes in hemoglobin or platelets, but there was "a suggestion of improvement in infections" (1). Although these drugs could be used to ease the blood-related symptoms of cancer patients, some oncologists also intend to use them for "dose intensification" in chemotherapy.

Primarily, CSF has been used to treat a depletion of white blood cells in patients with leukemia and urogenital cancer (2-5), to counteract the fever caused by chemotherapy (6), and to minimize blood-system damage (7).

Relatively few side effects have been seen, so far, from using these recombinant versions of natural agents. Some patients have experienced an increase in their diastolic blood pressure.

Sometimes, seizures have been reported with EPO use. G-CSF is generally well-tolerated, with some pain reported in the bone marrow. In addition, some headaches and flushing have occurred. Fever and bone pain are the most common side effects of GM-CSF, as well (1). Occasionally, at high doses, it causes anorexia, nausea and vomiting, however. It is often difficult to distinguish the side effects of these factors from those of conventional chemotherapy, or the symptoms of the cancer itself.

⊕ References

1.   Wittes R. [Ed.] Manual of oncologic therapeutics 1991/1992. Philadelphia: J.B. Lippincott, 1991:478.

2.   Heyll, A., et al. Granulocyte colony-stimulating factor (G-CSF) treatment in a neutropenic leukemia patient with diffuse interstitial pulmonary infiltrates. Ann Hematol.1991;63:328-32.

3.   Rave K and Brittinger G. Successful short-term treatment with granulocyte-macrophage colony-stimulating factor of neutropenia due to cytotoxic chemotherapy of chronic lymphocytic leukemia [letter]. Ann Hematol.1991;63:333.

4.   Hiddemann, W., et al. GM-CSF in the treatment of acute myeloid leukemia. Pathol Biol (Paris). 1992;39:959.

5.   Kotake T, et al. Effect of recombinant granulocyte colony-stimulating factor (rF-CSF) on chemotherapy-induced neutropenia in patients with urogenital cancer. Cancer Chemother Pharmacol.1991;27:253-7.

6.   Hamm JT. G-CSF for fever and neutropenia induced by chemotherapy [letter]. N Engl J Med.1992;326:269; discussion 270.

7.   Gianni AM, et al. The use of GM-CSF and peripheral blood stem cells (PBSC) minimises haematological toxicity following a myeloblastive course of chemo-radiotherapy. Pathol Biol (Paris)1992;39:956.

❧*I*NOSINE

••

Inosine is a natural chemical found in meat, meat extracts and sugar beets. It is a precursor of red blood cells. Several modified forms of this simple substance have been explored as antitumor agents and one is said to be highly active against mouse tumors (1).

Inosine and thymidine (one of the four major building blocks of DNA) were given as a way of protecting patients from the toxicity of the conventional antimetabolite, methotrexate. These two "protecting agents" blunted the toxic effects of this chemotherapeutic drug, without inhibiting its destructive effect on cancer cells. By giving these two more than six hours after the methotrexate treatment, there was "markedly decreased toxicity" in mice. There was a more than eight-fold increase in the amount of drug that could be delivered.

By giving these protectors, scientists were able to produce a 50 percent increase in life span, at doses that would have been too toxic for unprotected mice. They suggested in *Cancer Treatment Reports* that this finding could be used to give "much higher doses" of methotrexate (2).

In L1210 mice, inosine plus another chemical, sodium pyruvate, was found to be most effective among many combinations in restoring red blood cells to normal. The best therapy program used inosine-plus-sodium pyruvate ten to fifteen minutes before the administration of the conventional anticancer drug, BCNU. This combined treatment yielded 44 percent cures, whereas BCNU alone, in identical dose and schedule, produced no cures.

Median survival was 50 days for the inosine-pyruvate-treated mice, compared to 30 days for rodents treated with BCNU alone. Therefore, treatment with non-toxic doses of this red blood cell derivative, plus well-timed chemotherapy, resulted in significant therapeutic benefit and made red blood cells more normal (3).

In 1975, an initial clinical Phase I trial of inosine dialdehyde was carried out in 40 patients. There was some dose-related toxicity in all patients, including nausea and vomiting, local pain and changes in coagulation. There were no serious, dose-limiting blood disorders (as seen with most chemotherapy) although decreases in some blood counts were observed.

The most serious side effect was damage to the kidney, including a reversible kidney failure in one patient. There were responses (tumor shrinkages) in patients with three different kinds of cancer: seminoma, oat cell carcinoma, and melanoma, according to a study in *Cancer Chemotherapy Reports* (4). Elevated serum calcium returns to normal within one week of drug administration (5).

Inosine pranobex is another synthetic form of inosine, formed by merger with a benzoate salt. It has been reported to have both antiviral and antitumor effects in animals, due to its immune-stimulating ability. Early results have suggested beneficial effects in several diseases and infections including herpes simplex infection (the kind that causes cold sores), genital warts, influenza, and type B viral hepatitis.

It also seems useful for men with persistent generalized lymphadenopathy (constantly swollen lymph glands). Questions have been raised about the quality of these studies, however, and scientists have called for further long-term, well-controlled investigations (6).

Patients with cancer and other conditions associated with defective immunity—such as those receiving radiotherapy and surgery, or suffering from burns or AIDS—were treated for several months with three to four grams a day of another inosine derivative called inosiplex pranobex

(Imunovir®). They were then evaluated for the effects of the drug on their Natural Killer cells, T-cell count, and other parameters of the immune system.

Inosiplex treatment reduced complications, infections and deaths while generally enhancing the patient's immune system. The scientists concluded there were "important clinical benefits" for patients with a diverse group of diseases, which shared similar immunological defects (7).

Inosiplex also "significantly enhanced" the antitumor effect of the conventional drug 5-FU. This was shown both by test tube experiments on cancer cells, and by prolonging the survival of mice with Ehrlich ascites tumors (a laboratory model). Inosiplex by itself did not cause any great inhibition of cell growth but was beneficial when added to the conventional drug, 5-FU. Mean survival time was as follows:

Treatment Protocol	Days Survival (Mean)
Control group	18.2
Inosiplex alone	20.3
5-FU alone	31.9
5-FU + inosiplex	47.1

With the combination treatment, mice lived more than two-and-a-half times as long as the controls. There was obviously a significant value to the use of these two drugs together in mice, Japanese scientists reported in the *Cancer Letter* (8).

In a similar test, mice were inoculated with a million cancer cells. Then both interferon and inosine pranobex (Isoprinosin®), were injected three times a week for one month. Mean survival time was as follows:

INOSINE

Treatment Protocol	Days Survival (Mean)
Controls	26 days
Interferon alone	45 days
Interferon + Isoprinosine	64 days

Yet isoprinosine alone had no effect. "The final survial rate increased from one mouse out of 50 mice in the control group to 10 mice out of 50 in the interferon-treated groups and to 25 mice out of 50 with the combined treatment," according to this study in the *International Journal of Immunopharmacology* (9).

⊕ References

1.   Cysyk RL. Chemical assay for the antitumor agent inosine dialdehyde (NSC-118994) in biologic fluids. Cancer Chemother Rep.1975;59:685-7.

2.   Eleff M, et al. Analysis of "early" thymidine/inosine protection as an adjunct to methotrexate therapy. Cancer Treat Rep.1985;69:867-74.

3.   Cohen MH. Cure of advanced L1210 leukemia after correction of abnormal red blood cell deformability. Cancer Chemother Pharmacol. 1981;5:175-9.

4.   Kaufman J and Mittelman A. Clinical phase I trial of inosine dialdehyde (NSC-118994). Cancer Chemother Rep.1975;59:1007-14.

5.   Kaufman J, et al. Canine and human renal toxicity of inosine dialdehyde (NSC 118994). J Med.1977;8:239-51.

6.   Campoli-Richards D, et al. Inosine pranobex. A preliminary review of its pharmacodynamic and pharmacokinetic properties, and therapeutic efficacy. Drugs.1986;32:383-424.

7.   Glasky AJ and Gordon J. Inosiplex treatment of acquired immunodeficiencies: a clinical model for effective immunomodulation. Methods Find Exp Clin Pharmacol.1986;8:35-40.

8.   Namba M, et al. Potentiation of cytotoxic effects of 5-fluorouracil by inosiplex on cancer cells. Cancer Lett.1984;22:135-41.

9.   Cerutti I, et al. Isoprinosine increases the antitumor action of interferon. Int J Immunopharmacol.1979;1:59-63.

℞KRESTIN

Most Western doctors, asked to name the best-selling cancer drug in the world, would be stymied. The surprising answer is Krestin, or PSK®, a Japanese mushroom extract. Krestin was patented in Japan in 1973. Its anticancer properties were first reported at the chemotherapy congress in Athens that year. This product is manufactured by the Kureha Chemical Industry Co., Ltd, Tokyo, and marketed worldwide by Sankyo. With sales of nearly $360 million, in 1987 Krestin was the nineteenth top-selling drug in the world. Yet it is not sold in the US, because of difficulties of obtaining FDA approval for new, non-toxic treatments.

Technically speaking, Krestin is a polysaccharide from the fungus *Coriolus versicolor*, which, like the common field (or supermarket) mushroom is a member of the *Basidiomycetes* family. Krestin the drug comes as a brownish powder, tasteless but with a slight odor and is generally given orally.

Krestin can be combined with standard drugs, such as the antibiotic mitomycin-C (1). In such studies, it has been shown to be effective against a variety of tumors.

It not only boosts a suppressed immune system but also has a stabilizing, or homeostatic, effect, helping to bring an overcharged immune system back to normal, and earning it the title 'immunomodulator.' Killer T-cells are enhanced in experimental animals with cancer: this effect directly translates into cancer-killing activity.

Krestin also fights off the effects of immunosuppressive substances that are produced by the cancers of mice. Taken orally, Krestin shows a positive effect on the immune system (2). In mice, giving both Krestin and Mito-mycin C "significantly increased the survival rate of tumor-bearing mice and restored more effectively their immune functions" compared to mice that received one or the other agent, or none at all (3).

Starting in July, 1977 a very large study was carried out at 22 hospitals in Japan. Hundreds of patients recovering from stomach or colorectal cancer surgery were given Krestin and/or various drugs. Survival was significantly increased when patients received alternating doses of Krestin and the toxic drug carboquone, discovered by Japanese scientists five years earlier. Patients treated with this combination fared better than those receiving carboquone alone, or nothing at all.

"These differences were much more apparent among patients who received more than six courses of the regimen," said gastric surgeons at the Aichi Cancer Center in Japan (4). Results were then evaluated seven years after the start of the experiment. Again, the outcome was better for patients who received the immune stimulant in combination with the drug (5).

In 1981, scientists studied patients with acute leukemia "to determine if immunotherapy with Krestin can prolong the durations of complete remission and survival." Complete remission rates were higher and survival times were indeed longer in the Krestin group than in those receiving just chemotherapy. Crucial cell-mediated immunity was also enhanced (6).

These results suggested that Krestin was "useful for prolongation of the durations of remission and survival time in patients with acute leukemia."

Resistance to infection was depressed by both cancer itself and the conventional alkylating agent, cyclophosphamide. To find a way of preventing this, mice were first infected with a common bacteria (*Pseudomonas aeruginosa*) and then simultaneously given cyclophosphamide. When Krestin was also given, however, there was "an increase in survival rates," according to scientists at the Biomedical Research Laboratories of Kureha.

Resistance to infection was depressed by both the cancer and the standard cancer treatment, cyclophosphamide. But "such depression was prevented by [Krestin] administration" (7).

Conventional drugs, while killing cancer cells, often damage the chromosomes of normal cells, as well. But pathologists at Hokkaido University School of Medicine in Sapporo, Japan found that Krestin and another chemical derived from mushrooms, **lentinan,** "are not only useful for cancer treatment...but may also prevent the increase of chromosomal damage induced by anticancer drugs" (8).

Finally, 46 clinics in the Chubu district of Japan participated in a study of 262 stomach cancer patients in the mid-1980s. Some of these were given the conventional drug 5-FU while some also got Krestin.

Like other studies, this treatment alternated Krestin with the conventional drug. While a final follow-up will be carried out when all surviving patients have reached the five-year mark, preliminary results show that overall disease-free survival is higher in the Krestin-plus-5-FU group than in those receiving 5-FU alone (9).

⊕ References

1.   Oh-hashi F, et al. Effect of combined use of anticancer drugs with a polysaccharide preparation, Krestin, on mouse leukemia P388. Gann.1978;69:255-7.

2.   Tsukagoshi S, et al. Krestin (PSK). Cancer Treat Rev.1984;11:131-55.

3.   Fujii T, et al. Treatment with Krestin combined with mitomycin C,

and effect on immune response. Oncology.1989;46:49-53.

4.   Nakazato H, et al. [Clinical results of a randomized controlled trial on the effect of adjuvant immunochemotherapy using Esquinon and Krestin in patients with curatively resected gastric cancer. Cooperative Study Group of Cancer Immunochemotherapy, Tokai Gastrointestinal Oncology Group]. Gan To Kagaku Ryoho.1986;13:308-18.

5.   Ichihashi H, et al. [Clinical results of a randomized controlled trial on the effect of adjuvant immunochemotherapy using Esquinon and Krestin in patients with curatively resected gastric cancer—7-year survival—Cooperative Study Group for Cancer Immunochemotherapy, Tokai Gastrointestinal Oncology Group]. Gan To Kagaku Ryoho.1987;14:2758-66.

6.   Nagao T, et al. Chemoimmunotherapy with Krestin in acute leukemia. Tokai J Exp Clin Med.1981;6:141-6.

7.   Ando T, et al. Influence of PSK (Krestin) on resistance to infection of Pseudomonas aeruginosa in tumor-bearing mice. Cancer Chemother Pharmacol.1987;20:198-202.

8.   Hasegawa J, et al. Inhibition of mitomycin C-induced sister-chromatid exchanges in mouse bone marrow cells by the immunopotentiators Krestin and Lentinan. Mutat Res.1989;226:9-12.

9.   Nakazato H, et al. [An effect of adjuvant immunochemotherapy using krestin and 5-FU on gastric cancer patients with radical surgery (first report)—a randomized controlled trial by the cooperative study group. Study Group of Immuno-chemotherapy with PSK for Gastric Cancer]. Gan To Kagaku Ryoho.1989;16:2563-76.

ℐENTINAN

Lentinan is an immune booster, technically a polysaccharide derived from the edible—in fact, delicious—shiitake mushroom (*Lentinus edodes*) (1). Its anticancer properties were first described in *Nature* in 1969. In 1976, Japanese scientists isolated a fraction of lentinan that appeared particularly active in the test tube (2). It was patented in that same year by Ajinomoto, the huge Japanese chemical company.

Lentinan is rarely used alone. For example, it has been successfully employed, along with another immune booster, LPS (lipopolysaccharides), also known as endo-toxin, against breast cancer in mice. A single injection of lentinan-plus-LPS caused complete regression of these tumors twelve days later in about 90 percent of the animals. Other kinds of cancer responded almost as well (3).

In 1982, Japanese scientists found that lentinan helped stop the growth of liver cancer in mice. Untreated mice lived about 20 days. Mice that received toxic chemotherapy lived 22 days. Those receiving just lentinan lived over 25 days.

But the best results were in mice which received both chemotherapy and lentinan. These animals lived over 29 days. After about two weeks, the tumor's growth usually caused a breakdown of the immune system. But lentinan had a positive, "restorative" effect on immune function (4).

In August 1979, scientists at Osaka University began a major study with lentinan on people with advanced or recurrent stomach, colon-rectal and breast cancer. For gastrointestinal cancers, small doses of lentinan were administered intravenously in combination with conventional drug treatments. As a control, some patients received chemotherapy alone.

Lentinan added to the chemotherapy made the patients live longer—the ultimate criterion for an anticancer drug. Patients' immune responses were improved and blood abnormalities seen less frequently. Japanese scientists concluded that lentinan "should be effective for the patients with advanced or recurrent stomach or colorectal cancer in combination with chemotherapeutic agents" (5).

In a follow-up, two years later, they confirmed their earlier work and added that the drug was particularly effective in stomach cancer (6), which is widely prevalent in Japan. Other scientists have confirmed this finding (7).

Lentinan is now approved for this use by the Japanese regulatory authorities. Together with chemotherapy, lentinan also prolonged the lives of breast cancer patients. Osaka oncologists concluded:

"This result suggests that [lentinan] would also be effective for the patients with advanced or recurrent breast cancer as an agent for supportive therapy" (5).

Lentinan also prevents chemicals and viruses from triggering cancer (1) and is considered one of the most effective agents for controlling small metastases (8).

There are many studies of lentinan being done in Japan—far too many to discuss here—and almost without exception they are highly encouraging (9-27).

In a comprehensive review, its discoverer, Dr. G. Chihara of the National Cancer Center Research Institute of Tokyo, summed up Japanese experience.

Although derived from a natural source, lentinan has now been purified. Unlike chemotherapy, the anticancer action of the mushroom is entirely dependent on boosting the patient's immune system. Lentinan triggers the production of various factors associated with immunity and inflammation. This, in turn, causes important changes in the body. But most importantly, lentinan has "little toxic side effects" (1).

Other countries have been slow to follow Japan's lead. In America, Lentinan was initially evaluated in the early 1980s against lung cancer cells in mice. It caused a reduction in tumor growth rate in one of three experiments and an increase in life span of 48 percent at one dose level. Lentinan was "consistently curative" 50 to 70 percent of the time in three experiments. In subsequent experiments, 25 to 75 percent of the mice with lung cancer were cured in three separate experiments following early treatment (28).

Scientists reported in *Cancer Research* that even if lentinan therapy was begun after tumors were allowed to grow large, the results were dramatic: "complete tumor regression and cure" of 29 to 63 percent of the mice in three separate experiments.

As opposed to mice that only received surgery, survival rates were improved if the mice received lentinan in addition to surgery (28). Nevertheless, lentinan is not yet legally marketed in the United States.

⊕ References

1. Chihara G, et al. Current status and perspectives of immunomodulators of microbial origin. Int J Tissue React.1982;4:207-25.

2. Sasaki T, et al. Antitumor activity of degraded products of lentinan: its correlation with molecular weight. Gann.1976;67:191-5.

3. Abe S, et al. Combination antitumor therapy with lentinan and bacterial lipopolysaccharide against murine tumors. Gann.1982;73:91-6.

4. Moriyama M, et al. [Antitumor effect of polysaccharide lentinan on C3H/He mice bearing MH134 ascites hepatoma]. Gan To Kagaku Ryoho. 1982;9:1102-7.

5. Taguchi T. [Effects of lentinan in advanced or recurrent cases of gastric, colorectal, and breast cancer]. Gan To Kagaku Ryoho.1983;10:387-93.

6. Taguchi T, et al. [Results of phase III study of lentinan]. Gan To Kagaku Ryoho.1985;12:366-78.

7. Okuyama K, et al. Evaluation of treatment for gastric cancer with liver metastasis. Ca.1985;55:2498-505.

8. Chihara G. [Experimental studies on growth inhibition and regression of cancer metastases]. Gan To Kagaku Ryoho.1985;12:1196-209.

9. Wakui A, et al. [Randomized study of lentinan on patients with advanced gastric and colorectal cancer. Tohoku Lentinan Study Group]. Gan To Kagaku Ryoho.1986;13:1050-9.

10. Kosaka A, et al. [Synergistic action of lentinan (LNT) with endocrine therapy of breast cancer in rats and humans]. Gan To Kagaku Ryoho. 1987;14:516-22.

11. Shiio T, et al. [Suppressive effect of lentinan on pulmonary metastases in murine tumors]. Gan No Rinsho.1987;33:1427-30.

12. Taguchi T. Clinical efficacy of lentinan on patients with stomach cancer: end point results of a four-year follow-up survey. Cancer Detect Prev

Suppl.1987;1:333-49.

13. Akimoto M, et al. [Modulation of anticancer effects of immunochemotherapeutic agents in various nutritional environments]. Gan To Kagaku Ryoho.1988;15:827-33.

14. Minami A, et al. Augmentation of host resistance to microbial infections by recombinant human interleukin-1 alpha. Infect Immun.1988; 56:3116-20.

15. Vernie LN, et al. Cisplatin-induced changes of selenium levels and glutathione peroxidase activities in blood of testis tumor patients. Cancer Lett.1988;40:83-91.

16. Arlin ZA, et al. Philadelphia chromosome (Ph1)-positive acute lymphoblastic leukemia (ALL) is resistant to effective therapy for Ph1-negative ALL. Acta Haematol (Basel).1989;81:217-8.

17. Yamamoto S, et al. [NK activity and T cell subsets in percutaneous ethanol injection therapy of liver cancer—effect of lentinan with combined use]. Gan To Kagaku Ryoho.1989;16:3291-4.

18. Yamasaki K, et al. Synergistic induction of lymphokine (IL-2)-activated killer activity by IL-2 and the polysaccharide lentinan, and therapy of spontaneous pulmonary metastases. Cancer Immunol Immunother. 1989;29:87-92.

19. Cozzaglio L, et al. A feasibility study of high-dose cisplatin and 5-fluorouracil with glutathione protection in the treatment of advanced colorectal cancer [published erratum appears in Tumori 1991;77: following 93]. Tumori.1990;76:590-4.

20. Di RF, et al. Efficacy and safety of high-dose cisplatin and cyclophosphamide with glutathione protection in the treatment of bulky advanced epithelial ovarian cancer. Cancer Chemother Pharmacol.1990;25:355-60.

21. Kan N, et al. [Experimental study on the optimal treatment schedule for combination of BRM (immunostimulators, cultured killer cells or interleukin-2) and chemotherapy]. Gan To Kagaku Ryoho.1990;17:1421-7.

22. Kurokawa T and Tamakuma S. [Scanning electron microscopic observation of mouse ascitic carcinoma cells after intraperitoneal administration of lentinan]. Nippon Gan Chiryo Gakkai Shi.1990;25:2822-7.

23. Lien EJ. Fungal metabolites and Chinese herbal medicine as immunostimulants. Prog Drug Res.1990;34:395-420.

24. Maekawa S, et al. [A case report of advanced gastric cancer remarkably responding to mitomycin C, aclacinomycin A, SF-SP and lentinan combination therapy]. Gan To Kagaku Ryoho.1990;17:137-40.

25. Tanabe H, et al. [Studies on usefulness of postoperative adjuvant chemotherapy with lentinan in patients with gastrointestinal cancer]. Nippon Gan Chiryo Gakkai Shi.1990;25:1657-67.

26. Yoshino S, et al. [Effect of intrapleural and/or intraperitoneal lentinan therapy in carcinomatous pleuritis and peritonitis]. Gan To Kagaku Ryoho.1990;17:1588-91.

27.   Takeshita K, et al. [Diversity of complement activation by lentinan, an antitumor polysaccharide, in gastric cancer patients]. Nippon Geka Gakkai Zasshi.1991;92:5-11.

28.   Rose WC, et al. Immunotherapy of Madison 109 lung carcinoma and other murine tumors using lentinan. Cancer Res.1984;44:1368-73.

❦ℒEVAMISOLE

Levamisole (tetramisole) was introduced in 1966 as a broad-spectrum dewormer for animals and, occasionally, for people. Since the early 1970s it has been widely tested as an immune stimulant. This was based on an early report that in mice it augmented the effects of a vaccine against Brucella (an animal infection that can spread to people, causing fever, weakness and other symptoms).

Levamisole's mechanism of action is still unknown. It certainly stimulates white blood cells in a number of ways and augments hypersensitivity (allergic-type) reactions.

While generally ineffective as a solo performer, when added to chemotherapy it enhances the effects and increases survival. In addition to its influence on the immune system, levamisole may affect the way drugs are absorbed.

Levamisole by itself is a relatively weak agent. It had no effect in breast cancer, non-small-cell lung cancer or malignant melanoma. (Too small doses may have been employed, however.) Its main usefulness has been in a series of clinical experiments involving the treatment of Dukes' Stage C colon cancer (in which the lymph nodes are positive for cancer, but it has not yet spread to distant organs).

Initial US studies showed only a "borderline advantage" and a second, European tests showed "no detectable effect of levamisole alone." But scientists at the Mayo Clinic,

Rochester, MN have argued hard for the drug's inclusion in the treatment of this stage of colon disease.

In 1985, Dr. Charles G. Moertel and his colleagues at the Mayo Clinic reported on 335 patients with colorectal cancer who were given 5-FU plus levamisole, or other drugs. In an oddly-phrased statement, they wrote that "dosages were designed to produce definite toxicity in the majority of patients." And indeed, "5-FU plus levamisole produced mucocutaneous [mucous membrane and skin] reactions, diarrhea, and leukopenia [destruction of white blood cells]."

None of the regimens they tried, however, was "significantly superior to 5-FU alone." There was "no reasonable chance," they wrote, "that any combination regimen could produce as much as a 50 percent improvement when compared with 5-FU alone." They therefore stated that at the doses tested, "none of the combination regimens...can be recommended as standard therapy of advanced colorectal carcinoma" (1).

A second test, however, involved 401 patients with stage B (initial extension of the tumor) and stage C colorectal cancer, who had already been operated upon. These patients were given either levamisole or levamisole plus 5-FU for a year. "Levamisole plus 5-FU, and to a lesser extent levamisole alone, reduced cancer recurrence" compared to no treatment, Mayo doctors reported in 1989. These findings were "quite significant for levamisole plus 5-FU." Improvements in survival "reached borderline significance only for stage C patients treated with levamisole plus 5-FU."

The therapy was "clinically tolerable," the Mayo doctors wrote, and "severe toxicity was uncommon." These "promising results" led to a large national trial (2). These were reported in 1990.

Almost 1300 patients who had either locally invasive

(stage B2) or regionally involved (stage C) colon cancer were given either levamisole, levamisole plus 5-FU or nothing. Treatment with levamisole alone had no effect.

Among the patients with Stage C colon cancer, "therapy with levamisole plus fluorouracil [5-FU] reduced the risk of cancer recurrence by 41 percent," according to the Mayo doctors. The overall death rate was reduced by 33 percent." In the patients with Stage B2 colon cancer the results were "equivocal and too preliminary to allow firm conclusions."

The toxic effects of levamisole alone were infrequent, and generally consisted of mild nausea with some skin outbreaks and leukopenia (white blood cell damage). 5-FU, however, caused its usual symptoms: nausea, vomiting, diarrhea, dermatitis and leukopenia. The Mayo researchers concluded that "adjuvant therapy with levamisole and fluorouracil [5-FU] should be standard treatment for Stage C colon carcinoma" (3).

⊕ References

1.   Buroker T, et al. A controlled evaluation of recent approaches to biochemical modulation or enhancement of 5-fluorouracil therapy in colorectal carcinoma. J Clin Oncol.1985;3:1624-1631.

2.   Laurie J, et al. Surgical adjuvant therapy of large-bowel carcinoma: an evaluation of levamisole and the combination of levamisole and fluorouracil. The North Central Cancer Treatment Group and the Mayo Clinic [see comments]. J Clin Oncol. 1989;7:1447-1456.

3.   Moertel C, et al. Levamisole and fluorouracil for adjuvant therapy of resected colon carcinoma [see comments]. N Engl J Med.1990;322: 352-358.

❦ℳARUYAMA𝒰ACCINE

The Maruyama vaccine was one of the first modern immune stimulants to be used in the treatment of cancer. It is basically an extract of organisms that cause tuberculosis (*Mycobacterium tuberculosis* strain Aoyama B) and was first developed in the 1960s by the late Prof. Chisato Maruyama, then rector of the Nippon Medical School in Tokyo.

In 1981, the Japanese Health Ministry decided not to allow commercial production of the Maruyama vaccine, but did allow a company to continue supplying the product to this one medical school (*NCI Cancer Weekly* 6/24/91).

There are currently two forms of the vaccine: SSM, or Specific Substance of Maruyama; and Z-100, a highly concentrated form of SSM. SSM has been used on more than 280,000 patients in Japan. Z-100 is said to have 10 to 100 times the concentration of the original Maruyama vaccine and to be effective in restoring the white blood cell count, when lowered by radiotherapy, towards normal. The number of new users of both vaccines currently stands at between 4,000 and 5,000 per month.

The Maruyama vaccine has been the object of great controversy in Japan. The vaccine's manufacturer, Gerya Shinyaku Kogyo Co., had applied to the Health Ministry in May, 1990 for approval to use the vaccine, not for treating cancer itself, but for ameliorating the side effects of radiotherapy. In June, 1991, the Central Pharmaceutical Affairs Council urged Health and Welfare Minister Shinichiro Shimojo to approve Z-100 for this purpose.

Such approval would have, in effect, allowed any Japanese clinician to administer this concentrated vaccine to cancer patients, at their request. Such approval has not yet been granted, however.

There are several dozen articles in the peer-reviewed medical literature describing the benefits of the Maruyama vaccine. For example, in 1981, Japanese doctors described a remarkable case of metastatic lung cancer (derived originally from testicular cancer) that responded to sole treatment with SSM.

The patient had "completely satisfactory results and showed no recurrence over a period of 4 years."

There was a close correlation between changes in the white blood cell count and a blood chemical called alpha-2 globulin. Interestingly, in this case, in the first three months of treatment, there was an initial and contradictory *increase* in the size and numbers of the tumors. This was followed "by shrinking, disappearance, and finally healing" (1).

The ability of SSM to induce the in-body production of interferon was studied in mice. It was then compared to another preparation derived from tuberculosis bacteria, called PPD.

It is known that PPD cannot stimulate interferon production in mice that have not first been stimulated by the standard tuberculosis vaccine, **BCG**. But SSM was able to do so (2).

A unique feature of SSM is that it intensifies the production of collagen. Collagen has many roles in the body: it helps create the small blood vessels as well as muscles and nerve fibers (3).

When SSM was given, the proliferation of collagen was "accelerated remarkably," and its fibers "enclosed the cancer cells and prevented cancer cell proliferation."

SSM's influence on various kinds of white blood cells

was investigated in mice with leukemia and ascites tumors. SSM's effects were found to be due to T lymphocytes, but not macrophages or Natural Killer cells, according to scientists at the University of Texas Medical Branch in Galveston (4,5). SSM may also stimulate the production of another cytokine, interleukin-3 (6).

In a study in guinea pigs, tumor growth was more greatly suppressed in animals injected intravenously and subcutaneously than in control animals. Once again, study of the tumor cells showed that "collagen fibers enclosed the cancer cells and prevented cancer proliferation," according to scientists at the Institute of Vaccine Therapy of the Nippon Medical School (7).

As a side note, SSM also had a beneficial effect on type B hepatitis. Signs of the disease are said to have disappeared in 32 percent of patients after one year of treatment and in 65.2 percent of patients within two years. No notable side effects were observed (8).

⊕ References

1.   Fujita K, et al. A case of metastatic lung cancer healed clinically with an extract from human tubercle bacilli (Maruyama vaccine—SSM). Cancer Detect Prev.1981;4:337-46.

2.   Hayashi Y, et al. Interferon-inducing activity of an immunotherapeutic anticancer agent, SSM, prepared from Mycobacterium tuberculosis strain Aoyama B. Microbiol Immunol.1981;25:305-16.

3.   Kimoto T. Collagen and stromal proliferation as preventive mechanisms against cancer invasion by purified polysaccharides from human tubercle bacillus (SSM). Cancer Detect Prev.1982;5:301-14.

4.   Suzuki F, et al. Importance of Lyt 1+ T-cells in the antitumor activity of an immunomodulator, SSM, extracted from human-type Tubercle bacilli. J Natl Cancer Inst.1986;77:441-7.

5.   Pollard RB, et al. Release of a mitogenic factor by splenic Lyt 1+ T-cells from mice treated with SSM, an immunomodulator extracted from human type tubercle bacilli. Anticancer Res.1990;10:285-90.

6.   Sasaki H, et al. Induction of interleukin 3 and tumor resistance by

SSM, a cancer immunotherapeutic agent extracted from Mycobacterium tuberculosis. Cancer Res.1990;50:4032-7.

7. Nagae H. [Effects of SSM, an extract from human type tubercle bacilli, on syngenic guinea pig tumors]. Nippon Ika Daigaku Zasshi.1990; 57:235-43.

8. Fujisaki S, et al. [The effect of extract from human tubercle bacilli (SSM) on HBeAg positive type B chronic hepatitis]. Nippon Ika Daigaku Zasshi.1991;58:165-72.

❦ℳONOCLONALS

Monoclonal antibodies are laboratory creations. They are produced by fusing B lymphocytes with cells from multiple myeloma, a blood cancer that produces new misshapen cells at a furious rate. Once this laboratory marriage takes place, the new hybrid cells turn out anticancer substances in quantities great enough for them to be harvested as drugs (1).

More specifically, scientists inject human tumor cells into a mouse. The mouse's B cells react by becoming immunized and producing antibodies that fight that particular cancer. Those 'riled up' B cells are then fused with mouse melanoma cells. The result: cells that combine the anticancer proclivities of the B cell with the constant urge to reproduce of the myeloma. Further procedures are then used to isolate the one particular hybrid cell line that can do the most damage to the original human tumor from which it was derived.

Monoclonal antibodies have many uses. They can be used to:

• directly inhibit some tumors;

• join with other toxic substances (such as drugs, toxins, isotopes, cytokines, etc.) to send a lethal time bomb directly into the tumor;

• trigger a cascade of part of the immune system called complement, in turn releasing a host of other protective chemicals, sometimes resulting in the destruction of tumor cells;

• create prototypes for new kinds of cancer vaccines;

• purge bone marrow that has been removed from the body, for later reintroduction in bone marrow transplantation; and

• experimentally treat AIDS (2).

While certainly not a magic bullet, monoclonal antibodies are extremely useful tools for investigators (3). Since their creation in the 1970s, they have made major contributions to our understanding of how cells work. For example, they are now routinely used in the diagnosis of many kinds of cancer, especially those undifferentiated kinds that are hard to classify. This in turn can aid in staging and treatment. By making monoclonals radioactive, doctors can now use them to find obscure or hidden nests of cancer in the body.

Treatment trials with monoclonals alone have been a bit disappointing, however (4, 5). Clinical tests have been conducted with unmodified monoclonals in leukemia, lymphoma, melanoma, neuroblastoma and colorectal, ovarian and lung carcinomas (6). Long-lasting responses have only been in seen in lymphoma. There have also been some short-lived responses in leukemia (7).

Monoclonals which strongly activate complement can produce objective regressions of tumors in melanoma and neuroblastoma. In early trials, monoclonals that were combined with radioactive isotopes also produced some remissions in leukemia and lymphoma.

Trials are also underway combining monoclonals with a plant toxin called ricin A (4, 8). Experimental results suggest that these 'immunotoxins,' as they are called, may eventually become useful for treating cancer "as well as for other pharmacological purposes" (8).

It may be, however, that monoclonals linked to drugs "may find their greatest use in the eradication of small numbers of circulating tumor cells and micro-metastases remaining after removal of primary tumors" (9).

⊕ References

1.   Dillman R. Monoclonal antibodies for treating cancer. Ann Int Med. 1989;111:592-603.

2.   Lane HC and Fauci AS. Immunologic reconstitution in the acquired immunodeficiency syndrome. Ann Intern Med.1985;103:714-8.

3.   Chan SY and Sikora K. Monoclonal antibodies in oncology. Radiother Oncol.1986;6:1-14.

4.   Blythman HE, et al. Immunotoxins: hybrid molecules of monoclonal antibodies and a toxin subunit specifically kill tumour cells. Nature.1981;290:145-6.

5.   Boven E and Pinedo HM. Monoclonal antibodies in cancer treatment: where do we stand after 10 years? Radiother Oncol.1986;5:109-17.

6.   Dillman RO. Monoclonal antibodies in the treatment of cancer. Crit Rev Oncol Hematol.1984;1:357-85.

7.   Wittes R. [Ed.]. Manual of oncologic therapeutics 1991/1992. Philadelphia: J.B. Lippincott, 1991:478.

8.   Richer G, et al. [Immunotoxins (author's transl)]. Nouv Presse Med.1982;11:1321-4.

9.   Ghose T and Blair AH. Antibody-linked cytotoxic agents in the treatment of cancer: current status and future prospects. J Natl Cancer Inst.1978;61:657-76.

℞ℳTH-68

．．

The MTH-68 vaccine is a biological product used against cancer and viral diseases. It is a unique form of immunotherapy, developed by Laszlo K. Csatary, MD (pronounced Sha-tár-ee) of Ft. Lauderdale, FL, based on the idea that certain viruses can be used to interfere with the growth of cancer in humans. Csatary is convinced that much human cancer is actually viral in origin.

Interference between two viruses is a well-recognized phenomenon that has been intensively studied in the test tube and experimental animals, but somewhat less so in humans. It may occur because one virus stops the other from attaching itself to a target cell. Or once inside the cell, the first virus may prevent the other from maturing. Or a virus may stimulate the body's production of a protective factor, such as interferon, that prevents the opponent virus from proliferating.

But although the concept is well known, "few data exist for the usefulness of the interference phenomenon for treatment of viral disease in man," according to the Hungarian-American scientist (1).

In 1971, Csatary, then a physician at Jefferson Memorial Hospital in Alexandria, VA, read a report on regressions of leukemia and Burkitt's lymphoma after natural infections with measles. Csatary reported in the *Lancet* on the use of viruses in the treatment of cancer (2).

He wrote, "I am aware of the case history of a Hungarian chicken-farmer whose advanced and metastatic gastric carcinoma underwent regression coincidentally with an epidemic of viral fowl plague in the area of his dwelling."

This fowl plague is also known as Newcastle disease. It is caused by a destructive virus of birds (Paramyxovirus) originally discovered in Newcastle-on-Tyne, UK in 1927. In birds, it causes respiratory and nervous symptoms. While it is generally fatal in chickens, in humans it can only cause conjunctivitis ('pinkeye').

Csatary himself soon had occasion to test the effects of this virus. He was confronted with a relative who had metastatic and presumably incurable cancer of the prostate. Thinking of that Hungarian chicken-farmer, Csatary gave his relative intramuscular injections of live Newcastle disease virus.

"Radiological and clinical evidence indicates regression of all the tumors," he wrote in the *Lancet* (2). Two more patients were then treated by Csatary and his colleague, Dr. Laszlo N. Tauber. One had metastatic bladder cancer and the other had metastatic breast disease. There were clear signs of tumor regression after both were treated with live Newcastle virus.

Unfortunately, Csatary did not have the ability at the time to adequate analyze what was happening in these patients. "We feel we should have engaged the cooperation of colleagues equipped with adequate laboratory facilities," he wrote in 1971. But he proposed an interesting theory for why this vaccine was working.

There is a "balance in nature of viral-inducing and viral-destroying tumors," he suggested. To destroy cancer, a virus must first establish itself permanently in the tumor and thereby provide an easily recognizable target for the host's immune weaponry. He concluded that "inoculation of live viruses...may provide the tool by which the antigenicity [i.e., recognizability] of a tumor can be intensified so that it becomes vulnerable to immune rejection."

This approach was to form the foundation stone of Csatary's work for the next two decades. It is work that is now being tested in clinical trials currently underway in Hungary. And in fact this approach is being tried for other diseases as well, particularly herpes and hepatitis B infections, with apparent success.

In 1982, Csatary and colleagues at the Alexandria hospital and the Hungarian State Veterinary Research Institute in Budapest published a study of interference between herpes and influenza viruses (3).

Herpes can be a persistent, often tragic, infections of humans. But chickens are afflicted with a herpes infection of their own, called Marek's disease, first described in 1947 by the Hungarian veterinarian, Josef Marek (1867-1952). Marek's disease is a cancer-like illness of fowl characterized by the proliferation of white blood cells.

Csatary and his colleagues gave animals both Marek's disease and a human myxovirus, influenza A, in an attempt to study how they interfere with one another.

Coincidentally, in 1977 there was a severe human influenza A epidemic in Texas. In some poultry-producing areas, Marek's disease also happened to be rampant. It was noted that where the human disease was raging, the chicken disease "decreased significantly...in spite of the fact that the poultry flocks had not been vaccinated against Marek's disease virus" (1).

In a chance finding in the laboratory a similar thing happened. Chickens were being inoculated with human influenza A virus. But suddenly, both experimental animals and the uninoculated controls were inadvertently exposed to Marek's disease. The paradoxical result was that the chickens which had been exposed to *both* viruses recovered, but the birds which had only contracted Marek's disease all died.

In Csatary's first 1982 experiment, 50 healthy chickens were infected with Marek's disease virus. Nine days later, half of them were "superinfected" with a Texas strain of the human influenza A virus. In the group which only received Marek's disease, 17 out of 25 developed cancer-like changes. But in those which also received influenza, only 9 out of 25, or roughly half that number, got cancer. And several of the animals that developed cancer "showed less severe lesions."

In a second experiment, 90 chicks were infected with Marek's disease and then 40 of these were given a "super-infection" with the Texas strain of influenza A. Among those animals that got Marek's disease alone, over 89 percent died within 12 weeks. They all had typical cancer-like changes. But cancer only occurred in about 36 percent of the birds that also got a single injection of influenza virus. (Oddly, a single injection conferred more protection than repeated inoculations.)

Finally, a group of chicks was inoculated with Marek's disease. A second group was inoculated with influenza. And a third group served as uninoculated controls. The three groups were then kept together "exposing them to cross contaminations." All animals were examined after nine weeks.

The results were startling. By nine weeks, 21.7 percent of the group inoculated with Marek's disease had died. In the animals which simply picked up the disease from their inoculated cage-mates, 13.3 percent died of the disease. But in the third group, which had been immunized with human influenza virus, all survived until the end of the experiment "without developing Marek's disease lesions" (3).

In 1983, Csatary also published a study in a Hungarian journal on the interference between human hepatitis A virus and a bird virus. The bird virus was a weakened (attenuated), harmless (apathogenic) strain of avian bursa virus. Heptatitis A causes about 60 to 80 percent of all cases of this disease and no vaccine or special treatment is yet available (4).

Marmoset monkeys are an experimental model for

studying this illness, because most of the symptoms characteristic of this disease can be reproduced in these animals.

The goal of this experiment was to see if the course of the illness could be altered by giving them an inoculation of avian bursa vaccine. Superinfected moneys did not show the elevated liver enzyme (SGPT) that is a characteristic symptom of this disease nor did liver biopsies show pathological changes. Heptatitis was detected under the microscope in liver cells of the control animals, but not in the superinfected animals.

In 1985, Csatary and colleagues at the US National Institutes of Health (NIH) in Bethesda, MD and Rush Presbyterian-St. Luke's Medical Center in Chicago, IL published a wide-ranging paper in which the effects of 15 harmless viruses on four disease-causing viruses were studied. Among the "remarkable results":

• the 50 percent death rate caused in mice by a strain of rabies could be reduced to 15 percent by also giving a harmless avian encephalitis virus;

• clinical signs of the rabbit myxoma virus could be significantly delayed by using Newcastle disease vaccine; and

• the 72 percent death rate due to the Rous sarcoma virus in chickens could be reduced to 33.3 percent when the animals were pretreated with an avian bursa virus vaccine (5).

When Csatary began his studies, little was known about how such viruses could possibly interfere with cancer. Thus, it seemed a bit like magic. The last 20 years have seen an explosion in knowledge on such natural anticancer agents as interferon, interleukin and **tumor necrosis factor** (TNF). In 1988, however, scientists at the University of Illinois reported in the *Journal of the National Cancer*

Institute that Newcastle disease virus strains are "potent inducers of tumor necrosis factor (TNF)" in human white blood cells. Human cells that were resistant to the effects of TNF-alpha became susceptible to genetically engineered TNF when they were first treated with the bird virus. The same TNF had no effect on normal blood cells that had been pretreated with the bird virus.

It is likely that other immune stimulants, such as interferon and interleukins, are also induced by this therapy (6). This work has led to the development of an attenuated live virus vaccine. Since it is derived from the MTH-68 strain of the Newcastle disease virus of fowl, it is called the MTH-68/N vaccine.

While basic biological research continues (7, 8), there are large clinical trials underway in Hungary. One study is entitled "Treatment of Malignant Tumors with MHT-68/N." It is under the direction of Professor Sandor Eckhardt, MD. Since 1971, Prof. Eckhardt has been director general of the National Institute of Oncology, Budapest and is the 1990–1994 president of the prestigious International Union Against Cancer (UICC). He also served as Secretary-General of the 14th International Cancer Congress in Budapest in 1986 (9).

According to internal reports, signed by Dr. Eckhardt, the Phase I study with MTH-68/N showed that the treatment is not toxic and is devoid of side effects. A Phase II study, performed on terminal cancer patients, showed that "in some cases stabilization occurred which lasted for several months." In the majority of patients a favorable response was also noted in subjective factors, such as pain relief. The Phase II study included patients who received MTH-68/N by nasal drops and by inhalation.

All results were encouraging. According to a December 3, 1990 report from Dr. Eckhardt, in the majority of patients:

"Treatment with MTH-68/N either slowed or halted tumor progression. In a few cases, a clear-cut regression was noted. There was a striking improvement in subjective parameters of patients."

In addition, "their appetite and body weight increased, their general well-being increased and their performance status increased."

The treatment was well-tolerated, and an occasional fever did not necessitate withdrawal from the program. Dr. Eckhardt recommended using the treatment to prevent metastases (secondary growths) in patients undergoing radical surgery, as well as in combination with other treatments.

Naturally, these results must await final confirmation in peer-reviewed journals. Nevertheless, they are exciting findings, especially considering the source. Phase III trials are currently under preparation in a number of medical centers in Hungary. It is important to note that all of the patients treated by this method have either exhausted all conventional treatments or are those for whom no conventional treatment could have been offered.

Csatary's work on interference has been closely paralleled by other studies. In a Japanese clinical trial in the 1970s, the common mumps virus was shown to cause regression of some human cancers. Purified mumps virus (of the Urabe strain) was given intravenously to a total of 200 patients with cancer. The only side effects noted were a "transient mild fever in about half the patients." The beneficial clinical results included a decrease or disappearance of:

• ascites (excess fluid in the abdomen) in 26 out of 37 cases and edema (swelling) in 4 out of 4 cases of the lower limbs at high rates, usually within a week of the treatment;

- cancerous bleeding in 30 of 35 patients; and
- pain in most of the patients.

In addition, there was tumor regression in 26 patients with cancer of the breast, rectum, skin, thyroid gland, uterus, skin, and other sites. Mumps treatment caused desirable degenerative changes in tumor cells, but the Japanese scientists conceded that these "were not so great as those after chemotherapy or radiotherapy." White blood cells were found to have infiltrated into the area of the tumors. There was also fibrosis and the development of protective collagen (as with the **Maruyama vaccine**) around tumor tissues. The death of tumor cells was frequently observed (10-13).

⊕ References

1.   Csatary LK, et al. Interference between human hepatitis A virus and an attenuated apathogenic avian virus. Acta Microbiol Hung.1984; 31:153-8.

2.   Csatary LK. Viruses in the treatment of cancer. Lancet.1971;2:825.

3.   Csatary LK, et al. In vivo study of interference between herpes and influenza viruses. J Med.1982;13:1-7.

4.   Berkow R. The Merck manual of diagnosis and therapy (15th ed.). Rahway, NJ: Merck & Co., 1987:2696.

5.   Csatary LK, et al. In vivo interference between pathogenic and non-pathogenic viruses. J Med.1985;16:563-73.

6.   Csatary L. Virus vaccines for the treatment of cancer. Orvosi Hetilap.1990;131:2585-2588.

7.   Csatary LK, et al. Effect of attenuated viral vaccines on suckling mice infected with LCMV. Acta Microbiol Hung.1986;33:325-31.

8.   Szeri I, et al. Effect of chlorpromazine (CPZ) on the course of LCM virus infection in mice with developed and undeveloped immune system. Acta Microbiol Hung.1990;37:171-8.

9.   Weber G. Cover legend (explanation of picture of Prof. Eckhardt on cover). Cancer Res.1990;50:6769.

10. Asada T. Treatment of human cancer with mumps virus. Cancer. 1974;34:1907-28.

11. Okuno Y, et al. [Mumps virus therapy of neoplasms (1).]. Nippon Rinsho.1977;35:2867-72.

12. Okuno Y, et al. [Mumps virus therapy of neoplasms (2)]. Nippon Rinsho.1977;35:3820-5.

13. Okuno Y, et al. Studies on the use of mumps virus for treatment of human cancer. Biken J.1978;21:37-49.

℣ℳUROCTASIN

Muroctasin is an odorless, tasteless white powder, synthesized by Japanese scientists in 1981. It is derived from another drug called muramyl dipeptide, an immune stimulant derived from the cell walls of bacteria. Muroctasin is very similar to the parent drug, but more potent (1).

Muroctasin has also been reported to enhance resistance to infections. It helps build up various kinds of immunity and to increase the production of immune-enhancing colony stimulating factors (2). According to scientists at Daiichi Seiyaku Co., Ltd. of Tokyo, the patent holder, these effects may be due to the drug's ability to increase production of interleukin-1 in the body (3). It is thus of obvious interest for the treatment of cancer, since such natural substances can be powerful anticancer agents.

Muroctasin interacts with the various parts of the immune system in a complex way. It stimulates macrophage cells, which then release interleukin-1, which in turn triggers the production of **CSF** (colony stimulating factor) (4). Muroctasin can thus be called "a potent macrophage activator" (5).

The drug may also have special use in the treatment of people receiving chemotherapy. Resistance to infections, reduced by the conventional alkylating agent, cyclophosphamide, was restored by muroctasin. Antibiotics were also more effective when they were first potentiated by this drug. For that reason, scientists believe it may become an "important aspect in the future evaluation of therapy for infection in immuno-compromised patients" (1).

In Japan, 131 lung cancer patients whose white blood cells had fallen were enrolled in a study of muroc-tasin. They were divided into three groups: one received an injection of muroctasin once a day for six days, another received half that dose, while the third received nothing at all.

The white blood cells—especially neutrophils—of both treatment groups showed greater recovery than in the control group. Doctors at the Osaka Prefectural Habikino Hospital concluded that muroctasin is a good treatment of low white blood cell counts induced by chemotherapy (6).

These results were confirmed in a 'double blind' study of lung cancer patients at the National Kinki Central Hospital for Chest Diseases in Osaka. Doctors there demon-strated "the efficacy of muroctasin, at 200 micrograms doses levels only, in promoting early recovery." They sug-gested that this finding could be used to start chemother-apy earlier (7).

In a test at Kyoto University on urogenital cancer, it was found that a 100 microgram dose was also effective in boosting white blood cells. The researchers' conclusion: "muroctasin is useful for leukopenia [loss of white blood cells] after chemotherapy" (8).

Muroctasin has been carefully studied for its side effects. The most common one is a transient fever. In the Kyoto study of urogenital cancer, a mild fever and a local reaction at the injection site were the worst side effects experienced by 4 out of 25 patients. It showed no deleter-ious effects on behavior, spontaneous motor activity, convulsions, sleeping time, pain threshold, EEGs or other central nervous system symptoms in rodents. It did produce a significant elevation in body temperature in rabbits, however.

Nor did it show any significant effects on the lungs or heart in dogs. It did not cause spasms or affect stomach activity in the animals (9).

The drug is lethal to animals (LD_{50}) at between 200 and 800 milligrams per kilogram but showed little sign of toxicity at 90 milligrams per kilogram, which is considered the "critical dose of treatment" (10). Chronic toxicity in mice consisted of changes in the spleen and lungs, and some inflammation around the injection site (11).

⊕ References

1.   Otani T, et al. Stimulation of non-specific resistance to infection by muroctasin. Arzneimittel-forschung.1988;38:969-76.

2.   Yamaguchi F, et al. Production of colony-stimulating factor from macrophages by muroctasin. Arznei-mittelforschung.1988; 38:983-6.

3.   Akasaki M. Activation of immune responses by muroctasin. Arzneimittelforschung.1988;38:976-7.

4.   Akahane K, et al. Stimulation of macrophages by muroctasin to produce colony-stimulating factors. Arzneimittelforschung.1990;40:179-83.

5.   Nagao S, et al. Synergistic generation of tumoricidal macrophages by muroctasin and interferon-gamma. Arzneimittelforschung.1988;38:999-1002.

6.   Takada M, et al. [Restorative effect of muroctasin, MDP-Lys (L 18), on leukopenia caused by anticancer chemotherapy in lung cancer—comparative study by envelope method]. Gan To Kagaku Ryoho.1988; 15:3095-101.

7.   Furuse K and Sakuma A. Activation of the cytokine network by muroctasin as a remedy for leukopenia and thrombopenia. Arzneimittelforschung. 1989;39:915-7.

8.   Oishi K, et al. [Restorative effect of muroctasin; MDP-Lys (L18) [DJ-7041] on leukopenia in urogenital cancer patients treated with chemotherapy]. Hinyokika Kiyo.1989;35:527-36.

9.   Kojima H, et al. General pharmacological properties of muroctasin. Arzneimittelforschung.1988;38:1002-9.

10. Ono Y, et al. Acute toxicity of muroctasin in mice, rats and dogs. Arzneimittelforschung.1988; 38:1022-4.

11. Ono Y, et al. Chronic toxicity of muroctasin in mice. Arzneimittelforschung.1988;38:1028-30.

❧ $\mathcal{P}$SYCHOTHERAPY

Psychoneuroimmunology (PNI) is the use of the mind to influence the course of cancer and other diseases. PNI is pursued through a wide variety of techniques, such as encounter groups, mental imagery, positive thinking, motivational techniques, "mind development" courses, biofeedback, meditation, prayer and mutual support groups.

The link between psychology and cancer is very old. Several themes recur in the medical literature. For example, over the years many doctors have stated their belief that cancer patients tend to be chronically depressed, especially following a life setback. The Greco-Roman physician Galen, 2,000 years ago, noted that cheerful women were less prone to cancer than those who were depressed.

In 1701, a Dr. Gendron connected the "disasters of life" with the onset of breast cancer. In 1783, Dr. Burrows connected cancer with "the uneasy passions of the mind with which the patient is strongly affected for a long time." In his book *Cancer of the Breast*, Dr. Nunn stated that emotional factors contribute to the growth of tumors.

In fact, it remained the general medical belief throughout the nineteenth century that "mental misery, sudden reversals of fortunes, and habitual gloominess" contributed to cancer, according to the Simontons in their popular book, *Getting Well Again* (New York: Bantam, 1988).

In 1865, the famous physiologist Claude Bernard

warned that while it was necessary for science to analyze the various parts of the body, a living person had to be regarded as a harmonious whole. With the rise of surgery and radiation as the main cancer treatments, however, interest in the psychological dimension waned, at least among conventional doctors.

Only in the psychological literature, such as the works of Carl Jung, was the mind-disease link made, but most medical doctors were unfamiliar with this literature. In the late 1950s, psychologist Lawence L. LeShan wrote about the psychological and even the psychosomatic elements of various forms of cancer (1,2).

Scientists have focused on two particular predisposing mental states. The first is anger; the idea that suppressed rage predisposes to this disease. "Cancer patients seem to be unduly nice and cooperative people," was their unexpected conclusion. Interestingly, patients who were rated by their physicians as "uncooperative" or "unpleasant" tended to live longer (3, 4).

While this concept has been hotly debated, recent work shows that cancer patients do tend to be more "respectful" than the average person (5).

PNI was brought to public prominence by the work of Lawrence LeShan, Bernie Siegel and O. Carl Simonton, MD and his then-wife Stephanie Matthews-Simonton. Carl was chief radiologist at an air force base and Stephanie was a psychotherapist. Even as a medical resident, Carl says he noticed that patients "exerted some influence over the course of their disease."

People who survived tended to have a "positive stance toward life."

Bernie Siegel, MD is a well-known New Haven surgeon, who contends that patients who join support groups that involve visualization live longer than the norm. He formed "Exceptional Patient Groups," to help patients take some responsibilities for their own recovery.

The Simonton and the Siegel approaches have generated a great deal of attention in the media and an equal amount of controversy and opposition within the medical profession. Must of this has centered on doctors' fears that telling patients they are responsible for their health is tantamount to telling them they gave themselves cancer. Some feel this causes a tremendous and unnecessary burden of guilt.

Amidst all this debating, there have been few carefully controlled studies of this basic thesis. One of the most interesting was carried out by Dr. David Spiegel, MD, a psychiatrist at Stanford University on the effects of "psychosocial intervention" on the outcome of cancer.

"At the time—this was in the late 1970s—I did not believe there was such an effect," Dr. Spiegel has written (6). Spiegel's "treatment" of terminally ill breast cancer patients consisted of a once-weekly mutual support and discussion group among these patients. Those who served as untreated controls received no such support. While not surprisingly almost all of the patients eventually died in both groups, the effect on survival time was startling.

"The treatment group lived twice as long after the time they entered the study as the control group," Spiegel says. Survival on average was 18.9 months for the controls and 36.6 months for those in the program. The time between the recurrence of the illness and death was also significantly prolonged in the treatment group. And the more patients who participated in the group, the greater the effect.

At the same time, the Stanford researchers did not find that mood was associated with survival. Only participation in such a group seemed to matter. This was a striking, if unexpected, confirmation of Bernie Siegel's and the other pioneers' basic contention.

Other research has shown that, in general, psychological health is related to physical health and longevity. For example:

• The odds of dying at a certain age are related to "social integration," the feeling of belonging to a family or social network. Just "being connected" to other people reduces the chance of dying. Women who are highly integrated and sociable are about 60 percent less likely to die than women who are considered unsociable (7).

• The magnitude of this effect of social integration is formidable. It is in fact of the same importance as the relationship between smoking and death from lung cancer and cardiovascular disease, a two-fold increase.

• Involvement with women in general is healthy. It is good for men to be married, but it is also good for women to have women friends. "What that means is that it's good for your health to be associated with a woman, no matter what your own gender is," says Spiegel. "The converse is unfortunately also true—a relationship with a man does your health little good, regardless of your own gender" (6).

Spiegel concludes that support groups can clearly:

• improve the quality of life;

• teach patients to handle stress better; and

• cope with the often-taboo topics of death and dying.

Spiegel is a strong advocate of standard treatment, including cytotoxic drugs. He now advocates that group support become part of the conventional treatment for metastatic breast cancer (6).

 Hypnosis is another psychological approach that has been of value in decreasing the side effects of chemotherapy, particularly nausea and vomiting. (Compare **cannabis** and **electroacupuncture**.) Once a parlor sensation, hypnosis is now accepted as a serious medical tool, an effective relaxation technique which reduces drug-related nausea and vomiting, especially for children with cancer. It is an effective mode of treatment whose benefit as a self-relaxation technique is increasingly realized (8).

⊕ References

1. LeShan L. Psychological states as factors in the development of malignant disease: a critical review. Journal of the NCI.1959;22:1-18.

2. LeShan L. An emotional life history pattern associated with neoplastic disease. Annals NY Acad of Sci.1966;125:780-93.

3. Derogatis L, et al. Psychosocial coping mechanisms and survival time in metastatic breast cancer. JAMA.1979;242:1504-1508.

4. Greer S, et al. Psychological response to breast cancer: effect on outcome. Lancet.1979;2:785-787.

5. Goldstein D and Antoni M. The distribution of repressive coping styles among nonmetastatic and metastatic breast cancer patients as compared to non-cancer controls. Psych and Health.1989;3:245-258.

6. Spiegel D. A psychosocial intervention and survival time of patients with metastatic breast cancer. Advances: The Journal of Mind-Body Health.1991;7:10-19.

7. House J, et al. Occupational stress and health among men and women in the Tecumseh Community Health Study. Journal of Health and Social Behavior.1986;27:62-77.

8. Hockenberry MJ and Cotanch PH. Hypnosis as adjuvant antiemetic therapy in childhood cancer. Nurs Clin North Am.1985;20:105-7.

❦ SPLENOPENTIN

In 1981 a new hormone was described. At first it was called "thymopoietin III," because of its similarity to other hormones of the thymic gland. But in 1984 it was described as "splenin," a derivative of the spleen. The active part seems to be a five peptide (pentapeptide) fragment called "splenopentin" (also called DAc-SP5).

This fraction was quite active in immunological systems. For example, when mice were given a non-lethal dose of whole body radiation, their ability to produce antibodies was naturally reduced. But when they got splenopentin they "produced antibodies earlier and in a higher level than animals untreated," according to researchers at Humboldt University in Berlin, Germany (1).

Treated mice also showed significantly higher numbers of bone marrow-derived cells, as well as cells involved in forming other kinds of white blood cells, such as granulocytes and macrophages. They concluded that splenopentin "may be a useful substance for treating secondary forms of bone marrow depression" (2).

In an Italian study, 41 patients with Hodgkin's disease who had chemo- and/or radiotherapy, were then given either thymic hormone (17 patients) or splenopentin treatment (14 patients). All the patients had "severe immuno-deficiency...before starting thymic therapy."

In patients who had greatly reduced white blood cell counts either substance produced a significant increase in such cells. Hematologists at the San Bortolo Hospital in Vicenza also found a "significant decrease in incidence of herpes virus infection" in patients who received thymic therapy compared to a control group (18 percent vs. 53.8 percent) (3).

Splenopentin also can influence the course of the graft-vs.-host disease (GVHD), one of the major problems in bone marrow transplantation. German scientists found that "continuous treatment with splenopentin significantly prevented" some major symptoms of GVHD. There was no loss of spleen weight and much less suppression of antibody formation (4). But a later experiment showed that only a continuous treatment by splenopentin led to complete restoration of antibody formation (5).

Patients received injections of either a kind of splenopentin or a placebo during the peak of the pollen season. There were some slight, but normal, changes in the blood chemistry of patients receiving the drug. Doctors at Friedrich Schiller University in Jena, Germany concluded that it is a well-tolerated drug (6). Splenopentin has also been used in the treatment of psoriasis (7).

Both newborns and elderly adults normally suffer from immunodeficiencies. Jena scientists conducted a study to see if these immunodeficiencies could be influenced by splenopentin. Lymphocyte proliferation was inhibited in young people but increased among the elderly. There was no influence in newborns. Human splenopentin was more effective than that from cows (8, 9).

German scientists found that there were mixed results in using splenopentin in GVHD, however. While, it seemed to help in most cases, there was also one case in which it did not help at all and another in which the GVHD dramatically worsened. They concluded that before this peptide could be safely applied in bone marrow transplantation, measurements had to be found to allow for "an exact prediction about the influence of splenopentin" in each single case of GVHD (10).

⊕ References

1. Diezel W, et al. Effect of splenopentin (SP-5) on the antibody formation in immunosuppressed mice. Exp Clin Endocrinol.1986;87:215-8.

2. Weber HA, et al. Splenopentin (DAc-SP-5) accelerates the restoration of myelopoietic and immune systems after sublethal radiation in mice. Int J Immunopharmacol.1990;12:761-8.

3. Chisesi T, et al. The effect of thymic substances on T circulating cells of patients treated for Hodgkin's disease. J Biol Regul Homeost Agents. 1988;2:193-8.

4. Eckert R, et al. Prevention of graft-vs.-host reaction induced immunodeficiency by treatment with splenopentin (DAc-SP5). Allerg Immunol (Leipz).1989;35:279-85.

5. Eckert R, et al. Splenopentin-induced reconstitution of the immune response after total body irradiation: optimization of treatment regime. Exp Clin Endocrinol.1989;94:223-5.

6. Simon HU, et al. Phase-I study of diacetyl-splenopentin (BCH 069). Allerg Immunol (Leipz).1990;36:245-51.

7. Greiner J, et al. [Therapeutic use of splenopentin (DA SP-5) in patients with psoriasis arthropathica]. Dermatol Monatsschr. 1990;176:157-62.

8. Simon HU, et al. [Age-dependent sensitivity of human lymphocytes to the immunomodulating effect of bovine and human diacetyl splenopentin]. Allerg Immunol (Leipz).1990;36:351-8.

9. Evseev VA, et al. [Splenopentin—modulator of immunological and behavioral reactions in secondary immunodeficiency state induced by experimental alcoholism]. Biull Eksp Biol Med.1991;111:637-9.

10. Eckert R, et al. Splenopentin (DAc-SP5)—influence on engraftment and graft-vs.-host reaction after non-H-2 bone marrow transplantation in mice. Exp Clin Endocrinol.1990;96:307-13.

℣ $\int$TAPHAGE $\mathcal{L}$YSATE

Staphage lysate is a vaccine produced when a virus called bacteriophage attacks the microbe *Staphylococcus aureus*, commonly known as 'staph.' Staphage lysate has a beneficial effect on the immune system.

The use of staphage lysate in cancer was pioneered in the 1940s by a Medford, MA general practitioner named Robert E. Lincoln, MD. Lincoln noted that when this vaccine was "inhaled so that it was absorbed throughout the respiratory tract," it was "not only beneficial in sinus infection but improved or even cured a wide spectrum of illness," according to Raymond K. Brown, MD in *AIDS, Cancer and the Medical Establishment* (New York: Robert Speller, 1986).

Lincoln built a large practice around the use of this nontoxic substance. This led to an enormous controversy, which came to involve top US politicians and medical authorities. In 1952, Dr. Lincoln was expelled from the Massachusetts Medical Society and for a decade the Lincoln method languished on the American Cancer Society's unproven methods list (see *The Cancer Industry*, chapter 6).

In 1975, this innovative form of immunotherapy was quietly removed from the ACS list, through the efforts of Helen Coley Nauts (daughter of the discoverer of Coley's toxins) and Dr. Lloyd Old, vice president of Sloan-Kettering Institute.

In the 1980s, after the furor had died down, a few scientists began to take a second look at staphage lysate. In addition, says Brown, there has been "widespread and frequently surreptitious use" which has enabled it to survive as "a practical, versatile and safe" immunostimulant. Today's science may provide a rationale for the use of this product that was unavailable to either Lincoln or his critics.

For example, when staphage lysate was given to mice, scientists saw "significantly higher antibody levels" in the group that received the vaccine. This lasted "more than 14 days after injection" and demonstrated that staphage lysate boosts a crucial kind of immunity (1). It also induces the body to produce interferon, a non-toxic way of getting this powerful anticancer substance, which is quite toxic when given by injection (2).

In another study, mice were pre-treated weekly with staph for three weeks, in an 'induction' phase of the experiment. This was followed by injections of staphage lysate, in an 'elicitation' phase. Inducing just one phase or the other had no particularly beneficial effect. But the one-two combination resulted in prolonged survival from pneumonia. There was between 80 and 100 percent survival in mice given virulent staph microbes. Scientists at the Mason Research Institute of Worcester, MA suggested that "this enhancement of immune resistance" may possibly be related to the activation of white blood cells processed in the thymus gland as well as scavenger-type macrophages (3).

Patients with a severe inflammation of the sweat glands reported:

"noticeable improvement in odor, consistency and amount of drainage and considerable decreases in pain,"

---

according to doctors at Pennsylvania State University in Hershey, PA. Most also reported an improvement in the ability of such lesions to drain spontaneously, and a decrease in the frequency of inflammatory nodules of the sweat glands. "Early data suggests that staphage lysate is a useful adjuvant in the treatment" of these conditions, the scientists said (4).

But does staphage lysate fight cancer, as Lincoln claimed? To answer that question, University of Pittsburgh School of Medicine researchers gave female rats breast cancer. The mice were then given different preparations of staphage lysate. The size of the tumors was measured at different intervals and at the end of the experiment autopsies were performed to determine whether the cancer had grown and spread.

Rats receiving staphage lysate in two different ways "had significantly smaller tumors," they reported. Cancer spread to the lymph nodes 100 percent of the time in the controls, but only 40 percent in one of the staphage lysate groups. But lung metastases were seen in all groups (2). Staphage lysate appeared to be a fairly good protector against the growth and spread of breast cancer.

Negatives: At the same time, staphage lysate showed no antitumor effects in the previously-mentioned experiment at the Mason Research Institute of Worcester, MA (3). In addition, surgeons in Louisville, KY tested whether staphage lysate could be used to stimulate immunity. They could not confirm, they said, "the previously proposed hypothesis that staphylococcal vaccine improves the immune response to a bacterial challenge" (5).

⊕ References

1.   Esber HJ, et al. Staphage lysate: an immunomodulator of the primary immune response in mice. Immunopharmacology.1985;10:77-82.
2.   Mathur A, et al. Immunomodulation of intradermal mammary carcinoma using staphage lysate in a rat model. J Invest Surg.1988;1:117-23.
3.   Esber HJ, et al. Specific and nonspecific immune resistance enhancing activity of staphage lysate. J Immunopharmacol.1981;3:79-92.

4.   Kress DW, et al. A preliminary report on the use of Staphage Lysate for treatment of hidradenitis suppurativa. Ann Plast Surg.1981;6:393-5.

5.   Brown G, et al. Staphylococcal lysate fails to elicit nonspecific immune enhancement in a simulated surgical infection. Amer Surg.1984; 50:663-665.

❦ THYMIC FACTORS

The thymus, a gland in the chest that shrinks or even disappears as one grows older, produces a variety of polypeptides (protein-like substances) collectively called thymic factors. These bear confusingly similar names, such as thymopentin, thymopoietin and thymosin.

The various thymic factors influence the maturation and growth of T-cells, which are crucial in the body's defense against cancer and have been proposed as a way of boosting immunity and protecting the body during the administration of conventional toxic chemotherapy.

Animal studies have been very promising. For example, Hungarian scientists gave mice, which had been experimentally immunosuppressed by conventional anticancer drugs, fragments of the thymic hormone thymopoietin. They found that these fragments could partially or totally restore the animals' immune systems. But the results varied greatly depending on the particular drug used and the thymic fragment chosen. This also means that the proper thymopoietin fragment should always be chosen for combination therapy with various types of cytotoxic drugs, according to scientists at Budapest's Gedeon Richter Ltd. pharmaceutical company (1).

In another laboratory trial, in mice with lung cancer, a combination of thymosin (alpha) and interferon led to a "dramatic and rapid disappearance of tumor burden."

There was long-term survival in a high percentage of animals receiving this treatment as opposed to standard chemotherapy. This treatment "strongly stimulated natural killer [cell] activity" (2).

In a study of 41 patients with Hodgkin's disease, doctors at S. Bortolo Hospital in Vicenza, Italy found that thymosin enhanced the immune system. In particular, they observed "a significant decrease in incidence of herpes virus infection" in patients who had thymic therapy compared with the incidence of this infection in those who just received chemotherapy (18 versus 53.8 percent) (3).

But clinical results with these factors have been mixed. For example, patients with small-cell lung cancer who received intensive and generally successful chemotherapy were given either thymosin or (as a control) no thymosin during the initial six weeks of chemotherapy. The chemotherapy was then continued for two years. These two weeks of thymosin administration did not increase the complete response rate. But patients receiving thymosin did have "significantly prolonged survival times relative to the other treatment groups."

This benefit was due to an increase in the time before relapse occurred in patients who experienced a complete response to chemotherapy. How thymosin brought about this increased survival is not clear "but may relate to restoration of immune deficits due to disease or treatment," doctors reported in *JAMA* (4, 5).

Thymosin seems to work best in conjunction with other biological response modifiers. In a report to the New York Academy of Medicine, scientists reported that a form of thymosin "significantly restores the boosting capacity" of interleukin-2 and interferon. They speculate that this could result from the differentiation of Natural Killer (NK) cells, which then become sensitized to interferon. They were able to correlate the restoration of NK activity to the regulation of tumor growth. These results may be relevant to both cancer patients and people with AIDS (6).

The growth of melanoma has been linked to dysfunction of the thymus and the immune system in general. Russian scientists have used a thymosin-like substance to boost the immune system. This resulted in an "improved clinical course of the disease." The tumors "did not disseminate in patients retaining normal immune status" (7).

German doctors studied 25 patients with cervical, uterine and ovarian cancer, all of whom had shown a deficiency in their thymus-mediated immunity. They gave them a course of immunotherapy with a drug called thymopentin (Timunox®, Cilag Biotech). In the control group, which just received chemotherapy, the percentage of T-cells decreased greatly, "whereas in the immunotherapy group the percentage of these populations remained unchanged."

About a year and a half later "no differences concerning the survival time between both groups could be observed." There was only a slightly positive effect in advanced ovarian cancer.

However, the OB-GYN doctors at the University of Bonn in Venusberg believe that "these results do support the use of immunotherapy with thymopentin in combination with chemotherapy, especially in advanced cancer patients" (8).

Doctors in Biella, Italy saw a similarly protective effect for thymopentin in women with breast cancer. The drug protected them from some of the destructive effects of conventional anticancer chemotherapy. This was especially so when the "treatment was administered continuously from the start to the end of chemotherapy" (9).

Negative: Enthusiasm over such studies must be tempered by a 1984 report on 105 patients with advanced non-small-cell lung cancer who were receiving a chemotherapy regimen called VAP. This consists of the three conventional drugs, vincristine, doxorubicin and cisplatin. About half the patients received VAP alone, while the other half received VAP plus thymosin. About half of the VAP-treated patients had responses, mostly partial remissions of the tumors.

But only about one-quarter of those receiving VAP plus thymosin had such responses. Median survival time was also somewhat better in the VAP group. Quite surprisingly, "the addition of thymosin immunotherapy appeared to have a negative effect on the activity of VAP" (10). And in a 1985 report in *Cancer*, there was "no difference in survival or recurrence rate between patients treated with or without thymosin" (11).

⊕ References

1.   Denes L, et al. Selective restoration of immunosuppressive effect of cytotoxic agents by thymopoietin fragments. Cancer Immunol Immunother.1990;32:51-4.

2.   Garaci E, et al. Combination treatment using thymosin alpha 1 and interferon after cyclophosphamide is able to cure Lewis lung carcinoma in mice. Cancer Immunol Immunother.1990;32:154-60.

3.   Chisesi T, et al. The effect of thymic substances on T circulating cells of patients treated for Hodgkin's disease. J Biol Regul Homeost Agents. 1988;2:193-8.

4.   Cohen MH, et al. Thymosin fraction V and intensive combination chemotherapy. Prolonging the survival of patients with small-cell lung cancer.JAMA.1979;241:1813-5.

5.   Richman SP, et al. Cancer immunotherapy. Can Med Assoc J.1979; 120:322-4.

6.   Garaci E, et al. Enhanced immune response and antitumor immunity with combinations of biological response modifiers. Bull NY Acad Med. 1989;65:111-9.

7.   Labunets IF, et al. [Disorders of immune system function and their correction in melanomas with regional metastases]. Vopr Onkol.1989; 35:416-23.

8.   Mallmann P and Krebs D. [The effect of immunotherapy with thy-

mopentin on the parameters of cellular immunity and the clinical course of gynecologic tumor patients]. Onkologie.1989;3:15-21.

9. Cartia GL. [Evaluation of the effects of thymopentin on the incidence of leucopenia in patients treated with chemotherapy for breast carcinoma]. Minerva Med.1990;81:815-7.

10. Bedikian AY, et al. Prospective evaluation of thymosin fraction V immunotherapy in patients with non-small-cell lung cancer receiving vindesine, doxorubicin, and cisplatin (VAP) chemotherapy. Am J Clin Oncol.1984;7:399-404.

11. Shank B, et al. Increased survival with high-dose multifield radiotherapy and intensive chemotherapy in limited small cell carcinoma of the lung. Cancer.1985;56:2771-8.

☽TNF

Tumor necrosis factor (TNF) is one in a family of natural chemicals with powerful anticancer properties. These chemicals were first created by pretreating mice with the immune stimulant **BCG** and then giving them endotoxins, a substance found on the cell walls of bacteria.

The blood serum from such animals then contains a factor that causes dramatic, overnight "necrosis" or death of tumors. Scientists thus called this tumor necrosis factor (TNF). It is probably released from macrophages (1).

This 1975 discovery was ultimately derived from the work of Dr. William B. Coley (**Coley's toxins**) who noted that bacterial infections could cause the regression of tumors. TNF is a regulator of both inflammation and immunity and is presently in clinical trials as an anticancer drug at a number of centers (2, 3).

TNF—or rather the TNFs, for this is turning out to be a class of chemicals—are thus a group of proteins that are able to destroy tumor cells. They naturally occur in the body in small amounts, but now can be manufactured by recombinant DNA technology. While the results in animals have been dramatic, it is questionable whether they will show the same degree of response in humans. One problem is that TNFs, as powerful foreign proteins, can cause serious dose-limiting toxicity in people, including malaise and flu-like symptoms. Such side efects are similar to that seen with Coley's toxins, however, and probably do not lead to long-term damage to the immune system, such as is seen with conventional chemotherapy.

The treatment of cells with TNF or interferon results in "an antiviral state" and in the production of a common set of proteins. In fact, the induction by TNF is mediated through mechanisms that are both dependent and independent of interferon (4).

Tumor cells from 102 patients were exposed in the test tube to TNF, made by recombinant technology. Sixty-eight of these were also tested against interferon-gamma, also made by recombinant means.

Adding interferon-gamma reduced the dose of TNF required for significant antitumor activity "by about threefold." Based on such observations, scientists at the Arizona Cancer Center in Tucson concluded that recombinant TNF warrants more advanced clinical trials in selected solid tumors, with an emphasis on colorectal and lung cancer. They also felt that combining TNF and interferon-gamma should be studied in endometrial and breast cancer (5).

Japanese scientists have investigated the combined effects of TNF with **lentinan** (a mushroom polysaccharide) and lipopolysaccharide (LPS). They found that when LPS was administered after the tumor had grown fairly large, hemorrhagic (bloody) necrosis of the tumor occurred within 48 hours. They called this a "high antitumor effect."

When TNF was administered to cancer-bearing mice, bloody necrosis of the tumor was also observed within 48 hours. There was a better antitumor effect compared to LPS alone. But when LPS was used with lentinan "the highest antitumor effect could be achieved" (6).

Certain immune boosters perform better when used against tumors from patients who had previously been treated with chemotherapy, researchers at Oncotech, Inc. wrote in *JNCI*. These include women who had responded to treatment of breast and ovary cancers. These agents include TNF, interferon gamma and ImuVert, but not IL-2 or interferon alpha. The Irvine, CA scientists speculate that a successful response to chemotherapy "produces massive release and processing of tumor antigens." This in turn leads to a state in which the human immune system is primed to respond to such innovative drugs with "potent, specific antitumor effects" (7).

⊕ References

1.   Oettgen HF, et al. Endotoxin-induced tumor necrosis factor. Recent Results Cancer Res.1980;75:207-12.

2.   Old LJ. Tumour necrosis factor. Another chapter in the long history of endotoxin. Nature.1987;330:602-3.

3.   Old LJ. Tumor necrosis factor. Sci Am.1988;258:59-60.

4.   Rubin BY, et al. Tumor necrosis factor and IFN induce a common set of proteins. J Immunol.1988;141:1180-4.

5.   Salmon SE, et al. Antineoplastic effects of tumor necrosis factor alone and in combination with gamma-interferon on tumor biopsies in clonogenic assay. J Clin Oncol.1987;5:1816-21.

6.   Moriya N, et al. [Antitumor effect of bacterial lipopolysaccharide (LPS) and a combination use of LPS and lentinan on C3H/He mice bearing MH-134 tumor]. Gan To Kagaku Ryoho.1983;10:1646-52.

7.   Weisenthal LM, et al. Effect of prior cancer chemotherapy on human tumor-specific cytotoxicity in vitro in response to immunopotentiating biologic response modifiers. J Natl Cancer Inst.1991;83:37-42.

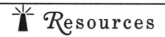
Resources

BCG:
Is approved by the FDA for treatment of carcinoma *in situ* of the bladder. Patients with damaged immune systems should not take it. Manufactured under the name TICE® BCG by Organon, Inc. 375 Mt. Pleasant Ave., West Orange, NJ 07052. Phone: 201-325-4500.

Bestatin:
Manufactured by Nippon Kayaku, 1-11-2, Fujimi, Chiyodo-ku, Tokyo, Japan 102. Phone: 03-3237-5111. Fax: 03-3234-8098. Approved by Japanese government on March 31, 1987.

Research on Bestatin:
Prof. George Mathé, Institut de Cancerologie et D'Immunogenetique, Hôpital Paul-Brousse, 14-16 Avenue Paul-Vaillant-Couturier, 94800 Villejuif, France. Phone: 1-46-77-0000. A Phase III adjuvant immunotherapy trial with bestatin for good-prognosis head and neck cancer patients. Details available from 800-4-CANCER.

Dr. N. Tatsumi, Department of Clinical and Laboratory Medicine Clinical Hematology Unit, Osaka City University Medical School Osaka, Japan

T. Yamasaki, Third Department of Internal Medicine Toyama Medical and Pharmaceutical University, Toyama, Japan

Coley's Toxins:
In the United States:

Burton A. Waisbren, MD, FACP, 2315 North Lake Drive, Room 815, Seton Tower, Milwaukee, Wisconsin 53211. Phone: 414-272-1929

In Germany:
Klaus F. Kölmel, Priv. Doz. Med., Universitäts-Haup Klinik von Sieboldstrasse 3, 3400 Gottingen, Germany. Phone: 011-49-551-396-081. Fax: 011-49-551-396-092.

In China:
The first hospital in the world devoted to the use of Coley's toxins in cancer was opened in 1990 in China:

Coley Hospital. Phone: 011-86-1-868-401. Dr. Guo Zheren MD, Chief surgeon, pediatric oncology
Beijing Children's Hospital, Nan Lishi Road,
Beijing, People's Republic of China

IMMUNE BOOSTERS RESOURCES

For current availability one should check with the Cancer Research Institute, 133 East 58th St., New York, NY 10022. Phone: 800- 223-7874. Mrs. Nauts, who is the director of communications for CRI, can be reached at 1225 Park Avenue, New York, NY 10128. Phone: 212-722-8547.

Colony Stimulating Factors (CSF): Amgen, Inc., Amgen Center, Thousand Oaks, CA 91320. Phone: 805-499-5725. Makes two forms of CSF.
Epogen® stimulates red blood cell production and is useful for AZT-treated HIV patients. Neupogen® is used to counteract the side effects of chemotherapy.
Immunex Corp., 51 University Street, Seattle, WA 98101.
Phone: 800-334-6273. Makes Leukine® to accelerate recovery in lymphoma and leukemia.
Hoechst-Roussel Pharmaceuticals Inc.. Route 202-206, PO Box 2500 Somerville, NJ 00876. Phone: 800-445-4774. Makes Prokine,® a similar product.

ImuVert: Patients seeking information on current status can call the current parent company, Air Methods, Inc., Boulder, CO.
Phone: 303-790-0587. Attn: Terry Schreier or Bill Critchfield.

Levamisole: Is marketed as Ergamisol® by Janssen Pharmaceutica, Inc., 40 Kingsbridge Road, Piscataway, NJ 08855. Phone: 800-253-3682.

There is a Phase III comparison trial underway for the treatment of colon cancer using chemotherapy plus levamisole, with or without an autologous tumor cell vaccine. Contact: Al Bowen Benson, III, Northwestern University Medical School, 303 East Chicago Avenue, Chicago, IL 60611. Phone: 312-908-9412.

Maruyama Vaccine: Available only in one place: the Nippon Medical School Hospital, Tokyo, Japan. Manufactured for them by Gerya Shinyaku Kogyo Company.

MTH-68: Phase III clinical trials are underway in Hungary.
For information on the status, one may contact:
Dr. Laszlo K. Csatary, MD, United Cancer Research Institute
PO Box 7147, Alexandria, VA 22307. Csatary may be out of the country.
One can try People Against Cancer (Box 10,Otho, IA 50569) for updated information and phone numbers. Phone: 515-972-4444.

Psychotherapy: Bernie Siegel, MD, Exceptional Cancer Patient Program (ECAP), 1302 Chapel Street, New Haven, CT 06511.
Phone: 203-865-8392. Fax: 203-497-9393.

David Spiegel, MD, Professor of Psychiatry and Behavioral Sciences
c/o Psychosocial Treatment Laboratory
Stanford University School of Medicine, Stanford, CA 94305.
Phone: 415-723-6643.

Simonton Cancer Center, 15601 Sunset Boulevard
Pacific Palisades, CA 90272. Phone: 213-459-4434. O. Carl Simonton, MD

Relaxation tapes for people with cancer and AIDS are available from:
Michael Ellner, c/o HEAL, 16 East 16th Street, New York, NY 10003.
Phone: 212-674-HOPE (212-674-4673). Fax: 212-243-1040.

In the New York area, Florence Klein, 2652 Cropsey Avenue, Apt. 5C,
Brooklyn, NY 11214. Phone: 718-996-8011. ECAP trained cancer
survivor. She is putting together a program modeled on Bernie Siegel's
groups.

Staphage Lysate: Manufactured by Delmont Laboratories, Inc., PO Box
269, Swarthmore, PA 19081. Phone: 800-562-5541.

Tumor Necrosis Factor:

A Phase II trial is underway at NCI comparing the effectiveness of heat
therapy with various substances including tumor necrosis factor for
malignant melanoma of the extremity.

Contact: Douglas L. Fraker, Surgery Branch, National Cancer Institute,
9000 Rockville Pike, Bethesda, MD 20892. Phone: 301-402-2575.

*L*ESS *D*OCUMENTED

All of the methods described so far in this book have been documented by publications in the peer-reviewed scientific literature. However, there are other methods of treating cancer that are not substantiated in this way. To the militant opponents of unconventional therapies known as quackbusters such treatments are self-evidently fraudulent. Fraud is always a possibility when money or power is at stake. However, there are other reasons why someone might be unable or unwilling to publish a detailed explanation of their results in the scientific literature:

• Writing scientific papers is a specialized skill and not every discoverer of a new method is able to write up results in the carefully-stylized form of a scientific paper.

• The researcher may lack the proper credentials or affiliation to convince editors of the importance of the work.

• Editors and peer reviewers who are used to "normal" science may unconsciously reject papers that threaten to effect radical changes in scientific paradigms.

• The discoverer might be hesitant to fully disclose his or her methods for commercial reasons or possibly because of some deep-seated fears or other personal problems. While this is certainly deplorable, it says little about the validity of the proposed method.

Below are several methods that fall into the gray zone of cancer therapies. They have not been adequately documented in the scientific literature. It is simply a cheap shot to dismiss these and similar treatments as quackery. They are in fact interesting, but less-documented developments that are crying out for further research.

We must always remind ourselves, in the words of Senator Harkin's Appropriations Committee, that "many routine and effective medical procedures now considered commonplace were once considered unconventional and counterindicated." In fact, as the Committee points out, even cancer radiation therapy "once was considered to be quackery." One can only hope that NIH's Committee on Unconventional Medical Practices, which was mandated by Congress, can break through the roadblock that has prevented a fair and impartial evaluation of such methods in the past.

❡ CANCELL

Cancell, also known as Entelev, is a nontoxic treatment for cancer developed in the 1930s by a man named Jim Sheridan. Sheridan graduated from Carnegie Tech in Pittsburgh, and then spent one year in graduate school there. Upon leaving Carnegie at the height of the Depression, he became an analytical chemist for the Dow Chemical Company in Michigan. The company later sent him back to law school and he became a patent attorney for the firm.

There is a great deal of mystery around Cancell. The idea for this drug came to Sheridan in a dream on the afternoon of September 6, 1936. It was a dream that only a scientist could have.

Sheridan saw a multilayered rainbow made up of the various respiratory enzymes of the oxidation-reduction ('redox') system. The dream suggested to the young chemist the possibility of controlling the production and flow of energy within the respiratory system, to either cause or cure cancer.

In Sheridan's developing view, the cancer cell exists at a "critical point" between a truly primitive cell (like yeast) and a normal human cell. The goal of Cancell is to push the cancer cell further down the 'redox' ladder, completely into the primitive state.

"Cancell tries to take away the last vestiges of normality" from cancer cells, "so they are no longer on the boundary line." He added,

---

"Once the cancer cell is definitely into the primitive stage, the body deals with it as the body does any other foreign object. It gets rid of it."

All descriptions of Cancell's ingredients and method of manufacture seem incomplete. However, Sheridan has said that Cancell contains a kind of natural catechol, a chemical that can inhibit respiration. It is similar, he says, to the chemical that turns cranberries red.

Sheridan claims that by 1942 he was already getting between 70 and 80 percent antitumor responses in mice. From 1950 to 1953, he worked at the Detroit Institute of Cancer Research (now the Michigan Cancer Foundation), in work funded by the Pardee Foundation.

Here begins a tale which is either paranoid fantasy or confirmation of the the most frightening conspiracy theories. For in 1953, just as human clinical tests were about to begin, they were blocked (Sheridan says) by representatives of the American Cancer Society.

Around this time, Sheridan, a devout Christian, began giving away the substance (then called Entelev) to all patients who asked for it. This has remained his policy for nearly forty years.

From 1961 to 1963, Sheridan worked at the Biosciences Division of the Battelle Institute in Columbus, OH, which tested anticancer compounds for the National Cancer Institute. Most anticancer compounds were expected to prove themselves in five days. But Cancell needed 28 days for significant results to appear in mice. Consequently, he was unable to prove the compound's value to NCI's satisfaction.

In April, 1982 Sheridan filed an Investigative New Drug (IND) application with the FDA and was quite surprised when on May 20, 1982 he received IND No. 20,258.

Shortly thereafter, however, Cancell was put on "clinical hold," a kind of bureaucratic limbo, by the agency. In 1986, FDA requested a study on the "minimum lethal dose." Sheridan claims that when he arranged for such a test to be done (at his own expense), the laboratory was scared off by the FDA. He also claims that the FDA began to visit and harass those with whom he associated in connection with the drug.

In the 1980s, Sheridan met a foundry owner in Michigan named Ed Sopcak. Sopcak took up where Sheridan left off, manufacturing 100 bottles a week in his garage. He would then give them away, even paying for the postage. He also answered calls from desperate cancer patients four hours a night, five nights a week. Sopcak has estimated that he has given away about 20,000 bottles of Cancell.

At times Sopcak has said that patients should go off all other medications before taking Cancell. Sheridan, in turn, has only warned patients not to take megadoses of vitamins C and E, while on his medication. Clinical results are generally seen in three to five weeks, they say, but sometimes take as long as three months.

Cancell "does not actually kill the cancer cell in the usual meaning of the word kill," Sheridan concludes. It is "effectively 'asking' the body to cure itself."

℣ CARNIVORA

Carnivora is an extract of *Dionea muscipula*, the meat-eating Venus Fly Trap plant. It was introduced into cancer therapy by Helmut Keller, MD of Germany. Keller was born in 1940 in Erlangen, and received his medical degree from that city's University in February, 1970. He then served in the Department of Oncology, at the Tumor Clinic Oberstaufen, and practiced pediatrics, internal medicine and surgery from October 1971 to March 1972. From June 1972 till December 1973 he was a researcher at Boston University. He has practiced general medicine and oncology in Germany since 1974.

In 1973, while still in Boston, he began testing juices pressed from the Venus Fly Trap, a kind of plant which his wife collected. Since Venus Fly Traps are such efficient digesters of protein, they are of considerable interest to biologists.

Keller had a hunch that the plants might be useful in digesting the abnormal proteins found in cancer. For the next few months, he applied plant extracts to human cancer cells growing in hamsters. Those animals that received a fly trap extract showed marked reduction in their tumors, he said. Keller dubbed his extract "Carnivora," meaning "meateater," from the plant's famous insect-devouring ability.

Since moving back to Germany, Keller has administered Carnivora to about 2,000 patients at his clinic in Germany. Morton Walker, an American medical writer, has suggested that President Reagan, Nancy Reagan and Yul Brenner all received Carnivora treatments.

Although Keller has not published his results in the regular peer-reviewed journals, what gives his claims more than ordinary credibility is the fact that the Venus Fly trap contains a powerful chemical called plumbagin. This is a non-toxic substance which has shown antimicrobial (1,2) and anticancer properties in scientific studies (3-5).

Support for Keller's thesis has also come from Munich's Technical University. Although scientists there were not looking for a cancer treatment, they observed that plumbagin from Venus Fly Traps produced both superoxides and hydrogen peroxide.

In other studies involving interferon, white blood cells were stimulated to produce hydrogen peroxide and thereby kill cancer cells. Together with certain enzymes in the plant, these chemicals were found to render proteins more digestible for the plant (6).

Clinical studies with plumbagin have also been conducted in India (4) and Brazil (3). The South American scientists found that plumbagin (isolated from a different local plant, *Plumbago scandens*) was responsible for a complete healing of skin lesions.

They concluded that this herb-based remedy could advantageously be substituted for surgery and radiotherapy, mainly for tumors of the external ear and the back of the nose. Radiotherapy, which is normally used in such cases, was judged harmful to cartilage (3).

Keller has conducted unpublished studies comparing Carnivora to cyclophosphamide, a standard form of toxic chemotherapy, according to Morton Walker. Cyclophosphamide reduced tumor weight by 99 percent, but was very poisonous to normal cells. Carnivora, on the other hand, reduced tumor weight by 59 percent, but there were no discernible harmful side effects.

In various other tests, Keller is said to have measured the activity of cancer cell metabolism and found that Carnivora was very active in inhibiting cancer activity.

Soviet studies found plumbagin so harmless that it was

recommended as a food preservative (1). While plumbagin is nontoxic, patients should never attempt to produce their own homemade Carnivora. This is because the extract contains endotoxins, which, if injected, might cause high fevers and other untoward reactions. Keller's Carnivora is said to be purified of these toxins.

The medicine contains one-third press juice; one-third alcohol and one-third purified water. Two milliliters is generally injected into the muscle daily until the doctor observes an increase in the ratio between two kinds of white blood cells. Another two milliliters are then administered to the patient through an intramuscular injection two or three times weekly as a maintenance dose.

By mouth, the patient generally takes 100 milliliters—30 drops of the extract—three to five times a day before meals and diluted in a glass of purified water or tea. Unmixed, it is said to taste like aged whiskey (it contains 60 proof alcohol). It can also be inhaled by means of a cold steam vaporizer.

In January 1990 Keller moved to the town of Bad Steben, where his clinic now offers in-house sleeping facilities for those coming from out-of-town or out of the country.

⊕ References

1. Ingre VG. [Harmlessness of plumbagine in a biological experiment]. Vopr Pitan.1978;4:74-7.

2. Farr SB, et al. Toxicity and mutagenicity of plumbagin and the induction of a possible new DNA repair pathway in Escherichia coli. J Bacteriol.1985;164:1309-16.

3. Melo AM, et al. [First observations on the topical use of Primin, Plumbagin and Maytenin in patients with skin cancer]. Rev Inst Antibiot (Recife).1974;14:9-16.

4. Krishnaswamy M and Purushothaman KK. Plumbagin: A study of its anticancer, antibacterial & antifungal properties. Indian J Exp

Biol.1980;18:876-7.

5.   Chandrasekaran B, et al. New methods for urinary estimation of antitumour compounds echitamine & plumbagin. Indian J Biochem Biophys.1982;19:148-9.

6.   Galek H, et al. Oxidative protein modification as predigestive mechanism of the carnivorous plant Dionaea muscipula: an hypothesis based on in vitro experiments. Free Radic Biol Med. 1990;9:427-34.

℞ *IAT*

IAT, or immunoaugmentative therapy, is "one of the most widely known unconventional cancer treatments," according to the Office of Technology Assessment (OTA). It is also one of the most bitterly contested. In fact, few people can involve themselves in this question, on one side or the other, without losing scientific detachment.

Essentially, IAT is an experimental form of cancer treatment consisting of daily injections of processed blood products. Supporters claim that IAT is a scientifically-valid method, essentially non-toxic, whose value is suggested by numerous case histories of dramatic improvement.

To detractors, IAT is a questionable method, unsupported by scientific studies, and potentially dangerous due to bacterial and viral contamination (1-3).

IAT is the alternative cancer therapy that has gotten the greatest attention from the US Congress. The controversy spilled into the streets of Washington, triggered the OTA report on unconventional cancer therapies (4), and indirectly led to the Ad Hoc Committee on Unconventional Medical Practices of the National Institutes of Health (*Washington Post*, 6/26/92).

IAT is essentially the work of one man, biologist Lawrence Burton, PhD, a New Yorker who now resides in Freeport, Bahamas. Much of the controversy over IAT stems ultimately from his actions and personality.

Burton attended Brooklyn College and New York University, from which he earned his PhD in 1955. From 1955 to 1965, he held various research and teaching positions at such institutions as California Institute of Technology (Cal Tech), NYU and St. Vincent's Hospital in New York City.

In the 1950s, Burton and co-workers at Cal Tech discovered what they claimed was a cancer-causing factor called "TIF" (tumor induction factor). TIF was unusual in that its ability to cause tumors seemed to cross the species barrier between fruit flies and mice. This was an unconventional thesis and the work on it was marked by serious controversy at the time (8).

Burton and his associate Frank Friedman were accused of improper laboratory procedures and the validity of their claim was questioned. One of Burton's erstwhile collaborators, contacted by the OTA in 1988, asserted that the work at Cal Tech raised "serious doubts about the validity of subsequent claims" (4). (This retrospective assessment came after Burton had gained international notoriety.)

Burton and Friedman left Cal Tech shortly thereafter and came to St. Vincent's, where they eventually rose to the rank of Senior Associates in the Hodgkin's Disease Research Laboratory, under the late Antonio Rottino.

At St. Vincent's, the two worked on cancer-inhibiting factors in mice (9,10). They later claimed to find this factor in human cancer tissue, as well (11).

Burton and his coworkers, especially Friedman and Robert Kassel (later of Sloan-Kettering Institute), published at least 17 scientific papers, most of them appearing in *Science, Cancer Research,* and publications of the New York Academy of Sciences and other major scientific societies (5-7, 9-22).

At St. Vincent's, Burton and his colleagues isolated what they said were two anticancer substances, called "V" and

"I," which they claimed caused dramatic reductions of 50 to 100 percent in lymph nodes and spleens of mice with cancer within 24 hours.

Daily administration of a combination of "I" and "V" were said to eliminate palpable disease in 26 of 50 mice with leukemia. The treated group also appeared to survive significantly longer than the controls.

At the New York Academy of Sciences, Burton repeated that "37 of 68 experimental animals survived for an average of 131 days without any evidence of leukemia. The leukemia gradually regressed." The average survival of untreated mice on the other hand was said to be 12 days (4). Burton concluded:

> **"The study of the biological action and interaction of these components in mice...has suggested the existence of an inhibitory system involved in the genesis of tumors and capable of causing specific tumor cell breakdown."**

In the mid-60s, Burton then made two spectacular public presentations of this factor and its alleged ability to destroy tumors. One was at an American Cancer Society (ACS) science writers' seminar, the other at the staid New York Academy of Medicine. At the Academy, "there was apparently skepticism and little interest in pursuing their research" (4).

At the ACS conference, however, after Burton made solid mouse tumors melt away in one hour, he was publicly accused of fraud by some of the other scientists there. Some contended that Burton had switched mice.

Others claimed that Burton had massaged the rock-solid tumors into a fluid state and then surreptitiously removed the residue with a needle. According to the organizer of the conference, the late Patrick McGrady, Sr., such claims were patently false (*The Cancer Industry*, chapter 12).

In the 1970s, Burton and Friedman left St. Vincent's to establish the Immunology Research Foundation (IRF) of Great Neck, NY. Here, they obtained four patents on their methods and took the first steps towards getting an Investigational New Drug (IND) permit from the FDA.

But the FDA would not allow the IND to proceed because of an alleged lack of information. And so, eventually, Burton and Friedman withdrew their IND. They closed the Great Neck clinic and in 1977 Burton—this time, without Friedman—moved the entire operation to Freeport, Grand Bahamas.

IAT is based on the injection of several blood fractions. Early in his career Burton adopted the view that immune therapy would work optimally when a balance was struck between the various activated components of the immune system. He attempted to exploit four blood substances, recovered by means of a centrifuge, which could be used to restore normal immune function in the person with cancer. Burton described these substances as :

• Deblocking protein (DP)—an alpha 2 macroglobulin derived from the pooled blood serum of healthy donors.

• Tumor antibody 1 (TA1)—a combination of alpha 2 macroglobulin with other immune proteins (IgG and IgA) derived from the pooled blood serum of healthy donors.

• Tumor antibody 2 (TA2)—also derived from healthy blood serum but differing in potency and possibly in composition from TA1.

• Tumor complement (TC)—a substance derived from the blood clots of patients with many types of cancer. This is described as a C3 complement, an immune factor said to be uniquely active in activating TA1 and TA2 (4).

Most of these terms are familiar to immunologists but questions have been raised about the exact way the Bahama scientist is employing them. To our knowledge,

Burton has not engaged in any dialogue with conventional scientists to help resolve these differences. There have also been repeated charges that Burton does not help other scientists to understand his techniques for isolating these four substances.

Another concern has been over viral or bacterial contamination of the serum. There was a major scare in 1985, when the Pan-American Health Organization and the Center for Disease Control prevailed upon the Bahamian government to close the IAT clinic because of alleged HIV contamination.

There is little doubt that this attack was abetted by certain officials at the National Cancer Institute. This furious and coordinated attack eventually even engaged the Reagan White House.

But the clinic was reopened in 1986, due in part to pressure from influential US Congressmen who took up the cause of IAT patients. In fact, there is good reason to doubt that such AIDS contamination ever took place (see *The Cancer Industry*, chapter 12).

Even though the serum is now carefully tested for contamination, the FDA still maintains an Import Alert against IAT products. Technically, it is illegal to bring such substances into the US, although patients routinely violate that ban without being hindered.

The initial purpose for establishing the Bahamian clinic was to serve as a research program to generate enough clinical data to gain acceptance for the method in the US and other countries. But neither the data nor the acceptance was forthcoming. Instead, the IAT clinic evolved into a fairly typical offshore cancer clinic: long on claims, short on scientific documentation.

Burton has supervised the treatment of several thousand patients. These tend to be loyal and satisfied medical consumers, generally better educated and more affluent than the norm. There are many anecdotal reports of improvement in symptoms and even of dramatic regression of tumors. But all attempts to scientifically verify these compelling stories have floundered, including the congressionally mandated investigations of the OTA.

Since he went to the Bahamas, this once well-published scientist hardly published any scientific articles. The one exception was an article with his sometimes medical director, Dr. R. J. Clement in an obscure journal, *Quantum Medicine*, which published only a few issues before it went out of business (23).

Their paper presented the favorable results of the treatment of 11 patients with peritoneal mesothelioma treated with IAT between May 1980 and February 1987.

Although the paper had its deficiencies, which critics were not slow to point out, the central claim is hard to dismiss out of hand. For Burton asserts that several of his mesothelioma patients have survived in good health for years on his treatment.

Mesothelioma, the asbestos-related cancer, is incurable and deadly. If these claims are false, then IAT is truly a delusion or fraud of monumental proportions. If they are true, however, then IAT is an astonishing discovery, with profound implications for the treatment of every cancer patient. Only good scientific studies can answer such a question. But in this bitter struggle neither side seems inclined to find an answer very soon.

⊕ References

1.   Curt G., et al. Immuno-augmentative therapy: a primer on the perils of unproved treatments. JAMA.1986;255:505-7.

2.   Nightingale, SL Immunoaugmentative therapy: assessing an untested therapy. JAMA.1988;259:3457.

3.   US Department of Health and Human Services, Public Health Service,

CANCER THERAPY

Centers for Disease Control. Isolation of Human T-lymphotrophic Virus Type II/Lymphadenopathy-associated virus from serum protein given to cancer patients. MMWR.1985;34:489-491.

4.   US Congress, Office of Technology Assessment, Unconventional Cancer Treatments. OTA-H-405, September 1990.

5.   Burton L. Carcinogenic effects of an extractable larval tumor agent. Trans NY Acad Sci.1955;17:301-8.

6.   Burton L and Friedman F. Detection of tumor-inducing factors in Drosophila. Science.1956;124:220-221.

7.   Burton L, et al. The purification of an inherited tumor-inducing factor in Drosophila melanogaster. Cancer Res.1956;16:880-884.

8.   Mitchell HK. Tumor-inducing factor in Drosophila. Science.1961;133:876. See also OTA Report, chapter 6.

9.   Burton L, et al. The activity of a tumor factor in Drosophila development. Cancer Res.1956;16:402-7.

10. Friedman, F and Burton L. Benign and invasive tumors induced in Drosophila by an inherited tumor-inducing factor. Cancer Res.1956;16:1059-1061.

11. Burton L., et al. A tumor-inducing factor in Drosophila melanogaster II. Its characteristics and biological nature. Ann NY Acad Sci.1957 68:356-367.

12. Friedman F, et al. Characteristics of an inherited tumor-inducing factor in Drosophila melanogaster. Cancer Res.1957;17:208-214.

13. Friedman F, et al. The etiology and development of a melanotic tumor in Drosophila. Pigment Cell Biology: Proceeding of the fourth conference on the biology of normal and atypical pigment cell growth. M. Gordon (Ed.). New York, NY: Academic Press, 1959.

14. Burton L., et al. The purification and action of tumor factor extracted from mouse and human neoplastic tissue. Trans NY Acad Sci 1959;21:700-7.

15. Kassel R, et al. Carcinogenic action of refined tumor factor isolated from mouse leukemia tissue. Proc Soc Exp Biol Med.1959;101:201-204.

16. Friedman F, et al. A rapid (24 hour) bioassay for detection of human and mouse tumor factor. Proc Soc Exp Biol Med.1960;103:16-19.

17. Friedman F, et al. The extraction and refinement of two antitumor substances. Trans . N Y Acad Sci. Ser II.1962;25:29-32.

18. Burton L, et al. Isolation of two oncolytic fractions from mouse leukemic tissue. Proceedings of the American Association for Cancer Research 1962;3:308.

19. Kassel R, et al. Synergistic action of two refined leukemic tissue extracts in oncolysis of spontaneous tumors. Trans NY Acad Sci Ser II.1962;25:39-44.

20. Burton L, et al. Methods for determination and alteration of titers of a complex of factors present in blood of neoplastic mice. Trans NY Acad Sci Ser II.1962;25:33-38.

21. Kassel R, et al. Utilization of an induced Drosophila melanoma in the

482

study of mammalian neoplasia. Ann N Y Acad Sci Ser II.1963;100:791-816.

22. Friedman F, et al. Necrosis liquefaction and absorption of C3H mammary tumors resulting from injection of extracts from tumor tissue. Abstract No. 78, Proceedings of the American Association for Cancer Research. 1965;6:20.

23. Clement RJ, et al. Peritoneal mesothelioma. Quantum Medicine. 1988; 1:68-73.

℣ℒIVINGSTON ℳETHOD

••

Virginia Livingston, MD, was an orthodox-trained physician who believed that cancer was caused by an ever-changing microbe she named *Progenitor cryptocides*. She claimed that this *P. cryptocides* would produce an important hormone called human chorionic gonadotropin (HCG). A high point of her scientific career came when this unlikely hypothesis was confirmed by respected academic scientists. (See *The Cancer Industry*, chapter 13.)

Dr. Livingston developed a large and successful practice in San Diego, whose centerpiece was a unique "autogenous vaccine" against *P. cryptocides*. On the first day of arrival at the clinic, patients were asked for urine samples. Dr. Livingston would then culture these samples for the patient's individual strain of the microbe. After about three weeks, the doctor would have a vaccine ready for injection back into the patient.

Most scientists denied the very existence of this microbe. Shortly before Dr. Livingston's death in 1990, California state health authorities prohibited her from using this unique treatment. The Livingston clinic carries on without her, but without the one treatment that made her program distinctive.

In her 1984 book, *The Conquest of Cancer*, Dr. Livingston explained the main features of her treatment program:

• All poultry products are eliminated from the diet, because they are allegedly heavily-infested with the *P. cryptocides*. White flour and sugar are forbidden, as are processed foods.

• Smoking and alcohol are forbidden.

• A suitable, mainly vegetarian diet is prescribed.

• Acutely-ill patients are treated with a whole-blood transfusion from a young, healthy individual, preferably a family member. No blood banks are used, since she thought most were contaminated with *P. cryptocides*.

• Gamma globulin is given as a source of antibodies.

• Splenic extract is injected two or three times a week, in order to increase the white blood count.

• BCG is administered in order to stimulate the patient's immune system against *P. cryptocides*.

• Small doses of nonspecific vaccines, either bacteria from teeth or tonsils or common respiratory bacteria, are given.
• Various vitamins, such as A, E, B_6, B_{12}, liver and intravenous vitamin C are given, when appropriate.

• The autogenous vaccine is administered both subcutaneously and orally.

• Antibiotics are administered with great attention paid to their effects on *P. cryptocides*.

• Since cancer patients are allegedly alkaline, measures are taken to acidify their blood and urine. The acidity of the uirne is routinely checked with Nitrazine paper, available in the pharmacy.

Dr. Livingston also claimed that a plant hormone, called abscisic acid, was "nature's most potent anticancer weapon." While there is extensive scientific research on this chemical, there is little standard literature on its use as an anticancer substance.

❦ METABOLIC TYPING

Metabolic typing is one of the names given to an unconventional approach to the cancer problem. It consists of various interpretations of ideas originally proposed by William Donald Kelley, DDS, a Texas orthodontist, who claims to have cured himself of pancreatic cancer through his own application of these methods. He later treated thousands of patients.

Nicholas J. Gonzalez, MD became interested in Kelley's work while a student at Cornell University Medical College in the late 1970s. Upon graduating, Gonzalez did postdoctoral work with Robert A. Good, MD, PhD, then president of Sloan-Kettering Institute, and investigated this method. He has claimed to apply the Kelley method in his practice in New York. (As part of a recent lawsuit, Dr. Kelley has disavowed any connection between their work and has stated that it is a "false premise" that Gonzalez is using the Kelley Program.)

Another practitioner of this method is Jack Taylor, DC, MS, a chiropractor, who uses a simpler form of the diet in his practice in Illinois.

In a lengthy unpublished monograph, *One Man Alone*, Dr. Gonzalez claims that when used properly this method achieved a remarkably high success rate, even in such seemingly incurable forms of cancers as carcinoma of the pancreas and liver. Gonzalez also claims this method is effective in treating other intractable diseases.

Although some scientists might object that "matched controls" are lacking, Robert G. Houston, author of *Repression and Reform in the Evaluation of Alternative Cancer Therapies*, argues that this study constitutes proof of the effectiveness of this method.

"The Gonzalez monograph," he writes, "documents results dramatic enough to constitute formal proof even with a single-arm study. Penicillin became a 'proven method' with only a few cases of dramatic recovery. The survival of five or more years for all five pancreatic patients on the full program is extremely significant statistically compared to the standard five-year survival of three percent. The odds against chance are forty million to one. Such is the nature of proof."

The basic idea behind this method is that the human species is divided into three genetically distinct subgroups. These are called:

• sympathetic dominants;

• parasympathetic dominants; and

• balanced types.

The terms "sympathetic" and "parasympathetic" refer to the two major divisions of the autonomic nervous system, the sympathetic and parasympathetic branches. Together, these systems of nerves are responsible for many of our bodily functions, the ones beyond our voluntary control, such as digestion, circulation and respiration. The two branches are often antagonistic to one another in their activity. Thus, when one is active, the other lies dormant, and vice versa.

"Sympathetic dominants" is the name given to people who allegedly have highly efficient sympathetic nervous systems. In them, the various tissues, glands and organs controlled by the sympathetic nerves (such as the heart) are particularly well-developed. As a corollary, the parasympathetic system in such individuals is said to be less-developed.

"Parasympathetics" are their diametrical opposites. The tissues, glands and organs controlled by this dominant system (e.g., the pancreas) are well-developed and efficient, but the sympathetically-controlled parts of the body are correspondingly less-developed.

In the third type, the "balanced" individuals, both branches are equally active, developed and efficient.

What makes an individual a sympathetic, parasympathetic or balanced type?

According to proponents of this theory, a person's national or geographic background determines his or her medical destiny. The sympathetic dominants of today are said to be the descendants of people who evolved in the subtropical parts of South America, Africa, Asia and Australia. Populations in these areas are presumed to have survived largely on plants, such as fruit, seeds and nuts.

On the other hand, the ancestors of today's parasympathetic dominants were northern people, as well as those who inhabited the cooler parts of Asia and America. These ancestors presumably survived on a meat-based diet and only occasionally consumed plants. The Eskimos are the epitome of parasympathetic types and lived almost entirely on meat before the introduction of the Western diet.

Those who have balanced types of systems are said to have ancestors who evolved in the middle latitudes and had access to a wide variety of foods, including many types of edible plants as well as meat.

Although a lot of genetic mingling has taken place in the intervening centuries, advocates of this theory claim that the basic types are still distinguishable, and that they still "breed true and have the same physiological makeup as their prehistoric ancestors," according to Dr. Gonzalez.

Thus, according to this theory, sympathetic dominants should eat a predominantly vegetarian diet, with up to 80 percent of calories coming from raw plant products. Vegetables with a high fat content (such as avocados) are avoided. The rest of the diet should consist of lightly-cooked vegetables, some cooked grains and some animal products.

Parasympathetics, by contrast, should get about 50 percent of their diet from fatty meat. They can eat large servings of beef, lamb or pork at least once a day. They also should eat generous helpings of dairy products, which are often considered unhealthy by other physicians.

Balanced types can consume a wide variety of foods. Plants should be fresh and unprocessed and meat meals should be alternated with vegetarian meals.

Dr. Gonzalez acknowledges that these beliefs are "far removed from what most medical researchers would accept as true." This is an understatement. These metabolic types are unknown to medical science and social scientists have generally given up trying to "type" people in this fashion.

Most doctors would also consider some of these recommendations—such as the "prescription" of fatty meat—as potentially dangerous for some people. However, a few doctors have based their medical practices on these concepts, because they believe it offers the key to understanding and treating chronic degenerative diseases which are not helped by conventional means.

In this system, accurate "typing" obviously becomes the essential step in diagnosing and treating the patient. The originator of these concepts used a very lengthy, complicated questionnaire and an elaborate computer program to find out which category each person belonged to. Others rely on blood and hair tests or simplified questionnaires.

In addition, this program often involves a detoxification of the body through various supplements and routines. These generally include:

• a huge array of vitamin, mineral and food supplements;

• a large number of pancreatic **enzymes;**

• a vigorous program of up to four (or more) coffee enemas

per day (see **Gerson Diet**);

• ancillary chiropractic adjustments.

Detoxification is the removal of toxins from the body, through the use of enemas, emetics, purges, sweat baths, etc. It is a very old idea. Ancient Egyptians (says Herodotus) purged regularly because they felt that diseases were caused by excess nutrients in the diet. In the nineteenth century it was widely believed that constipation produced a state of "autointoxication," literally self-poisoning.

Standard (so-called allopathic) medicine at first shared this philosophy and used a mercurial poison, laudanum, to irritate the bowel into discharging itself. In time, however, serious discussions of bowel movements were no longer to be found in standard journals.

One difficulty of evaluating this method is that it has introduced a great many new techniques and concepts at the same time. Scientists, however, are more comfortable when they evaluate single items at a time for specific effects in killing cancer cells or boosting immunity. Metabolic typing involves numerous factors in an ever-shifting pattern.

The best way to test this method would be to compare the outcome of various patients with matched controls treated by conventional methods. No such study has yet been done.

In 1990, the OTA attempted but failed to evaluate the 50 cases which Gonzalez had gathered in *One Man Alone*. Instead, OTA made the elementary error of failing to 'blind' the evaluators of the cases, thus opening the door to evaluator bias and prejudgment. OTA's experts included scientists favorable to and against unconventional cancer treatments. These predictably divided along 'party lines,' and a sterling opportunity was thereby lost.

❦𝒩AESSENS (714-X)

This is one of the most intriguing developments on the fringe of biology. Gaston Naessens is a microbiologist without the usual advanced degrees that go with that title. For nearly forty years he has been a thorn in the side of the cancer establishment, first in his native France, now in Sherbrooke, Québec. He was prosecuted and driven out of France in the 1950s when he proposed a treatment for leukemia called Anablast.

In the 1980s, he was similarly prosecuted for fraud in Canada, and even threatened with life imprisonment. This time he was acquitted, however.

Naessens has invented a special microscope, called a somatoscope, which can visualize living things at magnifications quite unattainable through an ordinary light microscope.

The ordinary light microscope permits an elargement of about 1800X, with a maximal resoltion of 0.1 microns (a micron is one millionth of a meter in length).

The more powerful electron miscroscope, on the other hand, can enlarge objects millions of times, with a resolution of 30 to 50 angstroms (an angstrom is one ten-billionth of a meter).

However, to be visualized by the electron microscope, the specimens must first be killed, dried and then fixed with stains, so what you finally see is basically the outlines of the object's skeleton.

Naessens has used a combination of laser and ultraviolet technology to develop an instrument that can observe *living* organisms at magnifications up to 30,000 and resolutions of as little as 150 angstroms. However, Naessens generally works at a lower range than this, in order to achieve greater clarity.

Using this somatoscope, Naessens claims to have made an astonishing discovery. He says he has observed "in all biologic liquids, and particularly in blood, an elementary particle endowed with movement and possessing a variable life cycle of many forms." He has called this particle a "somatid" and says he can isolate and culture it given the right growth media.

The main forms these organisms take, in addition to somatids, are spores and double spores. In normal individuals, the life cycle of this organism is controlled by blood inhibitors, which are mainly trace minerals and organic substances.

But if the individual is unduly stressed, this simple cycle can be diverted into another, elaborate life cycle which was originally identified by a German scientist in the 1930s. Within this group are a wide range of organisms that have been called, variously, pleomorphic organisms (see the **Livingston method**), "L-form" bacteria or "cell wall deficient organisms."

Why do not other scientists see these same organisms? First, Naessens says, they do not have his powerful instrument, which can visualize living organisms at high magnifications. Second, they are intellectually averse to the notion of everchanging microbes. Finally, debris from this microbe *is* seen by conventional microbiologists. But they usually dismiss these as "fibrin formations." "No one has ever explained the wide prevalence of these 'artifacts' in carefully prepared and usually sterile slides," he says.

Needless to say, Naessens's claims have roiled traditional microbiologists, many of whom have spent their careers neatly classifying bacteria and viruses. If Naessens is right, however, they won't have to rewrite their textbooks. They can throw them all away.

To our knowledge, aside from an occasional condemnation, nothing of a substantive nature has ever been published in a scientific journal on this method. However, not all authorities are negative.

A top official of a famous lensmaking company has written that the Naessens microscope is "a remarkable advancement in light microscopy, showing amazingly many details in the specimen."

And the director of the Georgia Institute of Technology's School of Applied Biology wrote in 1989 that Naessens's samples are "impressive...exciting...and remarkable." Naessens has now created a kit which can convert regular light microscopes into up-to-date somatoscopes. This should help disseminate his point of view and bring independent medical judgments on his remarkable claims.

Naessens also has developed a treatment for cancer and AIDS based on these discoveries. It is called 714-X and is a mixture of camphor and nitrogen, which is injected directly into the lymph system. Naessens claims that cancer cells are nitrogen-starved and that camphor helps deliver this nitrogen to them through the lymph system.

Does 714-X work? In his account of Naessens's 1989 trial for practicing medicine without a license, *Galileo of the Microscope*, author Christopher Bird quotes individuals who claim to have been cured of cancer and AIDS by Naessens. These are impressive stories.

On the other hand, prominent scientists have testified that what he is saying is impossible, although some of them admitted they formed their judgments without bothering to look through Naessens's microscope.

Many other individuals have looked through the somatoscope and seen what Naessens claims is there, a complex organism that takes many shapes. Without impartial scientific evaluation, however, it is difficult to see how this controversy can be resolved.

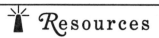

Resources

Cancell:

Ed Sopcak, PO Box 496, Howell, Michigan 48843. Phone: 313-684-5529, Monday through Friday, between 11 am and 2 pm Eastern Standard Time. Callers must be persistent as overworked volunteers staff the phones. To receive Cancell for free, patients must send a doctor's letter and a signed statement with proof that their condition is terminal. In addition, there is a videotape on Cancell called "At Whose Expense?" This is available from Backcountry Productions, 1117 6th Avenue, Longmont, CO 80501. Phone: 303-772-8358. Cost: $24.95 plus $3.00 S&H.

Carnivora:

Dr. Keller's clinic is: The Chronic Disease Control and Treatment Center, Am Reuthlein 2, D-8675 Bad Steben, Germany. Phone: 011-49-9288-5166; Fax: 011-49-9288-7815. The drug can be obtained from the Carnivora Research Company, Lobensteinerstrasse 3, D-8646 Nordhalben, Germany; Phone: 011-49-9267-1662; Fax: 011-9267-1040. Carnivora is available for purchase, depending on the laws of the country of import. In the United States, for instance, some patients have obtained Carnivora for their own use. The cost depends on the treatment regimen. A vial, used for about 25 treatments, costs several hundred dollars.

He prefers to begin treating the patient himself for four to six weeks in Bad Steben and then discharge the patient to the referring physician with a recommended schedule of treatment. In addition, Dr. Keller is willing to train physicians from around the world in the use of the drug, training to be conducted at Bad Steben.

Further information on what he calls "the Carnivora cure for cancer, AIDS and other pathologies" can be obtained from Morton Walker, DPM, 484 High Ridge Road, Stamford, CT 06905. Phone: 203-322-1551.

IAT (Immunoaugmentative Therapy):

Immunoaugmentative Therapy Centre, PO Box F-2689
Freeport, Grand Bahama Island, Bahamas
Lawrence Burton, PhD, primary contact.
Phone: 809-352-6455/6

Livingston Method:

Livingston Foundation Medical Center, 3232 Duke Street, San Diego, CA 92110. Phone: 619- 224-3515

Metabolic Typing:

Nicholas Gonzalez, MD, 737 Park Avenue, New York, NY 10021
Phone: 212-535-3993

Dr. Taylor's Wellness Center, Metabolic Assessment Program,
515 East Golf Road, Suite 107, Arlington Heights, IL 60005.
Phone: 800-398-6703

Naessens (714-X):
For information on the current availability of 714-X, patients are advised
to contact People Against Cancer, Box 10, Otho, IA 50569.
Phone: 515-972-4444. Fax: 515-972-4415. They can also try the Support
Committee for Gaston Naessens, 6912 Christophe Colomb, Montreal,
Quebec. H2S 2H2. Phone: 514-279-7570.

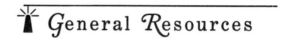

☀ General Resources

United States Organizations
American Cancer Society, 1599 Clifton Rd., NE, Atlanta, GA 30329
Phone: 404-320-3333 or 800-ACS-2345

Assn. of American Cancer Institutes, Elm & Carlton Sts., Buffalo, NY
14263. Phone: 716-845-3028 / Fax: 716-845-3545

Association for Brain Tumor Research, 3725 N. Talman Ave.,Chicago, IL
60618. Phone: 12-286-5571

Assn. of Community Cancer Centers, 11600 Nebel St., Ste. 201
Rockville, MD 20852. Phone: 301-984-9496

Assn. for Research of Childhood Cancer, PO Box 251, Buffalo, NY 14225
Phone: 716-681-4433

Breast Cancer Advisory Center, PO Box 224, Kensington, MD 20895
Phone: 301-718-7293. Fax: 301-949-1132

Breast Health Program of New York, 28 West 12th Street
New York, NY 10011. Phone: 212-645-0052. Leslie Strong, Med. Dir.

Cancer Federation, Inc., 21250 Box Springs Rd., No. 209
Moreno Valley, CA 92387. Phone: 714-682-7989

Cancer Guidance Institute, 1323 Forbes Ave., Ste. 200
Pittsburgh, PA 15219. Phone: 412-261-2211

Cancer Information Service, Boy Scout Bldg., Rm. 340
Bethesda, MD 20892. Phone: 301-496-8664 or 800-4-CANCER.

Corporate Angel Network, Westchester County Airport
Bldg. One, White Plains, NY 10604. Phone: 914-328-1313 / Fax: 800-328-4226. Provides free air travel for patients.

Damon Runyon-Walter Winchell Cancer Research Fund
131 East 36th St., New York, NY 10016. Phone: 212-532-7000

DES Action, USA, Long Island Jewish Medical Center
New Hyde Park, NY 11040. Phone: 516-775-3450

Intl. Society for Preventive Oncology, 217 East 85th Street, Ste. 303
New York, NY 10028. Phone: 212-534-4991

Komen Foundation (Breast Cancer), 6820 LBJ Fwy, Ste. 130, Dallas, TX
75240. Phone: 214-980-8841 / Fax: 214-980-4971

Latin American Cancer Research Project, 525 Twenty Third Street, NW
Washington, DC 20037. Phone: 202-861-3200. Fax: 1-202-223-5971

Leukemia Society of America, 733 3rd Avenue, New York, NY 10017.
Phone: 212-573-8484 / Fax: 212-972-5776

Make Today Count, 101½ S. Union St., Alexandria, VA 22314.
Phone: 703-548-9674

Natl. Alliance of Breast Cancer Orgs., 1180 Ave. of the Americas, 2nd Fl.
New York, NY 10036. Phone: 212-719-0154

National Cancer Care Foundation, 1180 Avenue of the Americas
New York, NY 10036. Phone: 212-221-3300

Natl. Coalition for Cancer Survivorship, 323 8th St. SW, Albuquerque,
NM 87102. Phone: 505-764-9956

National Leukemia Association, 585 Stewart Ave., Ste. 536
Garden City, NY 11530. Phone: 516-222-1944. Fax: 516-222-0457

Prostate Health Program of New York, 785 Park Ave.
New York, NY 10021. Phone: 212-988-8888

R.A. Block Cancer Foundation, H and R Block Bldg., 4410 Main
Kansas City, MO 64111. Phone: 816-932-8453

Reach for Recovery, c/o American Cancer Society
1599 Clifton Road, Atlanta, GA 30329. Phone: 404-320-3333

Skin Cancer Foundation, 245 Fifth Avenue, Ste. 2402, New York, NY
10016. Phone: 212-725-5176

Spirit and Breath Association, 8210 Elmwood Ave., Ste. 209
Skokie, IL 60077. Phone: 708-673-1384

Y-ME National Organization for Breast Cancer Info. and Support
18220 Harwood Ave., Homewood, IL 60430. Phone: 800-221-2141.
24-hour hotline: 708-799-8228

International Organizations
Argentina:
Latin American Association of Environmental Mutagens,
Carcinogens, etc., c/o Inst. Multidisciplinario Biol. Celular.
66 403 1900 La Plata, Argentina

Austria:
Intl. Academy of Tumor Marker Oncology, Lab. for Bio-analytic
Schwarzes Panier Strasse 15, A-1090 Wien, Austria
Phone: 43-1-4085433 / Fax: 43-1- 4089908

Belgium:
Anti-Cancer Service, Avenue de la Chasse 94, Bte 16, B-1040
Bruxelles, Belgium

Comité de Cancérologues de la Communauté européenne
Prof Christian de Duve, ICP, Avenue Hippocrate 75
BP 7550, B-1200, Bruxelles, Belgium
Phone: (32 2) 764 7538 / Fax: (32 2) 764 5322

European Cancer Center for Developmental and Supportive Therapy
Rue Héger-Bordet 1, B-1000 Bruxelles, Belgium

European Institute of Ecology and Cancer, Rue des Fripiers 24 bis
B-1000 Bruxelles, Belgium. Phone: (32 2) 219 08 30

European Lung Cancer Working Party, Inst. Jules Bordet, Service de
Médicine, Rue Héger-Bordet 1, B-1000 Bruxelles, Belgium

European Organization for Cooperation in Cancer Prevention Studies
Avenue R Vandendnessche, B-1150, Bruxelles, Belgium
Phone: (32 2) 762 04 85 / Fax: (32 2) 774 19 59

European Organization for Research and Treatment of Cancer, Avenue
Mounier 83, Boite 40, B-1200, Bruxelles, Belgium. Phone: (32 2) 774 16 40

European Society for Therapeutic Radiology and Oncology, Dept. of
Radiotherapy, Univ. Hospital, St. Raphaël, Capucijnenvoer 33
B-3000, Leuven, Belgium. Phone: (32 16) 21 22 13 / Fax: (32 16) 21 22 28

European Society of Surgical Oncology, Service de Chirurgie, Institut J. Bordet, Rue Héger-Bordet 1, B-1000 Bruxelles
Belgium. Phone: (32 2) 537 31 06

Intl. Society of Pediatric Oncology, Dept. d'Hématologie Pediatrique Hopital d'Universitaire St. Luc Avenue Hippocrat 10, B-1200 Bruxelles, Belgium. Phone: (32 2) 764 11 11, ext. 3332 / Fax: (32 2) 762 58 55

Vivre Comme Avant, Avenue Louise 223, B-1050 Bruxelles, Belgium
Phone: (32 2) 649 41 68

World Institute of Ecology and Cancer, Rue de Fripiers 24 bis
B-1000, Bruxelles Belgium. Phone: (32 2) 219 08 30

Brazil:
World Association for Gynecological Cancer Prevention, Av. S. Sopacabana 664, Apt. 606, Rio de Janeiro Zc-07, Brazil

Canada:
Intl. Assn. for Study of Lung Cancer, Ontario Cancer Institute
500 Sherbourne St., Toronto M4X 1K9, Canada

Denmark:
Assn. of European Cancer Leagues, c/o Danish Cancer Society
Rosenvaengets Hovedvej 35, DK-2100, København, Denmark
Phone: (45 1) 31 26 88 66 / Fax: (45 1) 31 26 45 60

Scandinavian Soc. of Mammography, Gentofte University Hospital, DK-2900, Hellerup, Denmark. (45 16) 51200

Egypt:
Medit. Soc. of Tumor Marker Oncology, Biochemistry Department
Ain Shams Univ., Abbasia, Cairo, Egypt

Middle East Fed. Against Cancer, Cancer Institute, 174 Tahrir Street
Cairo, Egypt

Finland:
Scand. Soc. for Head & Neck Oncology, University Central Hospital
Dept. of Otolaryngology, SF-20520, Turku, Finland.
Phone: (358 21) 611 611

France:
Eur. Soc. for Cancer Internal Medicine, Centre Antoine Lacassagne
36 Voie Romaine, F-06054 Nice, France

Intl. Agency for Research on Cancer, 150 Cours Albert Thomas, F-69372 CEDEX 08 Lyon, France. Phone: (33) 72 73 84 85 / Fax: (33) 72 73 85 75

Intl. Medical Sports Federation for Aid to Cancer Research, Chateau des Templiers, BP 231, F-34502 Béziers, France. Phone: (33) 28 86 16

International Society for the Campaign Against Cancer of the Breast, Hôpital Marie Lannelouque, F-92350 Le Plessis Robinson, France

European Soc. for Medical Oncology, Centre Antoine Lacassagne 36 Voie Romaine F-06054, Nice CEDEX France. Phone: (33) 93 81 71 33

Eur. Soc. for Psychosocial Oncology, Service d'Hématologie, Hotel-Dieu 1 Place du Parvis, Notre-Dame, F-75181 Paris CEDEX 04 France

Intl. Society Against Breast Cancer, 26 rue de la Faisanderie, F-75116 Paris, France. Phone: (33 1) 47 04 70 32

Oncological and Biological Centre for Applied Research, Le Village F-38370, St. Prim, France. Phone: (33) 74 56 58 00 / Fax: (33) 74 56 54 40

Org. Oncologique Méditerranéenne d'Enseignment et de Recherche Group Hospitalier Paul Brusse, 12-16 Avenue P V Coutourier, F-94800, Ville Juif, France. Phone: (33) 47 256 78 71

Germany:
European Tumour Virus Group, P.Ehrlich Inst., P.Ehrlich Strasse 51-59 D-6070 Langen, Germany. Phone: (49 6103) 755-102 / Fax: (49 6103) 755-123

International Psycho-oncology Project, Bergstrasse 10, D-2900 Oldenburg, Germany. Phone: (49 441) 1 31 47

Italy:
Eur. Soc. of Gynaecological Oncology, Galleria Storione, 2/A, I-35123 Padova, Italy. Phone: (39 49) 35724-36505

European Society of Mastology, Via Vivaio, 18, I-20122 Milano, Italy Phone: (39 2) 78 04 88 / Fax: (39 2) 78 10 19

European School of Oncology, Via Venzian 1, I-20133, Milano, Italy Phone: (39 2) 266 4662 / Fax: (39 2) 266 4662

World Comm. for Leukemia Research, Inst. di Anatomia e Istologia Patologica, Universita degli Studi di Padova, Via A Gabelli 35, 35100 Padua, Italy. Phone: 66 39 55

World Health Org. Melanoma Prog., Instit. Nazionale Tumori Via Veneziana 1, I-20133 Milano, Italy. Phone: (39 2) 29 39 92

GENERAL RESOURCES

Japan:
Asian and Pacific Fed. of Organizations for Cancer Research and Control
c/o Institute of Preventive Oncology, H1 Bldg., 1-2 Ichigaya-
Sadoharacho, Shinjuku-ku, Tokyo, 162, Japan. Phone: (81 3) 3267 2556

Netherlands:
European Assn. for Cancer Education, BOOG, Bloemsingel 1, 9713 BZ
Groningen, Netherlands. Phone: (31 50) 63 28 88 / Fax: (31 50) 63 28 83

Intl. Comm. for Protection Against Environmental Mutagens &
Carcinogens, Medical Biological Laboratory, TNO, PO Box 45, 2280 AA
Rijswijk, Netherlands

Norway
Latin Amer. Assn. of Environmental Mutagen Carcinogen & Teratogen
Societies, Institute of General Genetics, University of Oslo, PO Box 103d
Blindern, Oslo 3, Norway.

Spain:
Fed. of European Cancer Societies, Hospital 1 de Calubre Carretera de
Andulecia, Km 5 500, 280 Madrid Spain. Phone: (34 1) 269 56 90,
Fax: (34 1) 469 57 75

Sweden:
Nordic Cancer Union, c/o Cancerfonden, Swedenborgsgatan 20, Box
17096, S-114 62 Stockholm, Sweden. Phone: (46 8) 772 2800

Scandinavian Cancer Union, Riksforeningen mot Cancerfonden
Sturegatan 14, S-114 36 Stockholm, Sweden. Phone: 08 63 58 40

Switzerland
Eur. Org. for Research on Cancer, Birchstrasse 95, CH-8050 Zürich,
Switzerland. Phone: 312 44 56

International Union Against Cancer, Rue du Conseil General 3, CH-1205
Geneva, Switzerland. Phone: (41 22) 720 18 11 / Fax: (41 22) 720 18 10

European School of Oncology Found., Via Nassa 40, Lugano,
Switzerland. Phone: (41 91) 23 20 80 /Fax: (41 91) 23 26 01

International Society of Oncodevelopmental Biology & Medicine
Ludwig Institute for Cancer Research, Stadelhofer Strasse 22,
CH-8001 Zürich, Switzerland

UK:
European Assn. for Cancer Research, Cancer Research Campaign Labs.
U. Nottingham, Nottingham NG7 2RD, United Kingdom.
Phone: 0602 56101

Assn. for Intl. Cancer Research, Dept. of Chemistry, U. St. Andrews
St. Andrews KY16 9ST, UK. Phone: (44 344) 76161

Cancer Research Campaign, 2 Carlton House, Terrace
London SW1Y 5AR. Phone: (44 71) 930 8972

European Assn. for Cancer Research, Cancer Research Campaign Labs
University of Nottingham, Nottingham NG7 2RD UK
Phone: (44 602) 48 48 48, x3401/ (44 602) 58 66 30

European Oncology Nursing Society, & Intl. Soc. for Nurses in Cancer
Care, Mulberry House, Royal Marsden Hospital, Fulham Road
London SW3 6JJ UK. Phone: (44 71) 376 3623 / Fax: (44 71) 351 2191

Imperial Cancer Research Fund, CB DBE Box 123, Lincoln's Inn Fields
London WC 2A 3PX, UK.
Phone: (44 71) 242-0200 / Fax: (44 71) 405-1556

Intl. Soc. for Nurses in Cancer Care, Mulberry House, Royal Marsden
Hosp., Fulham Road, London SW3 6JJ UK. Phone: (44 71). 352 3171,
x2123 Fax: (44 71. 351 2191

Venezuela:
Fed. Latinoamericana de Soc. des Cancer, Canonigos a Esperanza 43,
Apt. 6702, Caracas 1010 Venezuela. Phone: (58 2) 561 99 22

Zimbabwe:
Afr. Org. for Research & Training in Cancer, Univ. of Zimbabwe
POB A178, Avondale, Harare, Zimbabwe

Information and Referrals on Alternative Treatments

American Assoc. of Orthomolecular Medicine, 7375 Kingsway
Burnaby, British Columbia, V3N3B5 Canada

American College of Advances in Medicine, 231 Verdugo Drive, Suite 204
Laguna Hills, CA 92653. Phone: 714-583-7666

Arlin J. Brown Information Center, PO Box 251, Ft. Belvoir, VA 22060
Phone: 703- 451-8638

Cancer Control Society, 2043 N. Berendo St., Los Angeles, CA 90027.
Phone: 213-663-7801

Comm. for Freedom of Choice in Medicine, 1180 Walnut Av., Chula Vista,
CA 92011. Phone: 800-227-4473 / Fax: 619- 429-8004

GENERAL RESOURCES

European Institute for Orthomolecular Sciences, PO Box 420, 3740 A.K.
Baarn, Holland

Found. for Advancement in Cancer Therapy, Box 1242, Old Chelsea Sta.
New York, NY 10113. Phone: 212-741-2790

Gerson Institute, PO Box 430, Bonita, CA 91908.
Phone: 619-267-1150 / Fax: 619-267-6441

Intl. Academy of Nutrition and Preventive Medicine, PO Box 18433
Asheville, NC 28814. Phone: 704- 258-3243 /Fax: 704-251-9206

Intl. Assn. of Cancer Victors & Friends, 7740 W. Manchester Ave., No.
110, Playa del Rey, CA 90293. Phone: 213-822-5032 / Fax: 213-822-5132

We Can Do!, 1800 Augusta, Ste. 150, Houston, TX 77057.
Phone: 713-780-1057

Of Special Note:
People Against Cancer is a non-profit, grassroots membership organization dedicated to cancer prevention and medical freedom of choice. It
counsels members about cancer therapy and distributes information
about innovative approaches. A regular membership costs $25.
People Against Cancer, Box 10, Otho, IA 50569.
Phone: 1-515-972-4444. Fax: 515-972-4415

GLOSSARY

Abscisic acid: a kind of plant hormone which inhibits the growth of plants. Counteracts growth-promoting substances.

Accutane: 13-cis-retinoic acid, a form of retinoic acid, used as a treatment for acne and experimentally for cancer.

Adjuvant: any substance added to a drug which affects the action of that drug in a predictable way.

Algae: an informal term for many simple plants which thrive in a damp or aquatic (freshwater or marine) environment.

Ames test: a simple assay using bacteria growing in a laboratory dish, to assess the mutation- or cancer-causing ability of a particular substance.

Amino acid: one of the building blocks of protein. About 20 amino acids commonly occur in proteins, of which about half are "essential" and must be obtained from food.

Antibody: an immune or protective protein which is created by B-cells in the presence of antigens and reacts with them in a demonstrable way.

Antigen: a foreign substance which, coming in contact with the appropriate tissues, elicits an immune response, especially the production of antibodies by B-type lymphocytes.

Autoimmune reaction: a hostile immune response to molecules the body normally regards as part of itself. This reaction by white blood cells can damage the adrenal cortex, thyroid gland, joints and other parts of the body and lead to serious disease.

B-cells: white blood cells (lymphocytes) that originate in the fetal liver and then migrate through the bone marrow, finally settling in either the lymph nodes or the spleen. B-cells are responsible for a major segment of immunity, producing antibodies to substances called antigens. Specialized forms of B-cells are called memory or plasma cells.

Bacteria: single-celled organisms classified as part of the Kingdom Monera. They vary in shape and size, but include rodlike (bacilli), spherical (cocci) and spirals (spirilli) forms. Reproduction is asexual, usually through simple fission.

Bacteriophage: a virus that parasitizes bacteria. The non-specific vaccine staphage lysate is produced through the activity of bacteriophage on staphylococcus microbes.

Biotechnology: the application of recent biological discoveries to the large-scale production of new organisms or their products. Often involves genetic manipulation or recombination.

Cachexia: a physical wasting syndrome associated with the late stages of cancer, AIDS and other diseases.

Cancer cell: a cell which has somehow escaped normal controls over growth and division. Cancer begins with a single cell which produces clones of itself (called daughter cells) which invade adjacent tissues and often interfere with their normal activity. Cancer cells have abnormal glucose requirements and produce lactic acid, which puts an extra burden on the liver. Cells which proliferate but stay together form benign tumors, not cancers. But those which disperse through the blood or lymph are called malignant, or cancerous cells.

Cancer: a disease, or rather group of diseases, characterized by a loss of cellular control mechanisms, the invasion of surrounding tissues, and a strong tendency to migrate (metastasize) to distant sites. Cancer may recur even after attempted removal and cause the death of the patient, unless adequately treated.

Carcinogen: any factor, but mainly synthetic chemicals, capable of transforming a normal cell into a cancerous one.

Carcinomas: malignant tumors arising in cells of epithelial origin. Encompassing most breast, lung, liver, etc. tumors, carcinomas are the most common type of cancer.

Carotene: yellow or orange pigments commonly found in plants, which can be converted into vitamin A in the liver.

Carotenoids: a large group of yellow, orange and red pigments located in those parts of plants where chlorophyll is absent. Includes xanthophylls as well as various carotenes.

Cartilage: after bone, the most important connective tissue of the human skeleton. Contains glycoproteins but lacks blood vessels and nerves.

Chemoprevention: the prevention of disease through the use of chemicals, drugs or food factors, such as vitamins.

Chemotherapy: the use of drugs, and especially of cytotoxic agents, in the treatment of cancer and other diseases.

Chlorophyll: a green pigment found in algae and most higher plants, which is responsible for capturing light in the process of photosynthesis.

Coenzyme: an organic molecule which serves as a cofactor in an enzymatic reaction by binding temporarily to that enzyme.

Coenzyme Q: a lipid-soluble coenzyme that plays a crucial role by transporting electrons during energy production in cells. Also known as CoQ or ubiquinone.

Colony Stimulating Factor: CSF, a hormone-like substance which stimulates the formation of white blood cells. Some forms of CSF stop leukemic cells from dividing.

Conjunctivitis: 'pinkeye,' an inflammation of the conjunctiva, the lining of the back of the eyelid. Can be caused by viruses, allergies and irritations.

Control: to verify an experiment by running a parallel test in which some crucial element is omitted. Also refers to the animal or person who receives the inert substance (placebo) in such an experiment.

Cytotoxic: anything poisonous, or lethal, to cells, such as conventional chemotherapy.

DNA: deoxyribonucleic acid. This double-stranded molecule forms the genetic material of all cells and of many viruses.

Edema: a swelling of tissues through an increase in tissue fluid. In cancer, edema can be caused by a blockage of the lymphatic system.

Endotoxin: a substance which is attached to the cell wall of certain bacteria. Also known as LPS (lipopolysaccharide). Capable of causing the symptoms of many infectious diseases. Has therapeutic potential.

Enzymes: protein catalysts which are responsible for the high rate and the specificity of most biochemical reactions. Higher forms of life are inconceivable without enzymes.

Essential fatty acids: substances required in the diet for normal growth. These include linoleic and gamma-linolenic acids.

Estrogens: a group of steroids, including the female sex hormones, which stimulate growth, e.g., of the mammary glands. Some tumors, called hormone-dependent cancers, grow under the influence of estrogen.

Fibrosis: the formation of tough, sinewy tissue as a repair or reactive process.

Folic acid: a water-soluble vitamin of the B-complex involved in many enzymatic reactions.

Free radicals: an atom or atom group which carries an unpaired electron but no charge. Free radicals are very short-lived but can cause serious damage to living tissues. They are counteracted by free radical scavengers, such as vitamin C.

Gene: the smallest physical unit of heredity normally found in a cell.

Genetic engineering: procedures by which genes are removed from genetic material of one species (e.g., humans) and then enzymatically inserted into the genes of other species (e.g., bacteria). Used in the manufacture of a modern class of drugs.

Graft-versus-host disease: reaction of the body's immune system to grafted or implanted tissues. Often leads to the rejection of the implant. A major problem in bone marrow transplantation, which is only partially overcome through the use of immunosuppressive drugs.

Heparin: an anticoagulant found in most connective tissues.

HIV: Human immunodeficiency virus. The presumed cause of acquired immunodeficiency syndrome (AIDS).

Homeopathy: an alternative medical system which treats symptoms of a disease with minute doses of a compound which, in larger doses, produces those very symptoms in healthy people.

Immunity: the ability of an organism to resist infection or the attacks of other harmful agents. An essential tool of survival in all species. In animals, immunity consists of two parts, innate immunity, which includes physical and chemical barriers, and adaptive immunity, which includes responses to particular substances, such as antigens.

Initiation: the first stage in the induction of a tumor by a carcinogen. Causes subtle changes in a cell so that it becomes cancerous when exposed to a promoter.

Interferons: proteins produced by virally-infected cells, as well as by non-infected white blood cells, which are able to prevent the further replication of viruses.

Interleukins: factors involved in communication among white blood cells. May also be produced by some non-white blood cells. Involved in activating T-cells and in making macrophages (scavenger cells) more effective. Interleukin-2 (IL-2) is used in the treatment of kidney cancer, melanoma and other tumors, but is highly toxic and rarely curative.

Keratocanthoma: a rapidly-growing tumor which generally occurs on exposed areas of the skin. May disappear spontaneously, even if untreated.

Lectin: proteins and other substances that can cause cells to clump together. Acts in some ways like an antigen. Lectins are often responsible for the toxic properties of seeds.

Leukemia: a malignant overproduction of white blood cells, which crowds out normal red blood cells and destroys platelet production. Death results mainly from indirect effects of this process.

Leukocytes: blood cells which have a nucleus, but lack hemoglobin. Includes several categories: granulocytes whose granules are visible under the microscope and agranulocytes (including both lymphocytes and monocytes).

Leukoplakia: white patches on the mucous membrane of the mouth, which cannot be wiped off and cannot be diagnosed as caused by any specific disease. Experimentally treated with vitamin A and its analogs.

Lipids: a broad category of organic compounds, including fats, waxes, steroids, the fat-soluble vitamins (A, D, E, K), prostaglandins, carotenes and chlorophylls.

Lipopolysaccharide: see Endotoxin.

Lipoprotein: a mixture of protein and lipids important in many biological reactions.

Lymph: clear fluid found in the vessels of the lymphatic system. Responsible for returning proteins from the tissue fluid to the blood.

Lymphoctyes: one kind of leukocyte (white blood cell) which plays a crucial role in immunity. There are two main varieties: T-cells and B-cells.

Lymphokines: soluble factors produced by lymphocytes. Those produced by T-cells are called interleukins.

Macrophage: scavenger (phagocytic) cell of the connective tissue not usually found in the blood. The two main types are (a) the wandering macrophages and (b) the static macrophages, which migrate to the site of an infection and engulf foreign particles.

Metabolism: the sum of all chemical and physical processes in a living body. More specifically, the term can refer to the combined action of a body's enzymes.

Metastasis: movement of cancer cells from a primary growth to a distant site, usually via the blood or lymph. Secondary growths in vital organs can be more dangerous than the primary tumor.

Microbe: any microscopic organism. Many microbes cause disease but others are 'friendly' and health-promoting.

Mitochondria: organelles (distinct structural parts) of human (and many other) cells and the source of energy in those cells. Varying in number per cell between one and several thousand, they usually show up on the electron microscope as spheres.

Mutagen: anything which increases the rate of alteration of the genetic material of a cell. Most mutagens are also carcinogens.

Myeloma: a malignant cancer of the myeloid (bone marrow) tissue. Causes anemia as its major symptom and mainly affects middle-aged and elderly persons.

Natural killer cell: a part of the innate immune system, a type of white blood cell which recognizes changes in infected or cancerous cells, binds to those cells and kills them. NK cells are activated by interferon.

Necrosis: the death of cells or tissues, resulting from a disease process.

Neoplasm: literally "new thing formed," scientific name for a tumor.

Nude mice: specially-bred mice which lack a thymus gland (athymic). They accept transplants of human tumor cells and are therefore widely used in cancer research.

Oncologist: a medical doctor who specializes in the treatment of cancer, especially through the use of chemotherapy.

Oncology: the science which studies the disease process of cancer.

Peptide: two or more amino acids linked together by a peptide bond. Long chains of peptides are usually called polypeptides.

pH: a measure of acidity and alkalinity, denoting the concentration of hydrogen ions in a solution.

Placebo: an inert substance, given in a clinical study, which is supposed to be identical in appearance to the drug under consideration. A placebo is used to distinguish between the true actions of the experimental drug and the power of suggestion.

Polysaccharide: a carbohydrate which, although somewhat like a sugar, lacks a sweet taste. Some examples are cellulose, starch and glycogen.

Promotion: second phase in the creation of an experimental tumor. A promoter may not be carcinogenic by itself but can stimulate a previously induced cell to become cancerous.

Prostaglandins: fatty acid derivatives which are continuously produced by many cells. Released into the bloodstream like hormones, but unlike hormones only effective over short distances.

Pulmonary: relating to the lung.

Redox reactions: oxidation-reduction reactions, generally involving the transfer of hydrogen atoms, and which are generally accelerated by enzymes.

Rhabdomyosarcoma: a tumor derived from skeletal (striated) muscle which mostly occurs in children.

Sarcoma: a malignant tumor arising in tissues of mesenchymal origin, such as connective tissue, bone, cartilage or striated muscle.

Streptococcus: a kind of non-spore-producing bacteria which forms long chains. Most are harmless but the pyogenic kind causes fever and diseases in humans, such as erysipelas. It can also destroy red blood cells. One of two bacteria used to produce Coley's toxins.

Syndrome: the signs and symptoms associated with a disease, which taken together constitute a picture of that disease.

T-cell: a lymphocyte formed in the bone marrow which then travels to the thymus for 'processing,' where it learns to recognize 'self' from 'non-self.' The T-cell then travels on to the spleen and lymph nodes. Some T-cells assist B-cells, others stimulate macrophages, while yet others suppress immune responses.

Terminal: relating to final stages of a deadly illness such as cancer.

Thymus gland: a two-lobed organ in the chest which reaches its largest size at puberty and then slowly diminishes. Responsible for the maturation of T-cells. The thymus produces various factors, such as thymopoietin and thymosin, which are hormone-like.

Toxicity: the state of being poisonous.

Transplantable tumor: an experimental tumor formed by the injection of cells from one animal to one of its genetic twins.

Trypsin: a protein-digesting enzyme which is secreted by the pancreas and breaks down protein into smaller units called peptides. Trypsin's activity is strongest at a pH of 7 to 8.

Vaccine: An immunologically-active substance that produces an immune reaction which is intended to prevent illness.

Virus: a minute infectious agent which is unable to multiply by itself, but can do so by using a living cell as its host. A virus can pass through the smallest bacterial filter and can only be seen with an electron microscope.

Vitamin A: A fat-soluble vitamin, the lack of which affects all tissues, but mostly the eyes. Infants and children are especially susceptible to vitamin A deficiencies.

Vitamin B complex: a group of 12 water-soluble vitamins, including biotin, cyanocobalamin, folic acid, nicotinic acid, pantothenic acid, pyridoxine and riboflavin.

Vitamin C: ascorbic acid. A water soluble sugar acid, which is especially abundant in fruit and tomatoes. Can be destroyed by cooking. Complete absence results in scurvy. Appears to also have an important role in cancer prevention and possibly treatment.

Vitamin D: a small group of fat-soluble vitamins, deficiency of which causes the disease rickets. Can be synthesized in the skin by exposure to ultraviolet light or if necessary supplemented in the diet with fish liver oil. Required for healthy bone and teeth.

Vitamin E: A group of fat-soluble vitamins obtained from seed oils, wheat germ, etc. Deficiency causes infertility and kidney degeneration.

Vitamin K: fat-soluble vitamins required for synthesis in the liver of a substance required for blood clotting. Produced by many plants and microorganisms, including some normally found in the gut.

Vitamin: an organic substance that is not normally made by an animal but has to be obtained from the environment in tiny amounts. Lack of a vitamin generally results in a specific deficiency disease.

INDEX

Antimicrobial, 78, 80, 100, 140, 474

Antimony, 163

Antimutation, 27, 147, 214-215, 306

Antinausea, 136, 374

Antineoplastons, 280-284, 294, 361, 367

Antioxidants, 28, 49, 53-54, 56, 61-62, 73-74, 77, 134, 137, 153, 174, 203, 208, 212, 214, 245, 264, 305

Antithrombotic, 61, 279, 331

Antiviral, 138, 254, 346, 417, 464

Anus, 190, 304, 342

Apes, 129

Aphrodisiac, 72, 143

Aplastic anemia, 211, 213

Apples, 121, 225, 264, 368

Apricots, 27, 63, 81, 267-268, 272, 292, 367-368

Aquaculture, 264

Arctium lappa, 146, 148, 161, 164

Argentina, 170-171, 496

Arginine, 284-287, 367

Arthritis, 102, 173, 229, 338, 341

As-101, 115-117, 123

Asafoetida, 175

Asbestos, 83, 481

Ascites, 62, 80, 100-101, 108, 203, 254, 259, 315, 325, 329, 418, 426, 433, 443

Ascorbic acid, 49, 54, 56, 58-63, 70-71, 77, 80, 106, 274, 293, 297

Asia, 153, 157, 172, 246, 487

Asian, 141, 156, 165, 180, 234, 265, 278, 367, 373, 499

Asparaginase, 307

Asparagus, 27, 197

Aspirin, 9, 22, 44-45, 73, 149, 177, 267, 288-290, 341, 344, 367-368

Asthma, 171, 268

Astragalus, 130-132, 166, 177, 180, 265

Astrocytoma, 413

Athymic (nude) mice, 132, 233, 281, 284

Australia, 171-172, 210, 289, 349, 487

Austria, 187, 192, 391, 496

Auto-antibodies, 116

Auto-immune disease, 232-233, 350

Autogenous vaccine, 483-484

Auto-intoxication, 489

Autologous vaccine, 467

Avocados, 197, 487

Ayur-veda, 132-134, 178

Azelaic acid, 48-49, 291-292

AZT, 22, 248, 467

Azuki beans, 197

B vitamins, 33, 41-42, 44, 46, 185, 250, 288, 291, 370

B-cell, 383, 390

Baboons, 60, 63

Bacille Calmette-Guérin (BCG), 162, 397, 399-400, 407, 432, 463, 466, 484

Bacilli, 162, 399, 433-434

Bacteria, 78, 81, 127-128, 138, 225, 234, 238-239, 245, 257-258, 291, 329, 336, 407, 411-413, 422, 426, 432, 445, 458, 463, 465, 476, 480, 484, 491

Bahamas, 368, 476, 479-481, 493

Bananas, 192

Bancha tea, 197-198

Baohuoside-1 (herbs), 143, 145

Barberry, 161-162

Barbiturates, 320

Barium, 190, 343

Barley, 196

Basil, 175

BCNU, 400, 416

Beans, 48, 81, 94, 185, 196-197, 224, 231-232, 274

Beardian thesis, 308-309, 368

Beef, 214, 227, 232, 244, 246, 264, 488

Beer, 198

Beetles, 46, 143-144

Beets, 80, 197, 416

Belgium, 79, 90, 103, 200, 261, 496-497

Benign tumors, 69, 119-120, 245, 302, 354, 390, 482

Benzaldehyde, 147, 272, 292-297, 368

Berberine, 163, 165

Berberis, 161-162

Pain-killer, 163, 190, 269
Pancreatic cancer, 308-309, 334, 485
Pancreas, 58, 94, 110, 230, 232, 293,
   308-309, 314, 380, 485-486, 488
Pantothenic acid, 154
Papayas, 34, 308-309, 361
Papillomas, 33-34, 43, 175, 390, 394
Paprika, 27, 49, 63, 81
Paraguay, 171
Parasites, 124, 128, 149, 162, 189,
   321, 346, 377
Parathyroid, 87, 361
Parsley, 81
Pau d'arco, 170-172, 181
Peaches, 267, 292, 372
Peanuts, 372
Peas, 185, 309
Pecans, 368
Pectin, 154, 225, 229, 264
Penis, 364
Pepper, 155-156, 175
Peppers, 27, 49, 81, 156, 197
Pepsin, 308
Peptides, 164, 203, 205, 278, 280,
   282-282, 323, 401, 404, 453-454
Perfumes, 275, 292
Peritonitis, 427
Periwinkle, 177
Peroxide, 111, 176, 336, 338, 474
Pharmaceuticals, 14, 82, 208, 325,
   338, 351, 370-372, 467
Photosensitizers, 386, 388,
   390-391, 395
Phototherapy, 330, 386-387, 389-394
Pigs, 71, 174, 177, 241, 274, 433
Pike, 85, 468
Pineapple, 27
Pistachios, 285
Plague, 128, 437
Platinum-containing drugs,
   166, 219
Pleurisy, 277
Plumbagin, 474-476
Plums, 63, 81
Podophyllium, 124
Poisoning, 28, 111, 128, 130, 147-
   148, 163, 165, 179, 202, 271, 274-
   275, 311, 329, 489

Pokeweed, 161-164
Poland, 73, 280-281
Pollutants, 50, 60, 67, 71, 257, 264
Polysaccharides, 127, 142, 145, 147,
   162, 164, 169, 176, 198, 228-229,
   249-251, 253-256, 258, 400, 420,
   422-423, 426-428, 433, 464
Polyunsaturated fats, 81, 217-218,
   221-222, 233
Pompano, 370
Potassium, 60, 93-96, 118, 123, 149,
   156, 161, 173, 189, 191-192, 194-
   195, 217, 370
Potatoes, 29, 81, 196-197, 324
Poultry, 79, 439, 484
Precancerous condition, 42-43, 45,
   83, 178, 230, 234, 305, 341, 360
Pregnant, 46, 50, 156, 173, 198, 216,
   273, 287, 308, 361
Premalignant condition, 43, 72, 230,
   232, 341, 360
Premenstrual, 76, 220, 222
Prevention, 3-4, 26, 31, 34, 37, 40,
   42, 45, 61-62, 77, 83, 85, 90,
   113-114, 153, 158, 179, 183, 186,
   188, 195, 199-200, 217, 224, 227,
   229, 259, 287, 290, 361, 412, 455,
   496-497
Provitamins, 29-30, 34, 36, 38
Progentior cryptocides, 483-484
Progesterone, 72, 326
Proliferation, 34, 47, 71, 90-91, 132,
   138, 140, 150, 153, 347, 351, 400,
   432-433, 439, 454
Promoters, 158, 160, 175, 200, 358
Prostacyclin, 278-279
Prostaglandins, 168,176, 218, 221-
   222, 232, 246, 265, 288, 315-316,
   332, 344
Prostate cancer, 29-30, 33, 118-120,
   218-219, 226, 228, 235-237, 288,
   303, 310-313, 346-348, 383, 438
Prostatitis, 167, 170
Psoralens, 387, 393
Psoriasis, 387, 454-455
Psychosocial, 324, 448-450, 452, 467-
   468, 498
Psyllium, 225, 228-229

The Cancer Industry:
The Classic Exposé on the Cancer Establishment
by Ralph W. Moss, PhD

This book shows why the billion dollar war on cancer is going nowhere. It details how drug companies influence cancer policy; how major industries keep the emphasis of cancer research away from prevention; how the American Cancer Society maintains a blacklist of unconventional practitioners; and how the government has collaborated in the suppression of new ideas.

"The revelations in this book about the ways in which the American people have been betrayed by the cancer establishment, the medical profession and the government are shocking. Everyone should know that the 'war on cancer' is largely a fraud, and that the National Cancer Institute and the American Cancer Society are derelict in their duties to the people who support them." —Nobel laureate Linus Pauling, PhD

"A sober and sobering account of...the medical and political aspects of cancer, written by an insider of extensive experience and remarkable courage."—Dean Burk, PhD, co-founder, National Cancer Institute

"This is a shocking, disturbing book."—Baltimore Evening Sun

"Without a doubt, this is one of the most unsettling books of the decade."
—West Coast Review of Books

"[Moss] delivers his argument with low-keyed logic and a slow, careful building-up of facts....Riveting!" —Denver Post

"Exceptionally well-written. Highly recommended."—Library Journal.

"Moss does not strive for sensationalism: he carefully cites sources as he assembles documentation that adds up to a blistering attack."
—Publishers Weekly

502 pages; $14.95 (Paragon House paperback, ISBN 1-55778-439-6)
Ask for it at your bookstore.

The Cancer Chronicles:
Serious Consideration of Alternative Ideas
A newsletter edited by Ralph W. Moss, Ph.D.

If you found *Cancer Therapy: The Independent Consumer's Guide* useful, you will want to subscribe to *The Cancer Chronicles*. Since 1989, the *Chronicles* has been the leading independent voice in the field of cancer alternatives.

- The *Chronicles* monitors the world scientific literature to bring you up-to-date news on advances in cancer therapy.
- The *Chronicles* details new discoveries in prevention and detection.
- The *Chronicles* covers the struggles of innovative practitioners and researchers.
- The *Chronicles* closely follows and takes part in the struggle for medical freedom of choice. It was an influential voice in the Office of Technology Assessment's report on Unconventional Cancer Therapies. It is currently closely following the National Institutes of Health's committee on unconventional medical practices.

Most of this information is simply not available elsewhere. It is reported in a very clear, simple but detailed style. If you are interested in the latest developments in non-toxic treatments for cancer, you need to subscribe to *The Cancer Chronicles*.

To subscribe, please send a check for $20 for six issues to: Equinox Press, 331 West 57th Street, Suite 268-B, New York, NY 10019. Make check out to Equinox Press.

You can also pay by MasterCard or Visa. Just write down your MasterCard or Visa Card number, together with the card's expiration date, and put your signature on the page. Please be sure to print your name and address clearly. Thank you.